Complex General Surgical Oncology

Carl Schmidt • Mary Garland Kledzik
Editors

Complex General Surgical Oncology

Preparing for Boards and Early Practice

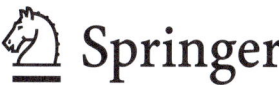

Editors
Carl Schmidt
Department of Surgery,
Division of Surgical Oncology
West Virginia University
Morgantown, WV, USA

Mary Garland Kledzik
Department of Surgery,
Division of Surgical Oncology
West Virginia University
Morgantown, WV, USA

ISBN 978-3-031-88953-0   ISBN 978-3-031-88954-7   (eBook)
https://doi.org/10.1007/978-3-031-88954-7

© The Editor(s) (if applicable) and The Author(s), under exclusive license to Springer Nature Switzerland AG 2025

This work is subject to copyright. All rights are solely and exclusively licensed by the Publisher, whether the whole or part of the material is concerned, specifically the rights of translation, reprinting, reuse of illustrations, recitation, broadcasting, reproduction on microfilms or in any other physical way, and transmission or information storage and retrieval, electronic adaptation, computer software, or by similar or dissimilar methodology now known or hereafter developed.
The use of general descriptive names, registered names, trademarks, service marks, etc. in this publication does not imply, even in the absence of a specific statement, that such names are exempt from the relevant protective laws and regulations and therefore free for general use.
The publisher, the authors and the editors are safe to assume that the advice and information in this book are believed to be true and accurate at the date of publication. Neither the publisher nor the authors or the editors give a warranty, expressed or implied, with respect to the material contained herein or for any errors or omissions that may have been made. The publisher remains neutral with regard to jurisdictional claims in published maps and institutional affiliations.

This Springer imprint is published by the registered company Springer Nature Switzerland AG
The registered company address is: Gewerbestrasse 11, 6330 Cham, Switzerland

If disposing of this product, please recycle the paper.

Preface

Welcome to the first edition of *Complex General Surgical Oncology: Preparing for Boards and Early Practice*. This work reviews relevant material for surgeons and others providing care to patients with many cancers. The content is tailored to residents with an interest in surgical oncology and fellows training in Complex General Surgical Oncology (CGSO) including preparation for qualifying (written) and certifying (oral) board exams. When possible, the authors provide key numbers or statistics meant to aid discussions with patients about treatment options and prognosis. We hope the guide is also useful to general surgeons and surgical oncologists in early practice.

Each chapter focuses on a cancer or group of related cancers. There is an additional chapter focused on palliative care in oncology. Content is presented in bullet point style rather than prose with an emphasis on diagnosis and management using evidence-based algorithms. The last section offers multiple review questions with suggested answers by the editorial team. Please email either or both of us if you have any suggestions for future editions, and we hope you enjoy the book!

Morgantown, WV, USA Carl Schmidt
Morgantown, WV, USA Mary Garland Kledzik

Contents

1	**Adrenal Tumors**...	1
	Deanna Cotsalas and Reese W. Randle	
2	**Anal Cancers**...	19
	Keri Mayers and Kevin Train	
3	**Biliary Cancers**..	29
	R. Connor Chick and Jordan M. Cloyd	
4	**Breast Cancer**..	41
	Kimberly S. Bailey and Gregory Stimac	
5	**Esophageal Cancer**...	71
	Rob Painter and Hari B. Keshava	
6	**Gastric Cancer**...	79
	Carl Schmidt and Mary Garland Kledzik	
7	**Gastrointestinal Stromal Tumor**................................	93
	Nicholas W. Miller, Dane C. Olevian, and Alan A. Thomay	
8	**Genetic Syndromes**...	117
	Jacob Swords, Carly Likar, and Mary Garland Kledzik	
9	**Hepatocellular Carcinoma**......................................	133
	Brian Sparkman, Kyeong Ri Yu, Apara Sai Jella, Leopoldo Fernandez, Jose Trevino, and Adam Khader	
10	**Large Intestine Cancers**.......................................	147
	Abhineet Uppal	
11	**Melanoma**...	161
	Jessica S. Crystal and Susan B. Kesmodel	
12	**Nonmelanoma Skin Cancers**.....................................	185
	Jason M. Lizalek and Juan A. Santamaria-Barria	
13	**Pancreatic Cancer**...	225
	Michael Sestito, Britney Niemann, and Brian A. Boone	

| 14 | **Palliative Interventions** . . . . 247 |

Sarah Mitchem, Frances Salisbury, Barbara Diane Gillis, Laura J. Ostapenko, and Katherine A. Hill

| 15 | **Peritoneal Surface Malignancies** . . . . 267 |

Jackson Baril and Trang Nguyen

| 16 | **Soft Tissue Sarcomas** . . . . 279 |

Cameron Keramati and Anthony Scholer

| 17 | **Small Intestine Cancers** . . . . 331 |

Mary Read and Laura M. Enomoto

| 18 | **Thyroid and Parathyroid Cancers** . . . . 339 |

Melissa LoPinto

Surgical Oncology: Review Questions and Suggested Answers 359

Index 367

Contributors

Kimberly S. Bailey Division of Surgical Oncology, Department of Surgery, West Virginia University, Morgantown, WV, USA

Jackson Baril Department of Surgery, Indiana University School of Medicine, Indianapolis, IN, USA

Brian A. Boone Department of Surgery, West Virginia University, Morgantown, WV, USA
Department of Microbiology, Immunology and Cell Biology, West Virginia University, Morgantown, WV, USA

R. Connor Chick Division of Surgical Oncology, Department of Surgery, The Ohio State University, Columbus, OH, USA

Jordan M. Cloyd Division of Surgical Oncology, Department of Surgery, The Ohio State University, Columbus, OH, USA

Deanna Cotsalas Department of Surgery, Atrium Health Wake Forest Baptist, Winston-Salem, NC, USA

Jessica S. Crystal Division of Surgical Oncology, Dewitt Daughtry Department of Surgery, University of Miami Miller School of Medicine, Miami, FL, USA

Laura M. Enomoto Graduate School of Medicine, University Surgical Oncology, University of Tennessee, Knoxville, TN, USA

Leopoldo Fernandez VCU School of Medicine, Department of Surgery, Richmond, VA, USA
Massey Comperhensive Cancer Center, Richmond, VA, USA
Central Virginia VA Health Care System, Richmond, VA, USA

Barbara Diane Gillis, MD Department of Surgery, University of Louisville School of Medicine, Louisville, KY, USA

Katherine A. Hill, MD, MS, FACS Department of Surgery, Division of General Surgery, Department of Medicine, Division of Geriatrics, Palliative Medicine & Hospice, West Virginia University, Morgantown, WV, USA

Apara Sai Jella VCU School of Medicine, Department of Surgery, Richmond, VA, USA

Cameron Keramati Department of Surgery, University of Texas Southwestern Medical Center, Dallas, TX, USA

Hari B. Keshava Division of Thoracic Surgery, Department of General Surgery, University of California, Irvine, CA, USA

Susan B. Kesmodel Division of Surgical Oncology, Dewitt Daughtry Department of Surgery, University of Miami Miller School of Medicine, Miami, FL, USA

Adam Khader VCU School of Medicine, Department of Surgery, Richmond, VA, USA
Massey Comperhensive Cancer Center, Richmond, VA, USA
Central Virginia VA Health Care System, Richmond, VA, USA

Mary Garland Kledzik Department of Surgery, Division of Surgical Oncology West Virginia University, Morgantown, WV, USA

Carly Likar West Virginia University, Department of Surgery, Morgantown, WV, USA

Jason M. Lizalek Division of Surgical Oncology, Department of Surgery, University of Nebraska Medical Center, Fred & Pamela Buffett Cancer Center, Omaha, NE, USA

Melissa LoPinto Department of Surgery, West Virginia University, Morgantown, WV, USA

Keri Mayers West Virginia University Ruby Memorial Hospital, Morgantown, WV, USA

Nicholas W. Miller West Virginia University, School of Medicine, Morgantown, WV, USA

Sarah Mitchem, MD Department of Obstetrics and Gynecology, Charleston Area Medical Center, Charleston, WV, USA

Trang Nguyen School of Medicine Department of Surgery, Washington University in St. Louis, Saint Louis, MO, USA

Britney Niemann Department of Surgery, West Virginia University, Morgantown, WV, USA

Dane C. Olevian West Virginia University, Department of Pathology, Morgantown, WV, USA

Laura J. Ostapenko, MD, MPP, DFPM Department of Anesthesiology and Perioperative Medicine, MaineHealth-Maine Medical Center, Portland, ME, USA

Rob Painter Division of Thoracic Surgery, Department of General Surgery, University of California, Irvine, CA, USA

Reese W. Randle Department of Surgery, Atrium Health Wake Forest Baptist, Winston-Salem, NC, USA

Mary Read Graduate School of Medicine, University Surgical Oncology, University of Tennessee, Knoxville, TN, USA

Frances Salisbury, MD Department of Obstetrics and Gynecology, West Virginia University, Morgantown, WV, USA

Juan A. Santamaria-Barria Division of Surgical Oncology, Department of Surgery, University of Nebraska Medical Center, Fred & Pamela Buffett Cancer Center, Omaha, NE, USA

Carl Schmidt Department of Surgery, Division of Surgical Oncology, West Virginia University, Morgantown, WV, USA

Anthony Scholer Department of Surgery, Division of Surgical Oncology, Jersey Shore University Medical Center Hackensack Meridian, Neptune, NJ, USA

Michael Sestito Department of Surgery, West Virginia University, Morgantown, WV, USA

Brian Sparkman VCU School of Medicine, Department of Surgery, Richmond, VA, USA

Massey Comprehensive Cancer Center, Richmond, VA, USA

Gregory Stimac Department of Surgery, West Virginia University, Morgantown, WV, USA

Jacob Swords West Virginia University, Department of Surgery, Morgantown, WV, USA

Alan A. Thomay West Virginia University, Department of Surgery, Morgantown, WV, USA

Kevin Train West Virginia University Ruby Memorial Hospital, Morgantown, WV, USA

Jose Trevino VCU School of Medicine, Department of Surgery, Richmond, VA, USA
Massey Comprehensive Cancer Center, Richmond, VA, USA

Abhineet Uppal, MD Emory University, Atlanta, GA, USA

Kyeong Ri Yu VCU School of Medicine, Department of Surgery, Richmond, VA, USA
Massey Comprehensive Cancer Center, Richmond, VA, USA

Adrenal Tumors

Deanna Cotsalas and Reese W. Randle

Introduction

- Adrenal tumors include both benign and malignant neoplasms arising from either the adrenal cortex or medulla. Here, we discuss the presentation, evaluation, and management of such tumors as well as the management of metastases to the adrenal glands.

Incidentalomas

- Evaluation of adrenal incidentalomas should focus on risk of malignancy and adrenal hormone production.
    - Imaging:
        - Useful to help stratify risk of malignancy.
        - Imaging Modalities.
            - Ultrasound can identify incidentalomas but characterizes adrenal nodules relatively poorly.
            - Adrenal protocol CT scan [5]:
                - Includes unenhanced CT and multiphase contrast-enhanced CT and thin cuts through the adrenal glands.
                - Size should be measured in three dimensions.
                - Density can be measured using Hounsfield units on unenhanced CT.
                - Absolute and relative washout is calculated and used to suggest an adenoma or indeterminate lesion.

- Higher washout (>50%) suggests an adenoma but cannot definitively rule out a pheochromocytoma or malignancy.
  – MRI chemical shift analysis usually provides similar information to adrenal protocol CT.
  – FDG PET [1, 43]:
    - Used when CT results are inconclusive and additional testing is needed.
    - No increased uptake: most likely a nonfunctional adrenal adenoma.
    - Increased FDG uptake can result in the setting of a functional adrenal adenoma, such as a cortisol secreting tumor, pheochromocytoma, or adrenocortical carcinoma.
    - Specificity of increased uptake is low for adrenal tumors. However, the sensitivity for pheochromocytoma is 80—100% [6].
  – Dotatate PET:
    - Form of somatostatin receptor scintigraphy used to image neuroendocrine tumors, such as pheochromocytoma [11].
    - Utilized in the setting of suspected malignant pheochromocytoma with metastasis. Dotatate PET should be used to evaluate metastatic disease [6].
- Size [5]:
  – Risk of malignancy is low for primary adrenal tumors <4 cm in greatest dimension.
  – Any mass >4 cm should be evaluated for adrenal cortical cancer [45].
  – Risk of malignancy increases with increasing size [30].
    - Tumors <4 cm associated with 2% risk of malignancy.
    - Tumors 4–6 cm associated with 6% risk of malignancy.
    - Tumors >6 cm associated with risk of malignancy up to 25%.
  – Most patients with adrenal cortical cancer present with large tumors (>10 cm).
- Laterality.
  – Metastatic disease should be ruled out in cases of bilateral adrenal tumors [5].
  – Adenomas are more often identified on the left but can occur on either side [20].
- Density.
  – Hounsfield units <10 on unenhanced CT strongly suggests a benign, lipid-rich adenoma.
  – Hounsfield units >10 on unenhanced CT is indeterminate density which can be seen with lipid poor adenomas, adrenal cortical cancer, pheochromocytoma, and metastases. In these cases, if washout is >60%, it is more commonly benign than if washout is <60%.
  – Myelolipomas often contain macroscopic adipose tissue.
- Borders.
  – Benign incidentalomas are characterized as having smooth borders on CT and ultrasound imaging [13].

- Irregular borders on imaging or invasive borders, as well as heterogenicity, can be characteristic of a malignant process.
  - Appearance of the contralateral gland.
    - Should be specifically examined to rule out bilateral lesions.
    - If the contralateral adrenal gland appears atrophied, the incidentaloma might be producing cortisol.
  - Growth Rate [34].
    - Incidentalomas should be monitored with repeat imaging and hormone lab work at 6 months, 1 year, and the two-year mark.
    - If the neoplasm's growth rate is greater than 0.8 cm per year, then surgery should be recommended.
    - However, there are very few controlled studies looking at growth rate.
- Functional Evaluation.
  - The goal of a functional evaluation of adrenal incidentalomas is to confirm or exclude the possibility of overproduction of cortisol, aldosterone, and catecholamines which all have implications for successful management.
  - Hypercortisolism [45]:
    - Cushing's syndrome refers to the constellation of symptoms associated with autonomous adrenal production.
    - Autonomous cortisol secretion prevalent in 5–30% of incidentalomas [44].
    - Symptoms of Hypercortisolism [10, 36].
      - Sequela of prolonged exposure to cortisol includes central obesity, development of a "buffalo hump," fatigue, poor wound healing, purple striae emotional symptoms, erectile dysfunction, hirsutism, impaired immunity, and proximal muscle weakness and atrophy.
    - Biochemical Testing.
      - Low-Dose Dexamethasone Suppression Test [10, 14]:
        - 1 mg of dexamethasone is given at 11 pm the night before and a cortisol level is drawn at 8 am the next day.
        - If cortisol level is less than 1.8 mg/dl, then suppression is appropriate.
        - If cortisol is greater than 1.8 mg/dl, there is an inability to suppress endogenous cortisol production, and a secondary test should be performed to confirm.
        - Adrenocorticotrophic hormone (ACTH) should be suppressed.
      - A 24-h urinary free cortisol: urinary cortisol greater than 100 mcg/24 h suggests hypercortisolism.
      - Midnight salivary cortisol: Measured via salivary swab three consecutive nights at 12 am; elevated levels suggest hypercortisolism.
    - Hypercortisolism is an indication for excision.
    - Hypercortisolism secondary to ACTH-independent bilateral macronodular hyperplasia should be treated with unilateral adrenalectomy of the largest nodules to attempt remission of cortisol excess without causing adrenal insufficiency [51].

- Bilateral adrenalectomy can be considered to palliate symptoms of cortisol excess failed resection of pituitary Cushing's disease or unlocalized or metastatic ectopic ACTH production, but this should be performed only with multidisciplinary consultation and management due to the resulting adrenal insufficiency.
- When ectopic ACTH production can be localized and resection is feasible, excision is recommended to treat the resulting Cushing's syndrome.
- Patients with hypercortisolism need to be monitored for postoperative adrenal insufficiency and might need steroids.
- Aldosterone or Primary Aldosteronism.
  - Primary aldosteronism refers to overproduction and autonomous adrenal production of aldosterone and is known as Conn's syndrome.
  - Observed in up to 1% of incidentalomas [28].
  - Aldosterone-producing adenomas are typically unilateral and are less than 2 cm.
  - Symptoms of Primary Aldosteronism [53]:
    - Marked refractory hypertension despite several antihypertensives.
    - Hypertension onset at young age.
    - Hypokalemia can be observed in 20%.
  - Biochemical Testing [53]:
    - Plasma aldosterone concentration to plasma renin activity ratio >20.
    - Confirmatory test: lack of decreased aldosterone with sodium loading.
    - Adrenal venous sampling is often necessary to rule out bilateral adrenal hyperplasia or contralateral aldosterone overproduction [18].
  - Primary aldosteronism should be further evaluated with adrenal venous sampling to lateralize and confirm unilateral hypersecretion. Unilateral disease is an indication for ipsilateral adrenalectomy.
  - Patients with primary aldosteronism should be monitored for hyperkalemia postoperatively.
- Catecholamines or Pheochromocytoma.
  - It is important to rule out a pheochromocytoma any time an incidentaloma is identified.
  - About 7% of adrenal incidentalomas are later diagnosed as pheochromocytomas [7].
  - Biochemical Testing:
    - Plasma metanephrines are more sensitive:
      - Pheochromocytomas usually produce metanephrine levels >3–4 times normal.
      - Mild elevations and false-positive results are observed with tricyclic antidepressants, decongestants, amphetamines, reserpine, caffeine, and nicotine.

- Urine metanephrines (24 h collection) are more specific if elevated.
  - Pheochromocytomas should be resected only following adequate preoperative preparation with alpha blockade until they have orthostatic hypotension. They should also be counseled to stay hydrated and consume salt.
  - Patients with pheochromocytomas should be monitored closely for hypotension and hypoglycemia postoperatively.
- Biopsy is often contraindicated or not useful.
  - Biopsy should never be attempted prior to ruling out a pheochromocytoma.
  - Biopsy of masses suspicious for adrenocortical carcinoma can potentially rupture the tumor capsule and seed the peritoneum or retroperitoneum.
  - Biopsy is reasonable to consider to diagnose metastatic disease if the result will alter management, but only after a pheochromocytoma is ruled out.
- Incidentalomas with suspicious radiologic findings or evidence of excess hormone secretion should be resected [9].

Adrenocortical Carcinoma (ACC)

- ACCs are rare and often have a poor prognosis.
- Incidence: 0.5–2 cases per million populations per year [40].
- Risk Factors.
  - Genetic risk factors: Li-Fraumeni syndrome (TP53 mutation), Beckwith-Wiedemann syndrome (IGF2 mutation), multiple endocrine neoplasia type 1, Carney complex, neurofibromatosis type 1 [27], and Lynch syndrome [38].
  - Female (2:1 female-to-male ratio) [25].
  - Tobacco use [22].
- Presentation.
  - 14% of cases are found incidentally [40].
  - 60% associated with clinical evidence of hypersecretion syndromes
    - Most common is hypercortisolism.
    - Can produce multiple hormones in excess.
  - 20–40% are metastatic at presentation.
  - Signs and symptoms.
    - Hormonal symptoms:
      - Hypercortisolism: plethora, diabetes, osteoporosis, and muscle atrophy.
      - Hyperandrogenism: male pattern baldness, virilization, hirsutism, and menstrual abnormalities.
      - Excess estrogen: gynecomastia and testicular atrophy.
    - Flank pain.
    - Early satiety.
    - Abdominal fullness.

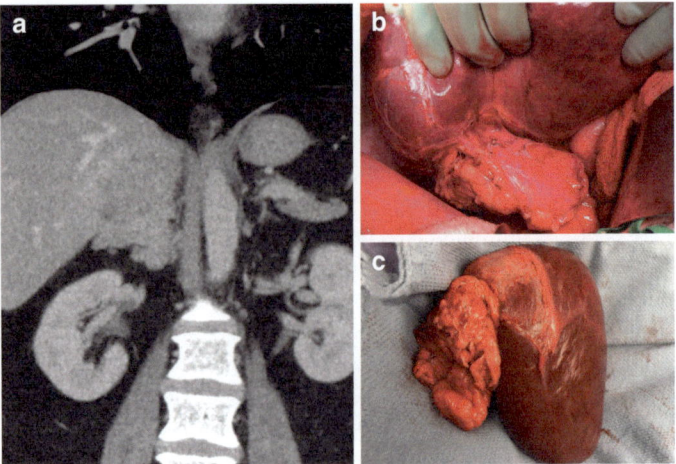

Fig. 1.1 Adrenocortical carcinoma. (**a**) depicts a CT scan showing a large right adrenal mass directly invading the liver with an atrophied left adrenal gland due to autonomous cortisol secretion from the adrenal mass. (**b**) shows the mass directly invading the liver during resection and (**c**) shows the final gross specimen

- Evaluation.
    - Detailed medical and family history.
    - Imaging (Fig. 1.1).
        - Risk of ACC is not determined by lab findings but by radiographic characteristics [53].
        - CT scan [45]:
            - ACC is heterogenous, high density with Hounsfield units greater than 10, irregularly shaped, and can have intramural necrosis.
            - In 30% of cases, calcifications are present.
            - On contrast-enhanced CT, there is irregular heterogenous peripheral enhancement and a nonenhancing central portion due to hemorrhagic or necrotic components.
        - MRI [45]:
            - On T1-weighted imaging: ACC is isointensive or hypointense when compared to the liver parenchyma.
            - On T2-weighted imaging: ACC is hyperintense when compared to the liver parenchyma.
    - Biochemical evaluation [45].
        - Adrenocorticotropic hormone [24]: In cases of adrenocortical carcinoma, morning ACTH levels can be normal or low in the setting of a cortisol producing tumor.
        - Aldosterone: Can be tested with plasma renin activity to determine if elevation is independent of renin.
        - Androgen production [24]: Elevated dehydroepiandrosterone sulfate (DHEA-S) levels are suspicious for ACC.

- Functional evaluation should also include metanephrine levels to rule out pheochromocytoma.
 - Biopsy should not be attempted for diagnosis if the mass is going to need to be removed regardless due to the risk of capsule rupture and peritoneal seeding. Biopsy should never be performed without first ruling out pheochromocytoma.
- Histology/Pathology [25].
 - The tumor is often tan or yellow in appearance with areas of hemorrhage or necrosis.
 - Weiss Criteria used to determine malignancy. Histologically, the tumor must contain three out of nine of the following criteria [48]:
   - High nuclear grade (Fuhrman III or IV).
   - High mitotic rate (>5 mitoses per 50 high power field).
   - Atypical mitotic figures.
   - ≤25% clear cells
   - Diffuse architecture.
   - Tumor confluent necrosis.
   - Venous invasion.
   - Sinusoidal invasion.
   - Capsular invasion.
 - Staging [3] (Tables 1.1 and 1.2).

Table 1.1 TNM categories for adrenocortical carcinoma

Tumor	Nodes	Metastases
TX—Tumor cannot be assessed T0—No evidence of primary tumor T1—Primary tumor is 5 cm or less T2—Primary tumor is >5 cm T3—Primary tumor is invading surrounding adipose tissue T4—Primary tumor is invading adjacent organs or vessels	NX—Regional lymph nodes cannot be assessed N0—No evidence of nodal metastases N1—Regional nodal metastases are present	M0—No evidence of distant metastases M1—Distant metastases are present

Table 1.2 American Joint Commission on Cancer eighth edition Staging for Adrenocortical Carcinoma

Stage	TNM groupings	Description
I	T1, N0, M0	Tumor 5 cm or less, no nodal involvement or distant metastases
II	T2, N0, M0	Tumor larger than 5 cm, no nodal involvement or distant metastases
III	T1–2, N1, M0 T3–4, any N, M0	Tumor invading surrounding tissue or organs or evidence of regional nodal involvement, no distant metastases
IV	Any T, any N, M1	Distant metastases are present

- Treatment.
  - Although diagnosis requires histology, patients with suspected ACC should be clinically staged prior to developing a treatment plan.
  - Full hormonal evaluation should be performed to aid management, gauge the likelihood of adrenal insufficiency postoperatively, and rule out a pheochromocytoma.
  - Any excess hormone production identified preoperatively can be used as a tumor marker postoperatively.
  - Operative resection is the primary treatment for resectable tumors.
    - Minimally invasive approaches are controversial with large indeterminate adrenal masses [52].
    - Open approach is indicated for any known cases of adrenal cortical carcinoma.
    - Goal of resection is negative margins when possible. Positive margins are associated with advanced carcinoma and worse survival [42].
    - Locoregional lymphadenectomy (perihilar and para-aortic/paracaval nodes) is associated with longer disease-specific survival in patients with localized (stages I–III) ACC (HR 0.42 [0.26,0.68]) [21].
  - Systemic Therapy.
    - Mitotane is cytotoxic for adrenal cortical cells and the primary systemic treatment for ACC.
      - It can be used to decrease cortisol levels in the neoadjuvant setting.
      - Mitotane is used for adjuvant therapy in patients considered high risk for recurrence or those with large tumor size or aggressive features should be considered for adjuvant treatment.
      - Mitotane is used as primary therapy in patients with unresectable disease.
    - Mitotane can be used in combination with etoposide, doxorubicin, and cisplatin (EDP) for aggressive cases or for recurrent or advanced disease.
  - Radiation.
    - Historically, ACC was considered relatively insensitive to radiation therapy.
    - Adjuvant radiation might play a role for high-grade tumors or for patients following incomplete resection or tumor spillage.
- Prognosis.
  - Overall poor.
  - A five-year disease-specific survival was 82% for stage I, 61% for stage II, 50% for stage III, and 13% for stage IV (PMID 19025987, [16]).
- Surveillance.
  - Patients should initially be followed every 3 months following resection with imaging.
  - Hormone levels can be used as tumor markers in cases where the cancer was hormonally active.

Pheochromocytoma

- An adrenal tumor that arises from chromaffin cells within the adrenal medulla.
- Pheochromocytomas are rare, occurring in less than 1 in 100,000 population [17].
- Risk factors.
  - Nearly one-third of seemingly sporadic pheochromocytomas are associated with a genetic predisposition [17].
  - Genetic syndromes associated with pheochromocytomas:
    - Von Hippel-Lindau disease [39].
      - Approximately 20% will develop a pheochromocytoma.
      - Malignancy is rare.
    - Multiple Endocrine Neoplasia Type II [50].
      - Risk of pheochromocytoma correlates with the specific RET codon mutations 918, 634, and 883.
      - When it cooccurs with other manifestations, the pheochromocytoma should be addressed first.
    - Neurofibromatosis 1.
      - Approximately 1% of NF 1 patients will develop a pheochromocytoma.
      - Can be malignant.
    - Familial Paraganglioma Syndromes [15].
      - Identified by a germline mutations in SDHA, SDHAF1, SDHAF2, SDHB, SDHC, and SDHD, MAX, or TMEM127.
      - SDHB mutations are associated with a higher risk of malignant pheochromocytoma and paraganglioma.
- Presentation.
  - Most pheochromocytomas are initially identified incidentally [19].
  - Most pheochromocytomas are hormonally active, in contrast to paragangliomas.
  - Signs and Symptoms [53]:
    - Hypertension can be severe and episodic but not all patients will present with hypertension (not present in 15% of patients).
    - Other classic symptoms include tachycardia, cardiac arrhythmias, headaches, anxiety, weight loss, panic attacks, constipation, pallor, and excessive sweating.
    - Episodic symptoms can be precipitated by activity, defecation, alcohol ingestion, and general anesthesia.
    - Cardiac presentations can include heart failure and myocardial infarction.
- Evaluation.
  - Detailed medical and family history.
  - Imaging (Fig. 1.2).

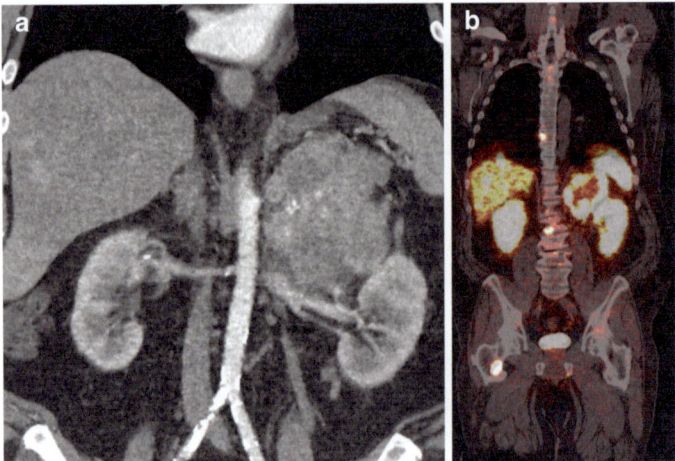

Fig. 1.2 Malignant pheochromocytoma. (**a**) depicts a CT scan showing a large irregular, heterogeneous left adrenal mass. (**b**) shows a dotatate PET scan showing uptake in the left adrenal mass as well as evidence of metastatic disease to the spine and hip

- When imaging pheochromocytomas, it is important to pay special attention to the contralateral adrenal gland and the sympathetic chain because they can present with bilateral or extraadrenal disease.
- CT adrenal protocol.
  - Provides anatomical information.
  - Might look cystic, solid, or partially necrotic.
  - Often mimic the appearance of other adrenal lesions [12].
- MRI.
  - Provides anatomical information, particularly helpful to evaluate vascular invasion.
  - High-intensity signal on T2-weighted images.
  - Can mimic the appearance of adrenocortical cancer.
- Imaging with *iodine-123 (^{123}I)-labeled metaiodobenzyl guanidine* (MIBG) [49].
  - Used for cases when a pheochromocytoma is biochemically suspected but CT or MRI does not confirm a mass.
  - MIBG is 82–88% sensitive and 82–84% specific for pheochromocytoma.
- *Gallium-68 DOTA,1-NaI(3)-octreotide* (Dotatate) PET scan.
  - Functional imaging specific to neuroendocrine tumors including pehochrmocytoma and paraganglioma.
  - May be superior to MIBG imaging for pheochromocytoma in cases of malignant pheochromocytoma and patients with a history of MEN2 [41].
  - Biochemical Evaluation [53].
    - Plasma-free metanephrines are sensitive and often exceed 3–4 times the upper limit of the normal range.

- False-positive results are common.
- Numerous medications including tricyclic antidepressants, decongestants, amphetamines, and reserpine, in addition to caffeine, nicotine, stress, and essential hypertension can all cause mild elevations.
  - Elevations in 24-h urine metanephrines are more specific than plasma-free metanephrines.
  - Although rare, some pheochromocytomas can be nonfunctional. Nonfunctional paragangliomas are much more common.
  - Chromogranin-A can serve as a nonspecific tumor marker for neuroendocrine tumors including pheochromocytomas which may be helpful for nonfunctional tumors.
- Biopsy should not be attempted for diagnosis or for any adrenal nodule prior to ruling out a pheochromocytoma due to the risk of precipitating a catecholamine crisis.
- Histology.
  - Pheochromocytoma of the Adrenal gland Scaled Score (PASS) score [46] is used to predict benign tumors and those with potential for aggressive malignancy:
    - Vascular invasion score = 1.
    - Capsular invasion score = 1.
    - Periadrenal adipose tissue invasion score = 2.
    - Large nests or diffuse growth score = 2.
    - Focal or confluent necrosis score = 2.
    - High cellularity score = 2.
    - Tumor cell spindling score = 2.
    - Cellular monotony score = 2.
    - Increased mitotic figures >3/10 high power fields; score = 2.
    - Atypical mitotic figures score = 2.
    - Profound nuclear pleomorphism score = 1.
    - Hyperchromasia score = 1.
  - If the factors add up to a PASS > or = 4, then there is more potential for malignancy.
- Staging [3] (Tables 1.3 and 1.4).

Table 1.3 TNM Categories for Malignant Pheochromocytoma and Sympathetic Paraganglioma [3]

Tumor	Nodes	Metastases
TX—Tumor cannot be assessed	NX—Regional lymph nodes cannot be assessed	M0—No evidence of distant metastases
T0—No evidence of primary tumor		
T1—Pheochromocytoma is 5 cm or less	N0—No evidence of nodal metastases	M1a—Distant metastases to bone
T2—Pheochromocytoma is >5 cm or sympathetic paraganglioma	N1—Regional nodal metastases are present	M1b—Distant metastases to nonregional lymph nodes, liver, or lung
T3—Primary tumor is invading surrounding tissue (adipose or organs)		M1c—Metastases to bone and multiple other sites

Table 1.4 American Joint Commission on Cancer eighth edition Staging for Malignant Pheochromocytoma and Sympathetic Paraganglioma

Stage	TNM groupings	Description
I	T1, N0, M0	Pheochromocytoma 5 cm or less, no nodal involvement or distant metastases
II	T2, N0, M0	Pheochromocytoma larger than 5 cm or sympathetic paraganglioma, no nodal involvement or distant metastases
III	T1–2, N1, M0 T3, any N, M0	Tumor invading surrounding tissue or organs or evidence of regional nodal involvement, no distant metastases
IV	Any T, any N, M1	Distant metastases are present.

- Treatment.
  - Surgical resection is the primary treatment for pheochromocytomas, but catecholamines must be adequately blocked before considering surgery.
  - Preoperative Preparation [32].
    - Adequate preoperative blockade prevents a catecholamine crisis during anesthesia and tumor manipulation. Classic preoperative blockade includes alpha receptor blockade.
    - Alpha-adrenergic Blockade.
      - Generally initiated at diagnosis and important for this blockade to occur at least 1–3 weeks prior to operation.
      - Classic alpha blockade includes phenoxybenzamine, a long-acting, nonselective α-adrenergic antagonist.
        - Dose is titrated to orthostatic hypotension.
        - Common side effects include severe congestion.
      - Selective alpha blockade with agents such as doxazosin and terazosin are often more widely available, less expensive, and easier to tolerate than phenoxybenzamine [37].
    - Calcium channel blockade—Useful for preparation in patients that are experiencing catecholamine-induced coronary vasospasm or those that are normotensive or only intermittently hypertensive and those that cannot tolerate alpha blockade due to hypotension.
    - Beta-adrenergic Blockade.
      - Should only be added after an alpha-adrenergic blockade for patients that remain tachycardic.
      - Use prior to adequate alpha blockade can precipitate a hypertensive crisis due to unopposed alpha receptor stimulation.
    - Patients should be encouraged to increase sodium intake and hydrate prior to surgical resection due to the decreased intravascular volume associated with chronic excess catecholamines.
  - Surgical resection requires a coordinated, multidisciplinary approach.
    - Anesthesia Considerations.

1 Adrenal Tumors

- Induction can precipitate a catecholamine surge, so invasive blood pressure monitoring is often established prior to induction.
- Tumor manipulation can also cause increased catecholamine release, and the decrease in catecholamines once the adrenal vein is ligated can be rapid and profound.
- Anesthesiologists must take drugs that stimulate catecholamine release into account and avoid use.
- Inhaled anesthetics are often used due to decreased cardiodepressant effects [53].
- Pheochromocytomas can be safely resected open or minimally invasively using laparoscopy or robotics and via a transabdominal or retroperitoneoscopic approach.
    - The surgeon should attempt to minimize tumor manipulation prior to ligating the adrenal vein.
    - Communication with anesthesia around the time of ligating the adrenal vein is vital.
- Postoperative Considerations [53].
    - The alpha-adrenergic blockade is discontinued following a complete resection.
    - Patients may require vasopressors immediately postoperatively, but these can usually be weaned rapidly with fluid resuscitation.
    - Patients should be monitored for hypoglycemia.
    - Genetic testing should be considered once pheochromocytoma is confirmed with pathology.
- Systemic Therapy.
    - Chemotherapy.
        - The most common chemotherapy regimen is cisplatin, vinblastine, and dacarbazine [29].
        - Sunitinib is a tyrosine kinase inhibitor that has some efficacy in treatment. It targets the vascular endothelial growth factor pathway [31].
    - Radiopharmaceutical Therapy [8].
        - *Iodine-131 meta-iodobenzylguanidine* (^{131}I-MIBG) is efficacious for palliative symptomatic control in patients with both inoperable and metastatic disease. This therapy is only an option if the patient has a positive ^{123}I-MIBG scan. The tumor must have avid tracer uptake. Imaging is required within 3–6 months of treatment.
        - *177-Lutetium-DOTATATE* (^{177}Lu-DOTATATE) is a second efficacious therapy for metastatic pheochromocytoma. Similar to ^{131}I-MIBG treatment, the tumor must have avid tracer uptake on dotatate PET scan [23]. Choosing which radiopharmaceutical therapy to use is based on the individual patient and a risk-benefit analysis of the side effects.
- Radiation Therapy.
    - External beam radiation therapy is utilized in patients with symptomatic localized disease progression [47] and may help with symptoms of local progression but often is not curative.

- Prognosis.
  - Those amenable to surgical resection without metastatic disease are curable. However, patients with metastatic disease at diagnosis or those that have recurrent pheochromocytoma have a 5-year survival rate of 34–60% [33].
  - Factors associated with shorter overall survival: increased tumor size, initial extraadrenal tumor location, and germline mutations of *succinate dehydrogenase B subunit* (SDHB) [2, 4].
- Surveillance [26, 35].
  - Resectable Disease (Postoperative Surveillance):
    - Patients should be monitored with history and physical, blood pressure measurements and hormonal markers in the first year postoperatively, anywhere from every 3 to 12 months. Can also consider imaging to surveil.
    - Postoperative years 1–3: Monitor with history and physical, blood pressure measurements, and hormonal markers every 6–12 months. Can also consider imaging to surveil.
    - Postoperative years 4–10: Patients should be monitored annually with hormonal markers. Imaging can also be considered.
  - Nonresectable Disease:
    - Every 3 months to 1 year: Patients should be under surveillance with history and physical, blood pressure measurements, and hormonal markers.
    - Imaging can be considered as well, especially if considering radionuclide therapies.

References

1. Akkuş G, Güney IB, Ok F, Evran M, Izol V, Erdoğan Ş, Bayazıt Y, Sert M, Tetiker T. Diagnostic efficacy of 18F-FDG PET/CT in patients with adrenal incidentaloma. Endocr Connect. 2019;8(7):838–45. https://doi.org/10.1530/EC-19-0204.
2. Amar L, Bertherat J, Baudin E, Ajzenberg C, Bressac-de Paillerets B, Chabre O, Chamontin B, Delemer B, Giraud S, Murat A, Niccoli-Sire P, Richard S, Rohmer V, Sadoul J-L, Strompf L, Schlumberger M, Bertagna X, Plouin P-F, Jeunemaitre X, Gimenez-Roqueplo A-P. Genetic testing in pheochromocytoma or functional paraganglioma. J Clin Oncol Off J Am Soc Clin Oncol. 2005;23(34):8812–8. https://doi.org/10.1200/JCO.2005.03.1484.
3. Amin MB, American Joint Committee on Cancer, American Cancer Society. AJCC cancer staging manual (Eight edition/editor-in-chief, Mahul B. Amin, MD, FCAP; editors, Stephen B. Edge, MD, FACS [and 16 others]; Donna M. Gress, RHIT, CTR-Technical editor; Laura R. Meyer, CAPM-Managing editor). American Joint Committee on Cancer, Springer; 2017.
4. Ayala-Ramirez M, Feng L, Johnson MM, Ejaz S, Habra MA, Rich T, Busaidy N, Cote GJ, Perrier N, Phan A, Patel S, Waguespack S, Jimenez C. Clinical risk factors for malignancy and overall survival in patients with pheochromocytomas and sympathetic paragangliomas: primary tumor size and primary tumor location as prognostic indicators. J Clin Endocrinol Metab. 2011;96(3):717–25. https://doi.org/10.1210/jc.2010-1946.
5. Bancos I, Prete A. Approach to the patient with adrenal incidentaloma. J Clin Endocrinol Metab. 2021;106(11):3331–53. https://doi.org/10.1210/clinem/dgab512.
6. Calissendorff J, Juhlin CC, Bancos I, Falhammar H. Pheochromocytomas and abdominal paragangliomas: A practical guidance. Cancers. 2022;14(4):917. https://doi.org/10.3390/cancers14040917.

7. Canu L, Van Hemert JAW, Kerstens MN, Hartman RP, Khanna A, Kraljevic I, Kastelan D, Badiu C, Ambroziak U, Tabarin A, Haissaguerre M, Buitenwerf E, Visser A, Mannelli M, Arlt W, Chortis V, Bourdeau I, Gagnon N, Buchy M, et al. CT characteristics of pheochromocytoma: relevance for the evaluation of adrenal incidentaloma. J Clin Endocrinol Metabol. 2019;104(2):312–8. https://doi.org/10.1210/jc.2018-01532.
8. Carrasquillo JA, Chen CC, Jha A, Pacak K, Pryma DA, Lin FI. Systemic radiopharmaceutical therapy of pheochromocytoma and paraganglioma. J Nucl Med. 2021;62(9):1192–9. https://doi.org/10.2967/jnumed.120.259697.
9. Chatzellis E, Kaltsas G. Adrenal Incidentalomas. In: Feingold KR, Anawalt B, Blackman MR, Boyce A, Chrousos G, Corpas E, de Herder WW, Dhatariya K, Dungan K, Hofland J, Kalra S, Kaltsas G, Kapoor N, Koch C, Kopp P, Korbonits M, Kovacs CS, Kuohung W, Laferrère B, et al., editors. Endotext. MDText.com, Inc; 2000. http://www.ncbi.nlm.nih.gov/books/NBK279021/.
10. Chaudhry HS, Singh G. Cushing syndrome. In: StatPearls. StatPearls Publishing; 2023. http://www.ncbi.nlm.nih.gov/books/NBK470218/.
11. Chen CC, Carrasquillo JA. Molecular imaging of adrenal neoplasms. J Surg Oncol. 2012;106(5):532–42. https://doi.org/10.1002/jso.23162.
12. Čtvrtlík F, Koranda P, Schovánek J, Škarda J, Hartmann I, Tüdös Z. Current diagnostic imaging of pheochromocytomas and implications for therapeutic strategy. Exp Ther Med. 2018;15(4):3151–60. https://doi.org/10.3892/etm.2018.5871.
13. Dietrich CF, Correas JM, Dong Y, Nolsoe C, Westerway SC, Jenssen C. WFUMB position paper on the management incidental findings: adrenal incidentaloma. Ultrasonography (Seoul, Korea). 2020;39(1):11–21. https://doi.org/10.14366/usg.19029.
14. Dogra P, Šambula L, Saini J, Thangamuthu K, Athimulam S, Delivanis DA, Baikousi DA, Nathani R, Zhang CD, Genere N, Salman Z, Turcu AF, Ambroziak U, Garcia RG, Achenbach SJ, Atkinson EJ, Singh S, LeBrasseur NK, Kastelan D, Bancos I. High prevalence of frailty in patients with adrenal adenomas and adrenocortical hormone excess: a cross-sectional multicentre study with prospective enrolment. Eur J Endocrinol. 2023;189(3):318–26. https://doi.org/10.1093/ejendo/lvad113.
15. Else T, Greenberg S, Fishbein L. Hereditary paraganglioma-pheochromocytoma syndromes. In: Adam MP, Mirzaa GM, Pagon RA, Wallace SE, Bean LJ, Gripp KW, Amemiya A, editors. GeneReviews®. Seattle: University of Washington; 2008. http://www.ncbi.nlm.nih.gov/books/NBK1548/.
16. Fassnacht M, Johanssen S, Quinkler M, Bucsky P, Willenberg HS, Beuschlein F, Terzolo M, Mueller H-H, Hahner S, Allolio B, German Adrenocortical Carcinoma Registry Group, European Network for the Study of Adrenal Tumors. Limited prognostic value of the 2004 International Union Against Cancer staging classification for adrenocortical carcinoma: proposal for a Revised TNM Classification. Cancer. 2009;115(2):243–50. https://doi.org/10.1002/cncr.24030.
17. Fishbein L, Nathanson KL. Pheochromocytoma and paraganglioma: understanding the complexities of the genetic background. Cancer Genet. 2012;205(1–2):1–11. https://doi.org/10.1016/j.cancergen.2012.01.009.
18. Funder JW, Carey RM, Mantero F, Murad MH, Reincke M, Shibata H, Stowasser M, Young WF. The management of primary aldosteronism: case detection, diagnosis, and treatment: an Endocrine Society Clinical Practice Guideline. J Clin Endocrinol Metab. 2016;101(5):1889–916. https://doi.org/10.1210/jc.2015-4061.
19. Gruber LM, Hartman RP, Thompson GB, McKenzie TJ, Lyden ML, Dy BM, Young WF, Bancos I. Pheochromocytoma characteristics and behavior differ depending on method of discovery. J Clin Endocrinol Metab. 2019;104(5):1386–93. https://doi.org/10.1210/jc.2018-01707.
20. Hao M, Lopez D, Luque-Fernandez MA, Cote K, Newfield J, Connors M, Vaidya A. The lateralizing asymmetry of adrenal adenomas. J Endocr Soc. 2018;2(4):374–85. https://doi.org/10.1210/js.2018-00034.

21. Hendricks A, Muller S, Fassnacht M, Germer CT, Wiegering VA, Wiegering A, Reibetanz J. Impact of lymphadenectomy on the oncologic outcome of patients with adrenocortical carcinoma – a systematic review and meta-analysis. Cancers. 2022;14(2):291. https://doi.org/10.3390/cancers14020291.
22. Hsing AW, Nam JM, Co Chien HT, McLaughlin JK, Fraumeni JF. Risk factors for adrenal cancer: an exploratory study. Int J Cancer. 1996;65(4):432–6. https://doi.org/10.1002/(SICI)1097-0215(19960208)65:4<432::AID-IJC6>3.0.CO;2-Y.
23. Jaiswal SK, Sarathi V, Memon SS, Garg R, Malhotra G, Verma P, Shah R, Sehemby MK, Patil VA, Jadhav S, Lila AR, Shah NS, Bandgar TR. 177Lu-DOTATATE therapy in metastatic/inoperable pheochromocytoma-paraganglioma. Endocr Connect. 2020;9(9):864–73. https://doi.org/10.1530/EC-20-0292.
24. Kiseljak-Vassiliades K, Bancos I, Hamrahian A, Habra M, Vaidya A, Levine AC, Else T. American Association of Clinical Endocrinology Disease State Clinical Review on the Evaluation and Management of Adrenocortical Carcinoma in an Adult: A Practical Approach. Endocr Pract. 2020;26(11):1366–83. https://doi.org/10.4158/DSCR-2020-0567.
25. Lam AK-Y. Adrenocortical carcinoma: updates of clinical and pathological features after renewed World Health Organisation classification and pathology staging. Biomedicines. 2021;9(2):175. https://doi.org/10.3390/biomedicines9020175.
26. Lenders JWM, Duh Q-Y, Eisenhofer G, Gimenez-Roqueplo A-P, Grebe SKG, Murad MH, Naruse M, Pacak K, Young WF, Endocrine Society. Pheochromocytoma and paraganglioma: an endocrine society clinical practice guideline. J Clin Endocrinol Metab. 2014;99(6):1915–42. https://doi.org/10.1210/jc.2014-1498.
27. Libé R. Adrenocortical carcinoma (ACC): diagnosis, prognosis, and treatment. Front Cell Dev Biol. 2015;3:45. https://doi.org/10.3389/fcell.2015.00045.
28. Libè R, Dall'Asta C, Barbetta L, Baccarelli A, Beck-Peccoz P, Ambrosi B. Long-term follow-up study of patients with adrenal incidentalomas. Eur J Endocrinol. 2002;147(4):489–94. https://doi.org/10.1530/eje.0.1470489.
29. Niemeijer ND, Alblas G, van Hulsteijn LT, Dekkers OM, Corssmit EPM. Chemotherapy with cyclophosphamide, vincristine and dacarbazine for malignant paraganglioma and pheochromocytoma: systematic review and meta-analysis. Clin Endocrinol. 2014;81(5):642–51. https://doi.org/10.1111/cen.12542.
30. NIH state-of-the-science statement on management of the clinically inapparent adrenal mass ("incidentaloma"). NIH Consens State Sci Statements. 2002;19(2):1–25.
31. O'Kane GM, Ezzat S, Joshua AM, Bourdeau I, Leibowitz-Amit R, Olney HJ, Krzyzanowska M, Reuther D, Chin S, Wang L, Brooks K, Hansen AR, Asa SL, Knox JJ. A phase 2 trial of sunitinib in patients with progressive paraganglioma or pheochromocytoma: the SNIPP trial. Br J Cancer. 2019;120(12):1113–9. https://doi.org/10.1038/s41416-019-0474-x.
32. Pacak K. Preoperative management of the pheochromocytoma patient. J Clin Endocrinol Metab. 2007;92(11):4069–79. https://doi.org/10.1210/jc.2007-1720.
33. Pacak K, Eisenhofer G, Ahlman H, Bornstein SR, Gimenez-Roqueplo A-P, Grossman AB, Kimura N, Mannelli M, McNicol AM, Tischler AS, International Symposium on Pheochromocytoma. Pheochromocytoma: recommendations for clinical practice from the First International Symposium. October 2005. Nature Clinical Practice. Endocrinol Metab. 2007;3(2):92–102. https://doi.org/10.1038/ncpendmet0396.
34. Papierska L, Cichocki A, Sankowski AJ, Cwikła JB. Adrenal incidentaloma imaging—the first steps in therapeutic management. Pol J Radiol. 2013;78(4):47–55. https://doi.org/10.12659/PJR.889541.
35. Patel D, Phay JE, Yen TWF, Dickson PV, Wang TS, Garcia R, Yang AD, Kim LT, Solórzano CC. Update on pheochromocytoma and paraganglioma from the SSO endocrine and head and neck disease site working group, part 2 of 2: perioperative management and outcomes of pheochromocytoma and paraganglioma. Ann Surg Oncol. 2020;27(5):1338–47. https://doi.org/10.1245/s10434-020-08221-2.

36. Pivonello R, De Martino MC, De Leo M, Lombardi G, Colao A. Cushing's syndrome. Endocrinol Metab Clin North Am. 2008;37(1):135–49., ix. https://doi.org/10.1016/j.ecl.2007.10.010.
37. Randle RW, Balentine CJ, Pitt SC, Schneider DF, Sippel RS. Selective versus non-selective α-blockade prior to laparoscopic adrenalectomy for pheochromocytoma. Ann Surg Oncol. 2017;24(1):244–50. https://doi.org/10.1245/s10434-016-5514-7.
38. Raymond VM, Everett JN, Furtado LV, Gustafson SL, Jungbluth CR, Gruber SB, Hammer GD, Stoffel EM, Greenson JK, Giordano TJ, Else T. Adrenocortical carcinoma is a lynch syndrome- associated cancer. J Clin Oncol. 2013;31(24):3012–8. https://doi.org/10.1200/JCO.2012.48.0988.
39. Rednam SP, Erez A, Druker H, Janeway KA, Kamihara J, Kohlmann WK, Nathanson KL, States LJ, Tomlinson GE, Villani A, Voss SD, Schiffman JD, Wasserman JD. Von Hippel–Lindau and hereditary pheochromocytoma/paraganglioma syndromes: clinical features, genetics, and surveillance recommendations in childhood. Clin Cancer Res. 2017;23(12):e68–75. https://doi.org/10.1158/1078-0432.CCR-17-0547.
40. Sharma E, Dahal S, Sharma P, Bhandari A, Gupta V, Amgai B, Dahal S. The characteristics and trends in adrenocortical carcinoma: a United States population based study. J Clin Med Res. 2018;10(8):636–40. https://doi.org/10.14740/jocmr3503w.
41. Sharma P, Dhull VS, Arora S, Gupta P, Kumar R, Durgapal P, Malhotra A, Chumber S, Ammini AC, Kumar R, Bal C. Diagnostic accuracy of (68)Ga-DOTANOC PET/CT imaging in pheochromocytoma. Eur J Nucl Med Mol Imaging. 2014;41(3):494–504. https://doi.org/10.1007/s00259-013-2598-1.
42. Skertich NJ, Tierney JF, Chivukula SV, Babazadeh NT, Hertl M, Poirier J, Keutgen XM. Risk factors associated with positive resection margins in patients with adrenocortical carcinoma. Am J Surg. 2020;220(4):932–7. https://doi.org/10.1016/j.amjsurg.2020.02.043.
43. Taïeb D, Sebag F, Barlier A, Tessonnier L, Palazzo FF, Morange I, Niccoli-Sire P, Fakhry N, De Micco C, Cammilleri S, Enjalbert A, Henry J-F, Mundler O. 18F-FDG avidity of pheochromocytomas and paragangliomas: a new molecular imaging signature? J Nucl Med. 2009;50(5):711–7. https://doi.org/10.2967/jnumed.108.060731.
44. Terzolo M, Stigliano A, Chiodini I, Loli P, Furlani L, Arnaldi G, Reimondo G, Pia A, Toscano V, Zini M, Borretta G, Papini E, Garofalo P, Allolio B, Dupas B, Mantero F, Tabarin A, Italian Association of Clinical Endocrinologists. AME position statement on adrenal incidentaloma. Eur J Endocrinol. 2011;164(6):851–70. https://doi.org/10.1530/EJE-10-1147.
45. Thampi A, Shah E, Elshimy G, Correa R. Adrenocortical carcinoma: a literature review. Transl Cancer Res. 2020;9(2):1253–64. https://doi.org/10.21037/tcr.2019.12.28.
46. Thompson LDR. Pheochromocytoma of the Adrenal gland Scaled Score (PASS) to separate benign from malignant neoplasms: a clinicopathologic and immunophenotypic study of 100 cases. Am J Surg Pathol. 2002;26(5):551–66. https://doi.org/10.1097/00000478-200205000-00002.
47. Vogel J, Atanacio AS, Prodanov T, Turkbey BI, Adams K, Martucci V, Camphausen K, Fojo AT, Pacak K, Kaushal A. External beam radiation therapy in treatment of malignant pheochromocytoma and paraganglioma. Front Oncol. 2014;4:166. https://doi.org/10.3389/fonc.2014.00166.
48. Weiss LM, Medeiros LJ, Vickery AL. Pathologic features of prognostic significance in adrenocortical carcinoma. Am J Surg Pathol. 1989;13(3):202–6. https://doi.org/10.1097/00000478-198903000-00004.
49. Wiseman GA, Pacak K, O'Dorisio MS, Neumann DR, Waxman AD, Mankoff DA, Heiba SI, Serafini AN, Tumeh SS, Khutoryansky N, Jacobson AF. Usefulness of 123I-MIBG scintigraphy in the evaluation of patients with known or suspected primary or metastatic pheochromocytoma or paraganglioma: results from a prospective multicenter trial. J Nucl Med. 2009;50(9):1448–54. https://doi.org/10.2967/jnumed.108.058701.
50. Yasir M, Mulji NJ, Kasi A. Multiple endocrine neoplasias type 2. In: StatPearls. StatPearls Publishing; 2023. http://www.ncbi.nlm.nih.gov/books/NBK519054/.

51. Yip L, Duh QY, Wachtel H, Jimenez C, Sturgeon C, Lee C, Fernandez DV, Berber E, Hammer GD, Bancos I, Lee JA, Marko J, Wiseman LFM, Hughes MS, Livhits MJ, Han MA, Smith PW, Wilhelm S, Asa SL, Fahey TJ, McKenzie TJ, Strong VE, Perrier ND. American Association of Endocrine Surgeons Guidelines for Adrenalectomy. JAMA Surg. 2022;157(10):870–7. https://doi.org/10.1001/jamasurg.2022.3544.
52. Zeiger MA, Siegelman SS, Hamrahian AH. Medical and surgical evaluation and treatment of adrenal incidentalomas. J Clin Endocrinol Metab. 2011;96(7):2004–15. https://doi.org/10.1210/jc.2011-0085.
53. Zeiger MA, Thompson GB, Duh Q-Y, Hamrahian AH, Angelos P, Elaraj D, Fishman E, Kharlip J, American Association of Clinical Endocrinologists, & American Association of Endocrine Surgeons. The American Association of Clinical Endocrinologists and American Association of Endocrine Surgeons medical guidelines for the management of adrenal incidentalomas. Endocr Pract. 2009;15 Suppl 1:1–20. https://doi.org/10.4158/EP.15.S1.1.

Anal Cancers

Keri Mayers and Kevin Train

Premalignant Neoplasms

- Human papilloma virus (HPV) is the primary cause of anal squamous cell carcinoma (SCC) and is often preceded by the development of squamous intraepithelial lesions (SIL)
  - HPV infection is nearly ubiquitous in sexually active adults
    - If the patient is immunocompetent, most infections are asymptomatic and clear within 2 years
    - About 15 HPV types are considered "high risk" and associated with the development of anal cancer
      - Most common cancer association: type 16 (~80%) and type 18
      - Most common low-risk genital warts association: types 6 and 11
  - Elevated risk for SIL
    - HIV infection
    - Men who have sex with men (MSM)
    - Women with history of cervical dysplasia
    - Solid organ transplant recipients with history of CIN or anal receptive intercourse
  - Incidence/prevalence ranges widely due to heterogenous populations studied
- SIL terminology
  - Previously graded as anal intraepithelial lesions (AIN) 1–3
  - Updated to a two-tier system with the LAST project
    - LSIL—previously AIN 1

- Abnormal cells extend less than 1/3 the thickness of the epithelium
- HSIL—previously AIN 2 and 3
- Abnormal cells extend greater than one-third the thickness of the epithelium.
  - Equivocal samples can be differentiated by p16 staining (marker of cell proliferation).
    - P16 positive = HSIL
- Natural history
  - LSIL lesions often spontaneously regress
    - 50% regression at 2 years
    - Not considered a precursor for anal cancer but can be a marker for concomitant HSIL
  - HSIL lesions are less likely to regress
    - Generally considered a precursor for anal SCC
    - Progression of HSIL to cancer is about −13% over 5 years if untreated
- Screening
  - No well-defined recommendations or guidelines at this time
    - Very limited evidence to support initial screening with anal PAP vs standard anoscopy vs high-resolution anoscopy (HRA)
- Treatment
  - Goal is to eliminate HSIL and visible lesions
  - Treatment of LSIL is optional but can be offered for cosmesis or to prevent progression to large condylomata
  - Perianal HSIL
    - Topical imiquimod or 5% FU
    - Compliance limited by discomfort
    - Recurrence rate is high after stopping treatment
    - Focused topical treatment with trichloroacetic acid (TCA)
    - Local ablation: electrocautery, infrared coagulation, and excision
  - Anal canal HSIL
    - Trichloroacetic acid (TCA)
    - Local ablation
  - HPV vaccination is now available up to age 45
    - Does not treat existing infection but can prevent infection with additional strains
- Surveillance
  - No well-established guidelines but generally stratified by degree of SIL and patient risk factors
    - Limited evidence to support benefit of gross exam and standard anoscopy vs HRA *except* in the HIV (+) population (Table 2.1)
    - Q6—12-month examination probably sufficient for LSIL
    - Q3—6 months for HSIL and consider more frequent if patient is immunosuppressed

Table 2.1 Notable trials in aSCC

Trial	Design	Locoregional failure
Nigro (1974)	Three patients ChemoXRT with 30 Gy RT with 5-FU and MMC APR after 6 weeks	Two patients had complete response at APR One patient with complete clinical response refused surgery and was clinically negative at 1 year
ACT I (996, 2010 update)	577 patients assigned to radiation alone or radiation +5-FU/mitomycin	ChemoXRT lowered locoregional recurrence (HR 0.46) and cancer related death (HR 0.86)
ACT II (2013)	940 patients assigned to chemoXRT with mitomycin OR cisplatin and then with OR without two doses of maintenance chemotherapy	No difference in treatment response, overall survival, or disease-free progression between treatment arms *Incidental*: supported extended surveillance after treatment. 72% of patients with incomplete response at 11 weeks had complete response by 26 weeks
ANCHOR (2022)	4459 HIV (+) patients with biopsy-proven HSIL All patients underwent HRA q6 months Treatment arm received ablative or topical therapy for visible HSIL lesions	Progression to SCC was 57% lower in the treatment group *Incidental*: May support HRA over other surveillance methods for HIV (+) patients but was not compared to other methods
Keynote 158 (2022)	Phase 2 trial 112 patients with locally advanced or metastatic aSCC with failure of standard therapy Received Pembrolizumab 200 mg IV Q3 weeks x 2 years	11% with objective response 15% response in PD-1-positive tumors and 3% response in PD-1 negative tumors
NCI9673 (2017)	Phase 2 trial 37 patients with metastatic aSCC who failed standard therapy Received nivolumab 3 mg/kg every 2 weeks	24% with a response Two patients with a complete response

Anal Cancer

- Anatomy
  - Definitions
    - *Perianal skin:* contains hair follicles and glands; extends 5 cm from the anal verge
    - *Anal verge:* squamous epithelium that lacks hair follicles; extends from perianal skin to intersphincteric groove
    - *Anal canal:* extends from anal verge to palpable superior border of the anorectal ring (anal sphincter and puborectalis muscles)

- Lymphatic spread
  - Tumors *above* dentate will typically drain via superior rectal → inferior mesenteric (IM) lymphatics and/or middle/inferior rectal → internal iliac nodes
  - Tumors *below* dentate drain via inguinal and femoral lymphatics
  - Tumors at the dentate line can follow both
- Incidence:
  - Incidence rates are low (1.8 per 100,000) but increasing worldwide about 2%/year with increased findings of distant disease at time of diagnosis
  - Increasing mortality of 3.1% per year
- Workup and staging (Table 2.2)
  - Exam: digital rectal exam (DRE), anoscopy, and inguinal node exam
  - Imaging: CT chest abdomen and pelvis
    - PET CT can better define groin node or other metastatic involvements
      - Alternatively, FNA for questionable nodes
    - MRI can *help* define local extent of disease or if patient has iodine contrast allergy but not required
  - Additional: HIV testing (if status not known), gynecology referral for cervical testing, and fertility counseling if appropriate for age
  - Table 2.3 shows five-year outcomes according to stage

Table 2.2 TNM staging

T	Primary tumor	N	Regional lymph nodes	M	Distant metastases
Tx	Cannot be assessed	NX	Cannot be assessed	Mx	Cannot be assessed
T1	Tumor </= 2 cm in greatest dimension	N0	No involvement of regional lymph nodes	M0	No distant metastasis
T2	Tumor >2 cm but </= 5 cm in greatest dimension	N1	Involvement of regional lymph node(s)	M1	Distant metastasis
T3	Tumor >5 cm in greatest dimension	*N1a*	Involvement of inguinal, mesorectal, superior rectal, internal iliac, or obturator lymph node(s)		
T4	Tumor any size invading adjacent organs (i.e., vagina, urethra, bladder)	*N1b*	Involvement of external iliac lymph node(s)		
		N1c	Involvement of external iliac + any N1a lymph node(s)		

Paraaortic lymph nodes are considered M1 disease but included as locoregional disease for treatment, as they can be included in XRT treatment field

Table 2.3 A five-year outcomes by stage

TN stage	Overall survival (%)	Locoregional failure (%)
T2N0	82	17
T3N0	74	18
T4N0	57	37
T2N+	70	26
T3N+	57	44
T4N+	42	60

Table 2.4 Chemotherapy for locoregional disease

Preferred	Alternative

5-FU + mitomycin + RT
  5-FU: Continuous infusion 1000 mg/m^2/day IV days 1–4 and 29–32
  Mitomycin: 10 mg/m^2 IV bolus days 1 and 29 with RT
OR
  Mitomycin: 12 mg/m^2 on day 1 with RT
Capecitabine + mitomycin + RT
  Capecitabine: 825 mg/m^2 PO BID
  Mitomycin: 10 mg/m^2 IV bolus days 1 and 29 with RT
OR
  Capecitabine: 825 mg/m^2 PO BID days 1–5
  Mitomycin: 12 mg/m^2 IV bolus on day 1 with RT
	5 FU + cisplatin + RT
	  5-FU: continuous infusion 1000 mg/m^2/day IV days 1–4
	  Cisplatin: 75 mg/m^2 day 1
	  ***Repeat every 4 weeks with RT

- Management of locoregional disease
  - Initial management for perianal and anal canal SCC is primarily chemoradiotherapy (Nigro protocol)
    - Mitomycin/5-FU and radiation therapy (Table 2.4)
      - Alternative chemotherapy/radiosensitization
        - Mitomycin + capecitabine
        - 5-FU + cisplatin
    - XRT should total 45 Gy minimum, typically 54 Gy
      - Option for 9–14 Gy boost to larger primary tumor or positive nodes
      - Intensity-modulated RT (IMRT) is preferred over three-dimensional conformal RT (3D-CRT)
  - Exceptions
    - Well or moderately differentiated T1 and N0 *perianal* SCC
      - Local excision with 1 cm margins
        - Inadequate margins → reexcision if possible, otherwise chemoradiation
      - Can be extended to select T2, N0 disease if no sphincter involvement
      - In general, perianal SCC has better prognosis than anal canal SCC
    - "Superficially invasive" on biopsy report
      - Defined as negative margins, less than 3 mm basement membrane invasion, and maximal spread less than 7 mm
      - Can be managed with excision alone
  - Post-treatment evaluation
    - Complete response with chemoradiation ranges from 60% to 90%
    - Evaluate with exam and DRE 8–12 weeks after chemoradiation (Fig. 2.1)
      - Complete remission: enter surveillance
      - Persistent disease: Continue exams q4 weeks up to 6 months for full response
        - Avoid biopsies until >6 months to avoid XRT artifact

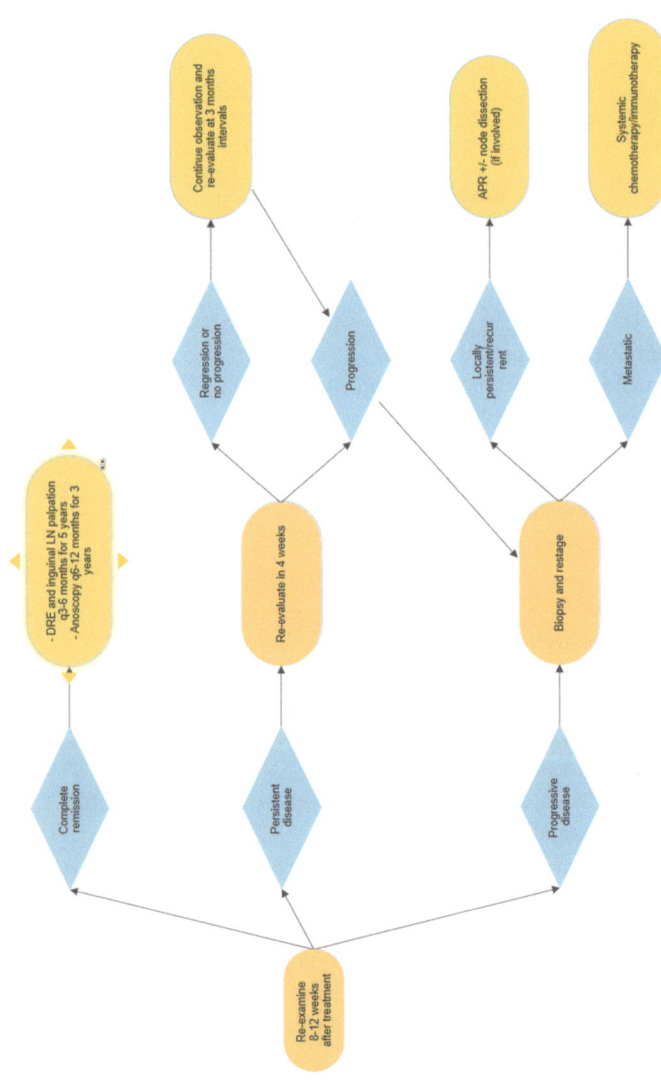

Fig. 2.1 Disease surveillance after chemo-radiation

- Progressive or non-regressing disease: Restage, then APR + groin dissection (if node positive)
  - Surgical management
    - For persistent, progressive, or recurrent disease → abdominoperineal resection (APR)
      - Include superficial inguinal node dissection if nodes are positive by biopsy
      - Consider flap coverage (i.e., VRAM)
        - Still prone to infection and/or dehiscence but can reduce time to complete wound closure by several weeks
    - APR occasionally required for radiation-related toxicity (i.e., extensive tissue necrosis, anal stenosis)
- Management of metastatic disease
  - Can treat primary site with 5-FU or capecitabine + RT for local control
  - Systemic therapy
    - First-line regimen
      - Carboplatin + paclitaxel
      - Alternatives
        - 5-FU + cisplatin
        - FOLFCIS
        - mFOLFOX6
        - Modified DCF
    - Second line
      - Nivolumab or pembrolizumab

Other Anal Tumors

- Anal adenocarcinoma
  - 20% of all anal cancers
  - Mass in anal canal with minimal mucosal component
    - Arises directly from the anal glands and is frequently associated with mucus discharge
    - Can be found in proximity to chronic fistula tracts (i.e., Crohn's disease)
    - Increased risk of lymph node metastases and overall lower survival than both anal canal SCC and rectal adenocarcinoma
    - Treatment like low rectal cancer
- Melanoma
  - Rare, represents 0.05% of all colorectal malignancy
  - Often a late diagnosis; very aggressive disease with poor overall prognosis
    - Generally presents with a pigmented, ulcerated mass, but 30% are amelanotic
  - Staging
    - Does not fall within the typical TNM staging system

- Pelvic MRI, PET, colonoscopy, complete dermatologic and ophthalmic exam—rule out other sites of disease
- No proven use for sentinel lymph node mapping
– Treatment
  - Targeted therapy if BRAF or c-KIT mutations present
  - Historically, APR offers no survival benefit vs. WLE
    – 21% five-year survival for APR and WLE
    – Treatment failure from distant metastases
- Perianal basal cell carcinoma
  – Also quite rare: 0.1% of all basal cell tumors and 0.2% of all perianal tumors
  – Frequently presents with other synchronous lesions
- Verrucous carcinoma (Buschke-Lowenstein tumor)
  – Large tumor, generally associated with HPV types 6 and 11
    - Can have areas of local invasion
    - A five-year malignant transformation of 40–60% if left untreated
  – Treatment
    - Typically wide excision to negative margins
    - Can consider chemoXRT or APR if local excision is not feasible or concern for invasive component

Questions

A 46-year-old woman with history of cervical dysplasia and prior pelvic radiation for Hodkin's lymphoma presents for widespread perianal skin change. She has no identifiable lesions within the anal canal. Representative biopsies all demonstrate HSIL.
- Topical treatment with imiquomod
- Routine surveillance, consider with HRA

A 36-year-old woman sees you for biopsy-proven anal canal cancer. She has no significant medical history, is monogamous with a single male partner, and currently feels well. On exam, she has a palpable left inguinal node.
- HIV testing
- Initial staging (CT chest/abdomen/pelvis, but consider PET for node)
- Discuss fertility implications, consider tissue banking
- Chemoradiation—include groin within radiation treatment field

A 50-year-old man sees you for follow-up 6 months after completing chemoradiation for T2N0 anal cancer. The anal canal lesion has completely resolved, but he has a left inguinal node that is newly palpable.
- Restage
- Consider PET +/− inguinal node FNA
- Once confirmed disease, unilateral groin dissection and continue surveillance of the primary tumor site

Scenario: A 64-year-old man completed chemoXRT 2 years ago for T3N0 anal canal SCC with complete remission. On surveillance, he has developed progressive stenosis of the anal canal. Most recent biopsies of this area were negative for

invasive disease, but it is becoming challenging to do an adequate physical exam and he is developing symptoms of impending obstruction.
- Divert
- Consider APR

Bibliography

1. Aberg JA, Gallant JE, Ghanem KG, et al. Primary care guidelines for the management of persons infected with HIV: 2013 update by the HIV medicine association of the Infectious Diseases Society of America. Clin Infect Dis. 2014;58:e1.
2. Barroso LF, Stier EA, Hillman R, Palefsky J. Anal cancer screening and prevention: summary of evidence reviewed for the 2021 centers for disease control and prevention sexually transmitted infection guidelines. Clin Infect Dis. 2022;74:S179.
3. Chin-Hong PV, Reid GE, AST Infectious Diseases Community of Practice. Human papillomavirus infection in solid organ transplant recipients: Guidelines from the American Society of Transplantation Infectious Diseases Community of Practice. Clin Transpl. 2019;33:e13590.
4. Deshmukh AA, Suk R, Shiels MS, et al. Recent trends in squamous cell carcinoma of the anus incidence and mortality in the United States, 2001–2015. J Natl Cancer Inst. 2020;112(8):829–38.
5. Dunne EF, Markowitz LE, Saraiya M, et al. CDC grand rounds: Reducing the burden of HPV-associated cancer and disease. MMWR Morb Mortal Wkly Rep. 2014;63(4):69–72.
6. Garland SM, Steben M, Sings HL, James M, Lu S, Railkar R, Barr E, Haupt RM, Joura EA. SOJ Infect Dis. 2009;199(6):805–14.
7. Goldstone SE, Lensing SY, Stier EA, et al. A randomized clinical trial of infrared coagulation ablation versus active monitoring of intra-anal high-grade dysplasia in adults with human immunodeficiency virus infection: an AIDS malignancy consortium trial. Clin Infect Dis. 2019;68:1204.
8. Hardt J, Mai S, Weiß C, et al. Abdominoperineal resection and perineal wound healing in recurrent, persistent, or primary anal carcinoma. Int J Color Dis. 2016;31(6):1197–203.
9. Ho GY, Bierman R, Beardsley L, et al. Natural history of cervicovaginal papillomavirus infection in young women. N Engl J Med. 1998;338(7):423–8.
10. James R, Glynne-Jones R, Meadows H, et al. Mitomycin or cisplatin chemoradiation with or without maintenance chemotherapy for treatment of squamous-cell carcinoma of the anus (ACT II): a randomized, phase 3, open-label, 2x2 factorial trial. Lancet Oncol. 2013;14(6):516–24.
11. Johnson LG, Madeleine MM, Newcomer LM, et al. Anal cancer incidence and survival: the surveillance, epidemiology, and end results experience, 1973–2000. Cancer. 2004;101(2):281–8.
12. Jongen VW, Richel O, Marra E, et al. Anal Squamous Intraepithelial Lesions (SILs) in Human Immunodeficiency Virus-Positive Men Who Have Sex With Men: Incidence and Risk Factors of SIL and of Progression and Clearance of Low-Grade SILs. J Infect Dis. 2020;222:62.
13. Kelly H, Chikandiwa A, Alemany Vilches L, et al. Association of antiretroviral therapy with anal high-risk human papillomavirus, anal intraepithelial neoplasia, and anal cancer in people living with HIV: a systematic review and meta-analysis. Lancet HIV. 2020;7:e262.
14. National Comprehensive Cancer Network. Anal carcinoma (Version 2.2023). https://www.nccn.org/professionals/physician_gls/pdf/anal.pdf
15. Northover J, Glynne-Jones R, Sebag-Montefiore D, et al. Chemoradiation for the treatment of epidermoid anal cancer: 13 year follow up of the first randomized UKCCCR anal cancer trial (ACT I). Br J Cancer. 2010;102:1123–8.
16. Palefsky JM, Lee JY, Jay N, et al. Treatment of anal high-grade squamous intraepithelial lesions to prevent anal cancer. N Engl J Med. 2022;386:2273.
17. Palesfky J, Lee J, Jay N, et al. Treatment of anal high-grade squamous intraepithelial lesions to prevent anal cancer. N Engl J Med. 2022;386:2273–82.

18. Pocard M, Tiret E, Nugent K, et al. Results of salvage abdominoperineal resection for anal cancer after radiotherapy. Dis Colon Rectum. 1998;41(12):1488–93.
19. Poynten IM, Jin F, Roberts JM, et al. The natural history of anal high-grade squamous intraepithelial lesions in gay and bisexual men. Clin Infect Dis. 2021;72:853.
20. Schofield AM, Sadler L, Nelson L, et al. A prospective study of anal cancer screening in HIV-positive and negative MSM. AIDS. 2016;30(9):1375–83.
21. Scholefield JH, Castle MT, Watson NF. Malignant transformation of high-grade anal intraepithelial neoplasia. Br J Surg. 2005;92(9):1133–6.
22. Stewart DB, Gaertner WB, Glasgow SC, et al. The American Society of Colon and Rectal Surgeons Clinical Practice Guidelines for Anal Squamous Cell Cancers (Revised 2018). Dis Colon Rectum. 2018;61:755.
23. Stewart D, Gaertner W, Glasgow S, et al. The American Society of Colon and Rectal Surgeons Clinical Practice Guidelines for Anal Squamous Cell Cancers (Revised 2018). https://fascrs.org/ascrs/media/files/downloads/Clinical%20Practice%20Guidelines/cpg_anal_squamous_cell_cancers_2018.pdf
24. Watson AJ, Smith BB, Whitehead MR, et al. Malignant progression of anal intra-epithelial neoplasia. ANZ J Surg. 2006;76(8):715–7.

Biliary Cancers

R. Connor Chick and Jordan M. Cloyd

Introduction

- Biliary tract cancers (BTCs) are a heterogenous group of cancers for which treatment and prognosis depend on anatomic location (Fig. 3.1)
  - Extrahepatic cholangiocarcinoma (ECC)
    - Distal cholangiocarcinoma (distal to cystic duct)
    - Perihilar cholangiocarcinoma (proximal to cystic duct)

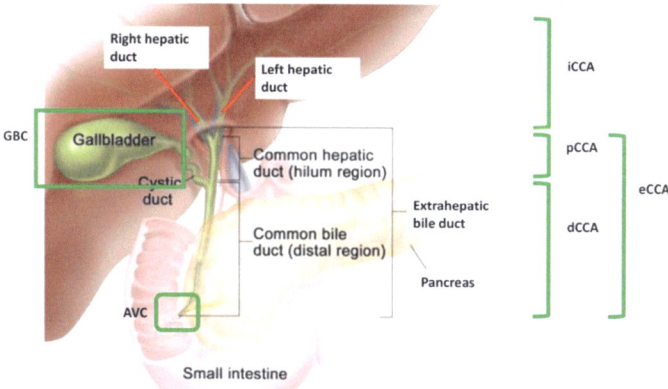

Fig. 3.1 Anatomic classification of biliary tract cancers, including intrahepatic (iCCA), perihilar (pCCA), distal (dCCA), and gallbladder (GBC). Extrahepatic (eCCA) includes both pCCA and dCCA [23]

- Gallbladder adenocarcinoma (GC)
  - Intrahepatic cholangiocarcinoma (ICC)
- Eighty percent are extrahepatic bile duct cancers, of which 60–70% are perihilar
- GC is often incidentally diagnosed either intraoperatively or incidentally on final pathology after cholecystectomy for other reasons (>70% of cases)
- ICC and ECC often diagnosed at advanced stages
- Epidemiology
  - ICC and ECC more common in Southeast Asia with >4 deaths per 100,000, less common in the West [1]
    - Risk factors include primary sclerosing cholangitis (PSC), choledochal cysts, parasitic infections (*Clonorchis sinensis*), hepatitis C, and anomalous pancreaticobiliary junction (PBJ)
    - Choledochal cysts (Fig. 3.1)—thought to be related to anomalous PBJ, induce low level chronic inflammation [2]
      - Todani classification of choledochal cysts [3] (Fig. 3.2)

CHOLEDOCHAL CYSTS

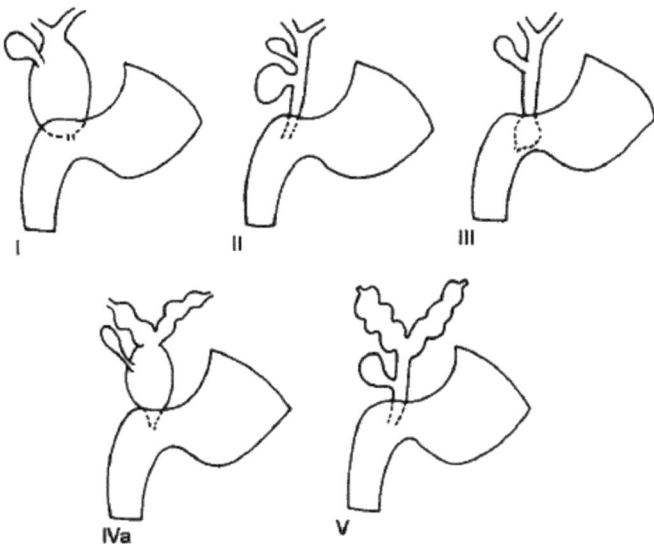

Fig. 3.2 Todani classification of choledochal cysts [3]

- GC more common among people of indigenous American descent and in southeast Asia
    - Other risk factors: obesity, large stones (>3 cm), and PSC
    - Segmental calcification = high risk for cancer
    - Porcelain gallbladder has no increased risk of malignancy
- Surgical resection (± chemotherapy) is a primary treatment for BTCs that are localized and resectable.
- Systemic therapy is the primary treatment for patients with metastatic or unresectable disease:
    - BTCs have a relatively high proportion of genetic mutations enabling an increasing number of targeted and immune-based treatment options available.
    - Numerous locoregional options are available to facilitate local control for those with unresectable cancers.

Diagnosis

Clinical Presentation

- ECC
    - Most often presents with jaundice, occasionally vague epigastric or right upper quadrant pain, acholic stool, dark urine, and pruritus [4]
- ICC often presents incidentally on cross-sectional imaging. Can present at later stages with nonspecific symptoms of pain, nausea, and jaundice.
- GC presents in three distinct scenarios:
    - Incidental (i.e., asymptomatic) pathologic finding after cholecystectomy
    - Incidental (i.e., asymptomatic) finding on cross-sectional imaging or intraoperative finding
    - With symptoms (e.g., jaundice, pain) secondary to large mass or metastatic disease

Genetics

- About 10% of BTCs will occur in association with a germline mutation [5]
    - BRCA2 > BRCA 1 > MLH1, MSH2, PALB2, RAD51d, BAP1, and ATM
    - Increased risk in patients with BRCA mutations and Lynch syndrome
- May be a role for somatic genetic testing in unresectable/metastatic disease to identify targetable mutations (in particular FGFR2, NTRK, IDH1, BRAF, and MMR genes)

Histology

- BTC: >90% adenocarcinoma, rarely squamous cell or signet ring [4]
  - Sclerosing (>70%)—dense desmoplastic stroma, risk for false-negative cytology
  - Nodular (20%)
  - Papillary (5–10%)
- Gallbladder almost exclusively adenocarcinoma (which also arises from epithelium)
  - Polyps and other benign lesions—very common (4–7% of the population) [6]
    - Cholesterol polyp—not a polyp at all, actually a lipid-laden nonmobile stone. Will not have Doppler flow
    - Adenoma—tubular, papillary, or mixed type, malignant potential
    - Adenomyomatosis—by definition is benign, located in fundus
    - Treatment versus surveillance based on size on US
      - If >2 cm polyp: treat as malignant
      - If 1–1.9 cm: simple cholecystectomy but increased risk
      - 6–9 mm: consider annual ultrasound
      - 5 mm or less: ultrasound in a year, if no change then stop surveillance

Anatomic Classification

- Cholangiocarcinoma
  - Distal ECC
    - Defined as distal to the cystic duct
  - Perihilar ECC
    - Defined as proximal to the cystic duct but distal to the second order biliary radicals
    - Bismuth-Corlette classification (Fig. 3.3)
      - I—distal to the confluence
      - II—involving the confluence but not either hepatic duct
      - IIIa/IIIb—involving the right (a) or left (b) hepatic duct
      - IV—involving both right and left hepatic ducts
  - ICC
    - Arising from biliary tracts proximal to the second order biliary radicals
- GC
  - Major factor is whether tumor is on peritoneal side or hepatic side [7] and location near the fundus or infundibulum

3 Biliary Cancers

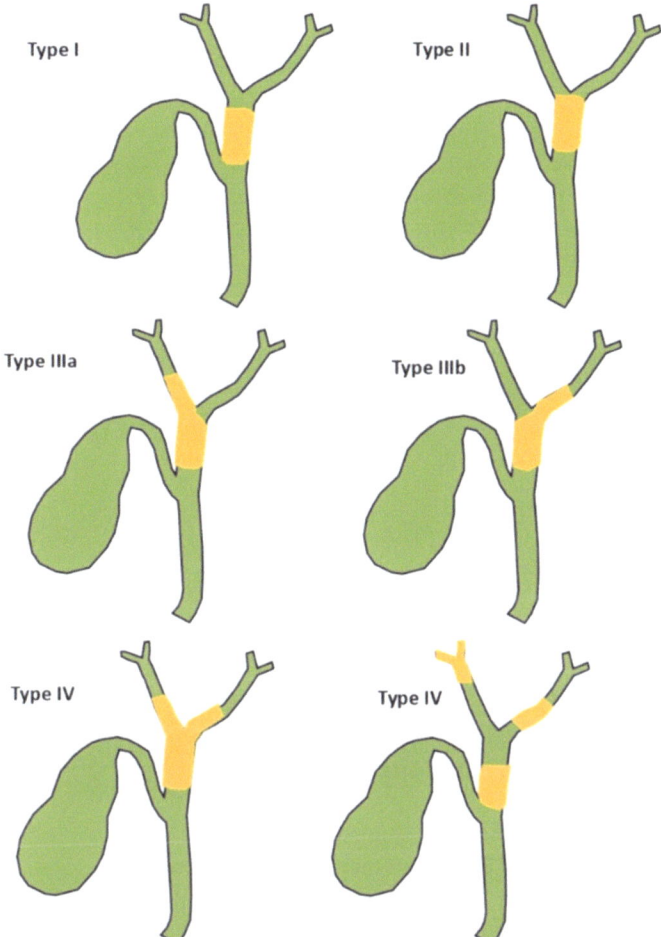

Fig. 3.3 Bismuth-Corlette classification of perihilar cholangiocarcinoma [24]

Evaluation and Staging

Labs

- Complete metabolic panel with LFTs, CBC, and coagulation tests
- CA 19–9 (except unreliable with concomitant jaundice)

Imaging

- Transabdominal US—useful for gallbladder pathology
- CT abdomen/pelvis with liver or pancreas protocol depending on tumor type
  - ECC can be localized based on upstream biliary dilation.
  - ICC has more variable appearance; classic finding is a focal segmental bile duct dilation proximal to an intrahepatic mass.
  - Primarily used for determining resectability, operative planning (vascular anatomy), and evaluation for metastatic disease.
- CT chest to evaluate for metastatic disease
- MRI liver—useful for evaluating liver lesions and/or ruling out metastatic disease
- MRCP—evaluate biliary anatomy and location of biliary tumor
- PET/CT—not routinely used except suspicion of metastatic disease
- Endoscopic cholangiopancreatography (ERCP)—as needed for diagnostic or therapeutic purposes
  - Brushings
  - Spyglass cholangioscopy
  - Biliary stenting
- EUS
  - Assess anatomic extent of tumor
  - FNA of biliary masses and/or porta hepatis lymph nodes, can help identify target mutations via next-generation sequencing

TNM Staging: Key Distinctions

- T stage is very different depending on subtype (Table 3.1)
  - T stage in distal ECC is based on depth of invasion
  - T stage in perihilar ECC and gallbladder cancer depends on relationship to surrounding structures in the porta hepatis
  - T stage in ICC depends on size, number of tumors, vascular invasion, and invasion of other structures
- Clinicopathologic stage (Table 3.2)
  - Relationship between TNM stage and clinicopathologic stage has become more complex as clinicopathologic stage is better correlated to prognosis.
  - Stages I–II are generally amenable to curative intent surgery
  - Stage III consists of locally and/or regionally advanced disease.
  - Stage IV in distal ECC and ICC represents metastatic disease. In perihilar and gallbladder cancer, stage IV includes the following:
    - Stage IVA: locally/regionally advanced disease
    - Stage IVB: metastatic disease

Table 3.1 T stage for biliary tract cancers [5, 8]

	Distal ECC	Perihilar ECC	Gallbladder	ICC
T1	Depth < 5 mm	Confined to bile duct	Invades lamina propria (T1a) or muscularis (T1b)	Solitary tumor without vascular invasion (T1a up to 5 cm, T1b >5 cm)
T2	Depth 5–12 mm	Invades surrounding adipose tissue (T2a) or liver parenchyma (T2b)	Invades perimuscular connective tissue on peritoneal side without involvement of serosa (T2a) or liver surface (T2b)	Solitary tumor with intrahepatic vascular invasion, or multiple tumors
T3	Depth > 12 mm	Invades unilateral branch of portal vein or hepatic artery	Perforates serosa, invades liver, or invades adjacent organ or bile duct	Perforates visceral peritoneum
T4	Involves celiac axis, SMA, and/or CHA	Invades main PV or both right/left PV, CHA, or second-order biliary radicals bilaterally with contralateral PV or HA involvement	Invades main portal vein or hepatic artery, or 2+ extrahepatic organs	Directly invades local extrahepatic structures

Table 3.2 AJCC prognostic groups for biliary tract cancers [5, 8]

Stage	Distal ECC	Perihilar ECC	Gallbladder	Icc
I	T1 N0 M0	T1 N0 M0	T1 N0 M0	T1a (IA) or T1b (IIA) and N0 M0
II	T1 N1 M0 (IIA) or T2 N0 M0 (IIA) or T2 N1 M0 (IIB) or T3 N0–1 M0 (IIB)	T2 N0 M0	T2a (IIA) or T2b (IIB) N0 M0	T2 N0 M0
III	T1–3 N2 M0 (IIIA) or T4 Nx M0 (IIIB)	T3 N0 M0 (IIIA) or T4 N0 M0 (IIIB) or Tx N1 M0 (IIIC)	T3 N0 M0 (IIIA) or T1–3 N1 M0 (IIIB)	T3 N0 M0 (IIIA) or T4 N0 M0 (IIIB) or Tx N1 M0 (IIIB)
IV	Tx Nx M1	Tx N2 M0 (IVA) or Tx Nx M1 (IVB)	T4 N0–1 M0 (IVA) or Tx N2 M0 (IVB) or Tx Nx M1 (IVB)	Tx Nx M1

Initial Therapy

Surgical Principles

- Distal ECC
  - Managed similar to pancreatic head cancer—often requires Whipple procedure (pancreatoduodenectomy)
  - Mid-bile duct cancers that are amenable to true extrahepatic bile duct resection without pancreas or liver resection are uncommon.
  - Porta hepatis lymphadenectomy indicated
    - Six lymph nodes recommended
- Perihilar ECC
  - Excision of bile duct plus major hepatectomy (typically formal anatomic resection), reconstruct with hepaticojejunostomy
  - As with any hepatectomy, consider arterial and portal inflow, venous outflow, biliary drainage, and future liver remnant (FLR)
  - Caudate resection often required due to direct invasion of biliary drainage
  - Involvement of both right and left ducts → unresectable; consider transplant if tumor <3 cm and confined to the liver
  - Porta hepatis lymphadenectomy indicated
    - Six lymph nodes recommended
- GC
  - Surgical management dependent on T stage
    - T1a: cholecystectomy alone
    - T1b+: "radical" cholecystectomy with porta hepatis lymphadenectomy
      - Consider anatomic IVb/V bisegmentectomy
      - Nonanatomic parenchyma-sparing resection (i.e., 2 cm margin around gallbladder fossa)
  - Consider sending cystic duct margin for frozen or resecting down to CBD—can be a common site of positive margin
    - If positive cystic duct margin, perform bile duct resection and hepaticojejunostomy
  - Consider diagnostic laparoscopy beforehand—30% will present with occult peritoneal metastasis, especially with known T2/T3 disease
- ICC
  - Hepatectomy with goal of R0 resection
  - As with any hepatectomy, consider arterial and portal inflow, venous outflow, biliary drainage, and future liver remnant (FLR)
  - Porta hepatis lymphadenectomy—one of very few indications for lymphadenectomy with hepatectomy for primary tumor
    - Six lymph nodes
    - Consider personalizing the lymphadenectomy based on location (left-sided tumors include lesser omentum nodes; right-sided tumors include retropancreatic lymph nodes) [9]

Liver Transplant

- Perihilar ECC
  - Mayo criteria: biopsy-proven cancer or malignant stricture with CA 19–9 > 100, tumor <3 cm, no distant metastasis, no evidence of nodal involvement by EUS-FNA or surgical lymph node biopsy [10]
  - Mayo protocol: Neoadjuvant EBRT + radiosensitizing chemotherapy +/− brachytherapy → staging laparoscopy → maintenance chemotherapy until transplant [11]
  - Each institution may have slight differences in own protocols
- ICC
  - Worse oncologic outcomes compared to perihilar
  - May be beneficial with best available neoadjuvant therapy and small, low-grade tumor with lower CA 19–9 [12]
  - Typically offered only as part of a clinical trial

Systemic Therapy

Systemic Therapy Options

- NCCN preferred regimen is gemcitabine + cisplatin + durvalumab (PD-L1 inhibitor) based on TOPAZ-1 trial [13]
- Alternative regimen is gemcitabine-cisplatin alone based on ABC-02 trial [14]
- Second-line preferred regimen is FOLFOX based on ABC-06 trial [15]
- BTCs have a relatively high rate of genetic mutations which make them susceptible to an increasing array of targeted therapies [5]
  - IDH
  - FGFR
  - MSI-H

Adjuvant Therapy

- Current standard of care adjuvant therapy following resection of BTC is adjuvant capecitabine (also known as Xeloda) based on BILCAP trial [16]
  - Grouped all BTCs together, not powered for subgroup analyses of individual cancer types or by prognostic factors (e.g., lymph node involvement)
  - Findings supported by the JCOG1202/ASCOT trial which showed improved survival with adjuvant S-1 (similar to Xeloda, used in Japan) [17]
- Ongoing ACTICCA-1 trial aims to compare adjuvant gemcitabine-cisplatin to capecitabine but previously published PRODIGE 12–ACCORD 18 Trial found no survival improvement with adjuvant gemcitabine-oxaliplatin compared to observation.

Neoadjuvant Therapy

- Upfront surgical resection is a preferred approach for resectable BTCs
  - Neoadjuvant therapy is primarily reserved for unresectable or those at risk for margin-positive resection [18].
  - Can be considered for biologically high-risk scenarios (clinically positive lymph nodes, markedly elevated tumor markers, satellite lesions, macrovascular invasion, etc.) [19]
- When used, neoadjuvant therapy generally consists of systemic therapy: gem-cis + durva for most BTCs.
- Increasing number of locoregional therapies (see below) which can be used for unresectable ICC with ~20% downstaging to resection.
- Ongoing Optimal Perioperative Therapy for Incidental Gallbladder Cancer (OPT-IN) trial randomizes patients with incidental GBC to neoadjuvant gemcitabine-cisplatin versus upfront surgery

Locoregional Therapies

Radiation Therapy

- Radiation can be considered based on nonrandomized SWOG S0809—adjuvant gemcitabine + capecitabine followed by capecitabine + RT for extrahepatic and gallbladder cancer [20].
- Unresectable tumors may be amenable to RT with concurrent 5-FU-based chemo (e.g., capecitabine).

Transarterial Therapies

- Rationale for liver-directed therapy is that death from ICC typically occurs from liver failure; these modalities can be effective in achieving disease control but uncommonly downstage unresectable disease to resectable [21].
- TACE (transarterial chemoembolization) can be considered for unresectable ICC.
- TARE (transarterial radioembolization) is also effective at achieving disease control.
  - MISPHEC trial of Gem-Cis + TARE with Y-90 downstaged 20% of patients and achieved disease control in 98% [22].

Hepatic Artery Infusion Pump

- Several nonrandomized prospective studies of HAI with floxuridine (FUDR) suggest good disease control and occasional downstaging to surgical resection [21].

Surveillance

- CT C/A/P every 3–6 months for 2 years and then every 6–12 months until 5 years
- Recurrences can occur locoregionally (along resection margin or regional lymph nodes) or distant (liver, lungs, peritoneum, lymph nodes most common)

References

1. Lafaro KJ, Cosgrove D, Geschwind J-FH, Kamel I, Herman JM, Pawlik TM. Multidisciplinary care of patients with intrahepatic cholangiocarcinoma: updates in management. Gastroenterol Res Pract. 2015;2015:1–14. https://doi.org/10.1155/2015/860861.
2. Brown ZJ, Baghdadi A, Kamel I, Labiner HE, Hewitt DB, Pawlik TM. Diagnosis and management of choledochal cysts. HPB (Oxford). 2023;25(1):14–25. https://doi.org/10.1016/j.hpb.2022.09.010.
3. De Vries JS, De Vries S, Aronson DC, et al. Choledochal cysts: age of presentation, symptoms, and late complications related to Todani's classification. J Pediatr Surg. 2002;37(11):1568–73. https://doi.org/10.1053/jpsu.2002.36186.
4. Lewis HL, Rahnemai-Azar AA, Dillhoff M, Schmidt CR, Pawlik TM. Current management of perihilar cholangiocarcinoma and future perspectives. Chirurgia. 2017;112(3):193. https://doi.org/10.21614/chirurgia.112.3.193.
5. Network NCC. Biliary tract cancers. Accessed June 30, 2023. https://www.nccn.org/professionals/physician_gls/pdf/btc.pdf
6. Riddell ZC, Corallo C, Albazaz R, Foley KG. Gallbladder polyps and adenomyomatosis. Br J Radiol. 2023;96(1142):20220115. https://doi.org/10.1259/bjr.20220115.
7. Krell RW, Wei AC. Gallbladder cancer: surgical management. Chin Clin Oncol. 2019;8(4):36. https://doi.org/10.21037/cco.2019.06.06.
8. Amin MB, American Joint Committee on Cancer, American Cancer Society. AJCC cancer staging manual. Eight edition/editor-in-chief, Mahul B. Amin, MD, FCAP; editors, Stephen B. Edge, MD, FACS and 16 others; Donna M. Gress, RHIT, CTR - Technical editor; Laura R. Meyer, CAPM - Managing editor. cd. American Joint Committee on Cancer, Springer; 2017. xvii, 1024 pages
9. Cloyd JM, Ejaz A, Pawlik TM. The landmark series: intrahepatic cholangiocarcinoma. Ann Surg Oncol. 2020;27(8):2859–65. https://doi.org/10.1245/s10434-020-08621-4.
10. Heimbach JK, Gores GJ, Nagorney DM, Rosen CB. Liver transplantation for perihilar cholangiocarcinoma after aggressive neoadjuvant therapy: a new paradigm for liver and biliary malignancies? Surgery. 2006;140(3):331–4. https://doi.org/10.1016/j.surg.2006.01.010.
11. Hewitt DB, Brown ZJ, Pawlik TM. Current perspectives on the surgical management of perihilar cholangiocarcinoma. Cancers. 2022;14(9):2208. https://doi.org/10.3390/cancers14092208.
12. Quaresima S, Melandro F, Giovanardi F, et al. New insights in the setting of transplant oncology. Medicina. 2023;59(3):568. https://doi.org/10.3390/medicina59030568.
13. Oh D-Y, Ruth He A, Qin S, et al. Durvalumab plus gemcitabine and cisplatin in advanced biliary tract cancer. NEJM Evid. 2022;1(8) https://doi.org/10.1056/evidoa2200015.
14. Valle J, Wasan H, Palmer DH, et al. Cisplatin plus gemcitabine versus gemcitabine for biliary tract cancer. N Engl J Med. 2010;362(14):1273–81. https://doi.org/10.1056/NEJMoa0908721.
15. Lamarca A, Palmer DH, Wasan HS, et al. Second-line FOLFOX chemotherapy versus active symptom control for advanced biliary tract cancer (ABC-06): a phase 3, open-label, randomised, controlled trial. Lancet Oncol. 2021;22(5):690–701. https://doi.org/10.1016/S1470-2045(21)00027-9.
16. Primrose JN, Fox RP, Palmer DH, et al. Capecitabine compared with observation in resected biliary tract cancer (BILCAP): a randomised, controlled, multicentre, phase 3 study. Lancet Oncol. 2019;20(5):663–73. https://doi.org/10.1016/S1470-2045(18)30915-X.

17. Nakachi K, Ikeda M, Konishi M, et al. Adjuvant S-1 compared with observation in resected biliary tract cancer (JCOG1202, ASCOT): a multicentre, open-label, randomised, controlled, phase 3 trial. Lancet. 2023;401(10372):195–203. https://doi.org/10.1016/s0140-6736(22)02038-4.
18. Akateh C, Ejaz AM, Pawlik TM, Cloyd JM. Neoadjuvant treatment strategies for intrahepatic cholangiocarcinoma. World J Hepatol. 2020;12(10):693–708. https://doi.org/10.4254/wjh.v12.i10.693.
19. Cloyd JM, Prakash L, Vauthey JN, et al. The role of preoperative therapy prior to pancreatoduodenectomy for distal cholangiocarcinoma. Am J Surg. 2019;218(1):145–50. https://doi.org/10.1016/j.amjsurg.2018.08.024.
20. Ben-Josef E, Guthrie KA, El-Khoueiry AB, et al. SWOG S0809: a phase II intergroup trial of adjuvant capecitabine and gemcitabine followed by radiotherapy and concurrent capecitabine in extrahepatic cholangiocarcinoma and gallbladder carcinoma. J Clin Oncol. 2015;33(24):2617–22. https://doi.org/10.1200/JCO.2014.60.2219.
21. Bressler L, Bath N, Manne A, Miller E, Cloyd JM. Management of locally advanced intrahepatic cholangiocarcinoma: a narrative review. Chin Clin Oncol. 2023;12(2):15. https://doi.org/10.21037/cco-22-115.
22. Edeline J, Touchefeu Y, Guiu B, et al. Radioembolization plus chemotherapy for first-line treatment of locally advanced intrahepatic cholangiocarcinoma. JAMA Oncology. 2020;6(1):51. https://doi.org/10.1001/jamaoncol.2019.3702.
23. Ricci AD, Rizzo A, Bonucci C, et al. PARP inhibitors in biliary tract ancer: a new kid on the block? Medicines. 2020;7(9):54. https://doi.org/10.3390/medicines7090054.
24. Hewitt DB, Brown ZJ, Pawlik TM. Current perspectives on the surgical management of perihilar cholangiocarcinoma. Cancers (Basel). 2022;14(9) https://doi.org/10.3390/cancers14092208.

Breast Cancer

Kimberly S. Bailey and Gregory Stimac

Introduction

- Most common malignancy of females in the United States and second highest cause of cancer death [1].
- Includes carcinoma in situ, invasive carcinoma, Paget's disease, phyllodes tumor, and inflammatory breast cancer.
- Common clinical staging studies include mammography, ultrasound, MRI, and PET/CT.
- Surgical options generally include partial mastectomy (aka lumpectomy) or mastectomy with or without sentinel lymph node biopsy or axillary dissection depending on stage and age of the patient.
- Adjunct treatments include chemotherapy, radiation therapy, immunotherapy, and endocrine therapy.

Diagnosis

- Symptoms may include a palpable mass or inflammation of the breast, but most breast cancers are now screen-detected.
- Most breast cancers are not painful.

K. S. Bailey (✉)
Division of Surgical Oncology, Department of Surgery, West Virginia University, Morgantown, WV, USA
e-mail: kimberly.bailey@hsc.wvu.edu

G. Stimac
Department of Surgery, West Virginia University, Morgantown, WV, USA
e-mail: gregory.stimac@hsc.wvu.edu

- Screening guidelines:
  - Average risk
    - 25–39-year-old women should have review of general medical and family history, clinical breast exam, risk assessment, risk reduction counseling, and education about concerning breast findings.
    - ≥40-year-old women should have the addition of annual screening mammogram with tomosynthesis. Consideration should be given to supplemental screening for those with heterogeneously dense or extremely dense breasts.
    - There is no consensus on when to stop performing annual screening mammograms, but comorbid conditions and a life expectancy of less than 10 years should be considered in discussion with the patient.
  - Increased risk
    - Includes individuals who:
      - Lifetime breast cancer risk of ≥20% (several risk models available)
      - Thoracic radiation therapy between the ages of 10 and 30
      - A 5-year risk of breast cancer of ≥1.7% by Gail model in those 35 years old and older
      - Atypical ductal hyperplasia (ADH), atypical lobular hyperplasia (ALH) or Lobular carcinoma in situ (LCIS) with ≥20% residual lifetime risk
      - Family pedigree suggestive of a genetic predisposition to developing breast cancer
    - No additional screenings prior to the age of 21
    - Consider referral to genetics counselor
    - Annual screening mammogram should begin 10 years earlier than age of youngest family member diagnosed with breast cancer but not before 30 years old or later than 40 years old.
    - Annual MRI with and without contrast
      - Contrast-enhanced mammography (CEM) or molecular breast imaging (MBI) for those who cannot undergo MRI
      - Consider whole breast ultrasound if CEM/MBI is not available
      - Start MRIs 10 years earlier than age of youngest family member diagnosed with breast cancer but not before 25 years old or later than 40 years old
    - Risk reduction
      - Chemoprophylaxis and/or lifestyle modification.
    - For individuals who have had thoracic radiation therapy (RT) between 10 and 30 years old, increased screenings should begin 8 years after RT, but not before age 25 with the exception of an annual clinical history and exam which should begin 8 years after RT.
    - There is limited data on screening mammograms for males at increased risk of breast cancer, but there is potential benefit.
  - Transgender individuals—No NCCN guidelines yet, below are condensed recommendations from the American College of Radiology
    - Data is still limited.

- Recommendations are based on sex assigned at birth, use and duration of gender-affirming hormone therapy (past or current), breast surgery, amount of breast development, age, and personal risk of breast cancer.
- Transgender men (assigned female at birth, male gender identity):
  - In the absence of mastectomy, patients are considered to have the same risk of developing breast cancer as cis-women and should follow standard screening guidelines as above
  - Risk of developing breast cancer decreases by 90% after mastectomy. No further need for screening
- Transgender women (assigned male at birth, female gender identity)
  - Screening is not recommended to those who have not used gender-affirming hormones
  - Screening mammogram should be considered for average risk patients ≥40 years old who have had ≥5 years of gender-affirming hormone therapy
  - Screening mammogram is usually appropriate for increased-risk patients 25–30 years old who have had gender-affirming hormone therapy but could also be considered for those who have not.
- Concerning findings on clinical exam
  - Palpable mass
    - ≥30 years old start with diagnostic mammogram with tomosynthesis or CEM +/− ultrasound
    - <30 years old
      - Start workup with ultrasound if clinically suspicious.
      - If not clinically suspicious, consider observation for 1–2 menstrual cycles. Get ultrasound if persistent.
  - Skin thickening with edema (Peau d'orange)
  - New nipple inversion
  - Palpable axillary lymphadenopathy
  - Unilateral, spontaneous, bloody nipple discharge
  - Erythema
  - Nipple excoriation
  - Scaling or eczema to the breast
  - Skin ulcers
  - Pain (focal)
- Imaging
  - Mammogram
    - Limited by breast higher breast density
    - Screening
      - Two images—craniocaudal (CC) and mediolateral oblique (MLO)
      - Tomosynthesis reduces callbacks and improves cancer detection but doubles radiation exposure
    - Diagnostic
  - Ultrasound

- Screening—routine use not recommended but can be helpful as an adjunct in individuals with dense breast tissue (4.3 additional cancers identified per 1000 exams performed)
- Diagnostic
- MRI
  - Screening—considered in the following:
    - Patients with lifetime risk of developing breast cancer ≥20%
    - Patients with dense breast tissue
    - Patients with a personal history of breast cancer and:
      - Dense breasts treated with breast conservation therapy (BCT) + RT
      - Diagnosed prior to age 50
      - Lifetime risk of second primary >20%
  - Diagnostic
- Can be used for staging evaluation to better define extent of disease, gauge response to neoadjuvant therapy, screen contra-lateral breast, or determine multifocal/centric disease at time of cancer diagnosis. More useful in patients with dense breast tissue and/or lobular cancers.
  - Can be used to identify otherwise unidentified disease in cases where there is a positive axillary node without known primary tumor
- Contrast-Enhanced Mammography (CEM)
  - Risk of iodinated contrast administration
  - Higher radiation exposure compared to standard mammography
- Molecular Breast Imaging (MBI)
  - Substantially higher whole-body radiation dose compared to mammography
- Breast Imaging Reporting and Data System—BIRADS
  - BIRADS 0—Needs additional imaging evaluation
  - BIRADS 1—Negative
  - BIRADS 2—Benign Finding
  - BIRADS 3—Probably benign finding
    - A 6-month follow-up generally recommended until 2–3 years of stability is established
    - ≤2% risk of malignancy
  - BIRADS 4—Suspicious Abnormality
    A. Low suspicion for malignancy 2–9%
    B. Moderate suspicion for malignancy 10–49%
    C. High suspicion for malignancy 50–94%
  - BIRADS 5—Highly suggestive of malignancy
    - ≥95% chance of malignancy
  - BIRADS 6—Known biopsy-proven malignancy
  - Density:
    A. Fatty replaced
    B. Scattered fibroglandular density
    C. Heterogeneously dense

- D. Extremely dense
- Metastatic workup (more below)
  - PET
  - CT chest/abdomen/pelvis + bone scan
- Biopsy
  - Core needle biopsy
    - Stereotactic
    - Ultrasound-guided
    - MRI-guided
  - Excisional biopsy
    - When core biopsy shows indeterminate, image/pathology discordance, ADH, papillary lesions with atypia, complex sclerosing lesions (including radial scar), and nonclassic LCIS
    - Consider for ALH, LCIS, flat epithelial atypia (FEA), columnar cell lesions (CCL), papillary lesions without atypia, and fibroepithelial lesions. Management of these lesions remains controversial with a range of upstaging rates after excisional biopsy.
  - Skin punch biopsy
    - Suspicion of inflammatory breast cancer
      - Peau d'orange
      - Skin thickening
      - Edema
      - Erythema
    - Suspicion of Paget disease
      - Nipple excoriation
      - Scaling
      - Skin ulceration
  - Aspiration
    - Proceed to core biopsy if mass persists
    - Resume screening if mass resolves with nonbloody cyst fluid obtained
    - Nontraumatic, bloody fluid should be sent to cytology
      - With negative cytology consider core needle biopsy vs short-term follow-up
      - Surgical excision if atypical or malignant cytology
- Environmental risk factors
  - Female sex
  - Dense breast tissue
  - Mantle radiation
  - Breast implants
    - Breast implant-related anaplastic large cell lymphoma (BIA-ALCL)
      - Effusion, enlargement, or mass
    - Breast implant-associated squamous cell carcinoma (BIA-SCC)
      - Ulceration

- Lifestyle risks—inactive, poor diet, excess alcohol intake, and outside of ideal body weight (BMI 20–25)
- Familial Risk Factors
  - 10% of breast cancer can be linked to a genetic mutation
    - 90% of hereditary breast cancer is due to mutations of the BRCA1 and BRCA2 genes.
    - Breast cancers caused by genetic mutations tend to occur at a younger age, are more likely to be bilateral, and are more likely to be associated with other cancers such as ovarian, prostate, pancreatic, and melanoma.
    - Male breast cancer is more likely to be associated with a genetic mutation.
  - Genetic mutations associated with breast cancer (Table 4.1)
    - BRCA1—tumor suppressor gene
    - BRCA2—tumor suppressor gene
    - TP53—tumor suppressor gene
    - PTEN—tumor suppressor gene
    - STK11—human protein kinase and tumor suppressor gene
    - CDH1—tumor suppressor gene
    - PALB2—tumor suppressor gene
    - CHEK2—tumor suppressor gene
    - ATM—spouses of carriers should also be tested as homozygous ATM carriers develop ataxia telangiectasia which is a neurological disorder leading to the formation of cancerous tumors and neurodegeneration
    - NBN—associated with Nijmegen breakage syndrome
    - BARD1—works with BRCA1 to repair damaged DNA
    - BRIP1—spouses of carriers should also be tested as homozygous BRIP1 carriers may develop Fanconi anemia leading to bone marrow failure syndromes, birth defects, and increased risk of head, neck, skin, GI and genital tract cancers.
    - RAD51C
  - When a mutation is discovered, further genetic testing for at-risk family members is recommended.
- Pathologic Principles
  - Noninvasive breast cancer vs invasive cancer
  - Histology
    - Common
      - Ductal/no special type (NST)—80% of breast cancers
      - Lobular - 2nd most common type
      - Mixed
      - Micropapillary
      - Metaplastic
    - Favorable
      - Cannot be high grade
      - Human epidermal growth factor receptor 2 (HER2) negative
      - Pure tubular

Table 4.1 NCCN Clinical Practice Guidelines in Oncology (NCCN Guidelines®) Genetic/Familial High-Risk Assessment: breast, ovarian, and pancreatic [8]

Gene	Breast cancer risk/Management	Epithelial ovarian cancer risk/management	Other cancer risk/management
ATM	20–40% lifetime risk. Annual mammograms starting at age 40. Consider breast MRI with contrast starting at age 30–35. Manage based on family history.	2–3% lifetime risk. Manage based on family history	5–10% lifetime risk of pancreatic cancer. May be associated with an increased risk of prostate cancer
BARD1	20–40% lifetime risk. Annual mammograms starting at 40 years. Consider breast MRI with contrast starting at age 40. Manage based on family history	No evidence of increased risk	No evidence of increased risk
BRCA1	>60% lifetime risk in women. CBE q6–12 months, MRI with contrast annually starting at age 25. Begin annual mammogram (staggered q6 months with MRI) at age 30. RRM. 0.2–1.2% lifetime risk in men.	39–58% lifetime risk. Transvaginal US of ovaries with CA-125 q6mo starting at ages 30–35. RRSO between ages 35 and 40 or upon completion of child bearing	≤5% lifetime risk of pancreatic cancer. Consider pancreatic cancer screening starting at age 50 (or 10 years younger than earliest pancreatic cancer diagnosis in the family) in those with first- or second-degree relatives with pancreatic cancer and same genetic variant. MRI/MRCP and/or EUS. 7–26% lifetime risk of prostate cancer
BRCA2	> 80% lifetime risk in women. CBE q6–12 months, MRI with contrast annually starting at age 25. Begin annual mammogram (staggered q6 months with MRI) at age 30. RRM upon diagnosis. 1.8–7.1% lifetime risk in men. Self-breast exams monthly, CBE q6–12mo starting at age 35. Consider annual mammogram starting at age 50 or 10 years before youngest male breast cancer in family.	13–29% lifetime risk. Transvaginal US of ovaries with CA-125 q6mo starting at age 30–35. RRSO between ages 35 and 40 or upon completion of child bearing (ovarian cancer diagnosis typically 8–10 years later in BRCA2 carriers compared to BRCA1 carriers)	5–10% lifetime risk of pancreatic cancer. Consider pancreatic cancer screening starting at age 50 (or 10 years younger than earliest pancreatic cancer diagnosis in the family) in those with first- or second-degree relatives with pancreatic cancer and same genetic variant. MRI/MRCP and/or EUS. 19–61% risk of prostate cancer. Begin prostate screening at age 40. Increased risk of lymphoma, leukemia, colon, gastric, gallbladder, and bile duct cancers and melanoma have been described.

(continued)

Table 4.1 (continued)

Gene	Breast cancer risk/Management	Epithelial ovarian cancer risk/management	Other cancer risk/management
BRIP1	Absolute risk unknown. Management is based on family history.	5–15% lifetime risk RRSO at 45–50 years	Unknown
PALB2	Absolute risk: 41–60% Annual mammogram and breast MRI with and without contrast at age 30 Discuss option of RRM Male breast cancer Absolute risk: 0.9% by age 70	Absolute risk: 3–5% Consider RRSO starting at ages 45–50	*Pancreatic cancer* Absolute risk: 2–5% Management: Screen P/LP variant carriers with a family history of pancreatic cancer Strength of evidence of association with cancer: Limited *Other cancers* Unknown or insufficient evidence
TP53 Li-Fraumeni Syndrome	Absolute risk: >60% Breast awareness starting at age 18 Clinical breast exam, q6–12 months starting at age 20 Ages 20–29 annual breast MRI screening with and without contrast Ages 30–75 annual breast MRI screening with and without contrast and mammogram Age > 75 management should be considered on an individual basis Discuss option of RRM Refer to NCCN guidelines for LFS management	No evidence of increased risk	*Pancreatic cancer* Absolute risk: ~5% Management: Screen P/LP variant carriers with a family history of pancreatic cancer *Other cancers* Classical LFS spectrum cancers (in addition to breast): soft tissue sarcoma, osteosarcoma, CNS tumor, and ACC Many other cancers have been associated with LFS, especially melanoma, colorectal, gastric, and prostate.

PTEN Cowden syndrome	Absolute risk: 40–60% (historical cohort data), >60% (projected estimates) Breast awareness starting at age 18 Clinical breast exam q6–12 months, starting at age 25 or 5–10 years before earliest known breast cancer in the family (whichever comes first) Annual mammography and breast MRI screening with and without contrast starting at age 30 or 10 years before the earliest known breast cancer in the family (whichever comes first). Age > 75, management should be considered on an individual basis. Risk reducing surgery should be based on family history.	*Thyroid, colorectal, endometrial, and renal cancers* See NCCN guidelines for Cowden syndrome management
CDH1	Absolute risk: 41–60% Annual mammogram and consider breast MRI with and without contrast starting at age 30. Discuss option of RRM	No evidence of increased risk	*Hereditary diffuse gastric cancer (HDGC)* See NCCN Guidelines for Gastric Cancer: Principles of Genetic Risk Assessment for Gastric Cancer
STK11	Absolute risk: 32–54% Annual mammogram and breast MRI with and without contrast starting at age 30 NCCN Guidelines for Genetic/Familial High-Risk Assessment: Colorectal—Peutz-Jeghers syndrome (PJS) Discuss option of RRM	No evidence of increased risk	*Pancreatic cancer* AAbsolute risk: >15% *Nonepithelial ovarian cancer (sex cord with annular tubules)* Absolute risk: >10% Management: NCCN Guidelines for Genetic/Familial *High-Risk Assessment: Colorectal—PJS* NCCN Guidelines for Genetic/Familial High-Risk Assessment: Colorectal – PJS

(continued)

Table 4.1 (continued)

Gene	Breast cancer risk/Management	Epithelial ovarian cancer risk/management	Other cancer risk/management
CHEK2	Absolute risk: 20–40% Annual mammogram at age 40 and consider breast MRI with and without contrast starting at ages 30–35 Evidence insufficient for RRM, manage based on family history	No evidence of increased risk	*Colorectal cancer* NCCN Guidelines for Genetic/Familial High-Risk Assessment: Colorectal (GENE-1) *Prostate cancer* Emerging evidence for association with increased risk. Consider prostate cancer screening starting at age 40 years (NCCN Guidelines for Prostate Cancer Early detection)
RAD51C	Absolute risk: 17–30% Annual mammogram and consider breast MRI with and without contrast starting at age 40	Absolute risk: 10–15% Recommend RRSO starting at age 45–50	*Other cancers* Unknown or insufficient evidence
RAD51D	Absolute risk: 17–30% Annual mammogram and consider breast MRI with and without contrast starting at age 40	Absolute risk: 10–20% Recommend RRSO at starting at age 45–50	*Other cancers* Unknown or insufficient evidence
CDKN2A	Evidence of increased risk: No established association	Evidence of increased risk: No established association	*Pancreatic cancer* Absolute risk: >15% *Melanoma* Absolute risk: 28–76% depending on other risk factors, including family history, geographic location, and other genetic modifiers Other cancers

Gene	Breast cancer	Other cancers

MSH2
MLH1
MSH6
PMS2
EPCAM
	MLH1, MSH2, MSH6, PMS2, and EPCAM
	Absolute risk: <15%
	Management: Insufficient data; managed based on family history
		MLH1
		  Absolute risk: 4–20%
		MSH2/EPCAM
		  Absolute risk: 8–38%
		MSH6
		  Absolute risk: ≤1–13%
		PMS2
		  Absolute risk: 1.3–3%
		Evidence of increased risk: No established association
			Pancreatic cancer
			Absolute risk: <5–10% (excluding PMS2)
			Management: Screen P/LP variant carriers with a family history of pancreatic cancer (insufficient evidence for PMS2)
			Colorectal, uterine, and others
			Refer to NCCN Guidelines for Genetic/Familial High-risk Assessment: Colorectal

NF1	Absolute risk: 20–40% Annual mammogram starting at age 30 and consider breast MRI with and without contrast from ages 30–50 Evidence insufficient for RRM, manage based on family history		Malignant peripheral nerve sheath tumors, GIST, and others Recommend referral to NF1 specialist for evaluation and management

ACC adenoid cystic carcinoma, *CBE* clinical breast exam, *CNS* central nervous system, *EUS* endoscopic ultrasound, *GIST* gastrointestinal stromal tumor, *LFS* Li-Fraumeni syndrome, *MRCP* magnetic resonance cholangiopancreatography, *MRI* magnetic resonance imaging, *NF1* neurofibromatosis 1, *P/LP* pathogenic/likely pathogenic, *PJS* Peutz-Jeghers syndrome, *RRM* risk-reducing mastectomy, *RRSO* risk-reducing salpingo-oophorectomy, *US* ultrasound

- Pure mucinous
- Pure cribriform
- Encapsulated or solid papillary carcinoma
- Adenoid cystic or other salivary carcinoma
- Secretory carcinoma
- Rare low-grade forms of metaplastic carcinoma
- Receptors
    - Estrogen receptor (ER)
        - 0 – <1% of nuclei stain → ER negative
        - 1–10% of nuclei stain → ER low positive
        - >10% of nuclei stain → ER positive
    - Progesterone receptor (PR)
        - 0 – <1% of nuclei stain → PR negative
        - 1–100% of nuclei stain → PR positive
    - Human epidermal growth factor receptor 2 (HER2)
        - Not useful in DCIS
        - Validated by immunohistochemistry (IHC) assay or dual-probe ISH assay
            - If IHC 0 or 1+ → HER2 negative
            - If IHC 2+ → equivocal
                - Reflex test with ISH on existing specimen or validate with new specimen
            - If IHC 3+ → HER2 positive
- Nottingham Grade
    - Overall grade is based on combination score of glandular (acinar)/tubular differentiation + nuclear pleomorphism + mitotic rate
- Luminal Types
    - Luminal A
        - ER and/or PR-positive, HER2 negative, and <20% Ki-67
        - Clinically low grade, slow growing, best prognosis, less incidence of relapse, and higher survival rate.
        - High response to hormone therapy
        - Limited chemotherapy benefit
    - Luminal B
        - ER-positive, +/− PR negative, >20% Ki-67
        - Intermediate/high grade
        - May benefit from hormonal therapy and chemotherapy
        - Worse prognosis with higher rate of recurrence, higher rate of relapse, and lower survival
- Special Types of Breast Cancer [2, 3]
    - Medullary carcinoma
    - Mutinous carcinoma
    - Tubular carcinoma
    - Inflammatory breast cancer
    - Paget's disease of the nipple

- Benign, borderline, and malignant phyllodestumor
- Mucinous cystadenocarcinoma
- Dermatofibrosarcoma protuberans
- Malignant mesenchymal tumor
- Mucinous carcinoma
- Invasive papillary carcinoma
- Adenoid cystic carcinoma
- Cribriform carcinoma
- Apocrine carcinoma
- Lobular pleomorphic carcinoma
- Micropapillary carcinoma
- Metaplastic spindle cell carcinoma

Evaluation and Clinical Stage

- Labs
  - ≥cT2 or cT1c HER2+
    - Complete blood count
    - Comprehensive metabolic panel
    - Hepatic function tests
  - Pregnancy test in all patients with childbearing potential
- The stage of the cancer is the most prognostic factor
- Survival—5 years [1]
  - 99.3% of patients with localized disease
  - 86.3% with regional advancement
  - 31.0% of patients with distant metastases
- Lymph node status and prognosis, 5-year overall survival [1]
  - 92% with unoccupied regional lymph nodes
  - 81% with 1–3 lymph nodes occupied
  - 57% when metastases were found in ≥4 lymph nodes
- Tumor dimensions and prognosis—5-year survival [1]
  - 99% with disease confined to the breast and a tumor <1 cm
  - 89% with a tumor measuring 1–3 cm
  - 86% with a tumor of 3–5 cm
  - A tumor with an originally large size predisposes to the involvement of regional lymph nodes
- T4 features, that is, invasion of the skin or chest wall, which is associated with a worse prognosis
- Clinical staging studies (Table 4.1)
- Axillary Imaging preop with biopsy as indicated
- CT scan chest, abdomen, and pelvis
- FDG-PET—18-fluorodeoxyglucose positron emission tomography
  - FES PET/CT for ER-positive disease
- MRI brain with contrast if suspicious CNS symptoms are present

- MRI spine with contrast if back pain/symptoms or cord compression present
- *TNM staging* (Tables 4.2, 4.3, 4.4, and 4.5)
    - T stage—tumor size and/or extension into local structures
    - N stage—nodal status of local and regional nodes
    - M stage—presence or absence of microscopic vs macroscopic distant metastasis
    - pTNM stage based on surgical resection
        - Qualifiers: y = after treatment; m = multifocal

Table 4.2 AJCC Cancer Staging Manual, Eighth Edition, Definition of Primary Tumor (T)—Clinical and Pathological [9]

T category		T criteria
TX		Primary tumor cannot be assessed
T0		No evidence of primary tumor
Tis		Cancer in situ
	Tis (DCIS)[a]	Ductal carcinoma in situ
	Tis (Paget)	Paget disease of the nipple *not* associated with invasive carcinoma and/or carcinoma in situ (DCIS) in the underlying breast parenchyma. Carcinomas in the breast parenchyma associated with Paget disease are categorized based on the size and characteristics of the parenchymal disease, although the presence of Paget disease should still be noted.
T1		Tumor ≤20 mm in greatest dimension
	T1mi	Tumor ≤1 mm
	T1a	Tumor >1 mm, ≤5 mm
	T1b	Tumor >5 mm, ≤10 mm
	T1c	Tumor >10 mm, ≤20 mm
T2		Tumor >20 mm, ≤50 mm
T3		Tumor >50 mm
T4		Tumor of any size with direct extension to the chest wall and/or to the skin (ulceration or macroscopic nodules) and invasion of the dermis alone does not qualify as T4.
	T4a	Extension to the chest wall (but not the pectoral muscles)
	T4b	Ulceration and/or ipsilateral macroscopic satellite nodules and/or edema (including peau d'orange) of the skin that does not meet criteria for inflammatory carcinoma
	T4c	Both T4a + T4b
	T4d	Inflammatory carcinoma

[a]Note: Lobular carcinoma in situ (LCIS) is a benign entity and is removed from TNM staging in the AJCC Cancer Staging Manual, eighth Edition

Table 4.3 Regional lymph nodes clinical (cN) [9]

cN category		cN criteria
cNX[a]		Regional lymph nodes cannot be assessed (e.g., previously removed)
cN0		No regional lymph node metastases (by imaging or clinical examination)
cN1		Metastases to movable ipsilateral Level I, II axillary lymph node(s)
	cN1mi[b]	Micrometastases (approximately 200 cells, larger than 0.2 mm, but none larger than 2.0 mm)
cN2		Metastases in ipsilateral level I, II axillary lymph nodes that are clinically fixed or matted; or in ipsilateral internal mammary nodes in the absence of axillary lymph node metastases
	cN2a	Metastases in ipsilateral level I, II axillary lymph nodes fixed to one another (matted) or to other structures
	cN2b	Metastases only in ipsilateral internal mammary nodes in the absence of axillary lymph node metastases
cN3		Metastases in ipsilateral infraclavicular (level III axillary) lymph node(s) with or without level I, II axillary lymph node involvement, or in ipsilateral internal mammary lymph node(s) with level I, II axillary lymph node metastases, or metastases in ipsilateral supraclavicular lymph node(s) with or without axillary or internal mammary lymph node involvement
	cN3a	Metastases in ipsilateral infraclavicular lymph node(s)
	cN3b	Metastases in ipsilateral internal mammary lymph node(s) and axillary lymph node(s)
	cN3c	Metastases in ipsilateral supraclavicular lymph node(s)

Note: (sn) and (f) suffixes should be added to the N category to denote confirmation of metastasis by sentinel node biopsy or fine needle aspiration/core needle biopsy, respectively
[a]The cNX category is used sparingly in cases where regional lymph nodes have previously been surgically removed or where there is no documentation of physical examination of the axilla
[b]cN1mi is rarely used but may be appropriate in cases where sentinel node biopsy is performed before tumor resection, most likely to occur in cases treated with neoadjuvant therapy

Table 4.4 Regional lymph node pathological (pN) [9]

pN category		pN criteria
pNX		Regional lymph nodes cannot be assessed (e.g., not removed for pathological study or previously removed)
pN0		No regional lymph node metastasis identified or ITCs only
	pN0(i+)	ITCs only (malignant cell clusters no larger than 0.2 mm) in regional lymph node(s)
	pN0(mol+)	Positive molecular findings by reverse transcriptase polymerase chain reaction (RT-PCR); no ITCs detected
pN1		Micrometastases; or metastases in 1—3 axillary lymph nodes; and/or clinically negative internal mammary nodes with micrometastases or macrometastases by sentinel lymph node biopsy
	pN1mi	Micrometastases (approximately 200 cells, larger than 0.2 mm, but none larger than 2.0 mm)
	pN1a	Metastases in 1—3 axillary lymph nodes, at least one metastasis larger than 2.0 mm
	pN1b	Metastases in ipsilateral internal mammary sentinel nodes, excluding ITCs
	pN1c	pN1a and pN1b combined

(continued)

Table 4.4 (continued)

pN category		pN criteria
pN2		Metastases in 4—9 axillary lymph nodes; or positive ipsilateral internal mammary lymph nodes by imaging in the absence of axillary lymph node metastases
	pN2a	Metastases in 4—9 axillary lymph nodes (at least one tumor deposit larger than 2.0 mm)
	pN2b	Metastases in clinically detected internal mammary lymph nodes with or without microscopic confirmation, with pathologically negative axillary nodes
pN3		Metastases in ten or more axillary lymph nodes; or in infraclavicular (level Ill axillary) lymph nodes; or positive ipsilateral internal mammary lymph nodes by imaging in the presence of one or more positive level I, Il axillary lymph nodes; or in more than three axillary lymph nodes and micrometastases or macrometastases by sentinel lymph node biopsy in clinically negative ipsilateral internal mammary lymph nodes; or in ipsilateral supraclavicular lymph nodes
	pN3a	Metastases in ten or more axillary lymph nodes (at least one tumor deposit larger than 2.0 mm); or metastases to the infraclavicular (Level Ill axillary lymph) nodes
	pN3b	pN1a or pN2a in the presence of cN2b (positive internal mammary nodes by imaging), or pN2a in the presence of pN1b
	pN3c	Metastases in ipsilateral supraclavicular lymph nodes

Note: (sn) and (f) suffixes should be added to the N category to denote confirmation of metastasis by sentinel node biopsy or FNA/core needle biopsy, respectively, with *no* further resection of nodes
ITC isolated tumor cell

Table 4.5 Distant metastasis (M) [9]

M category		M criteria
M0		No clinical or radiographic evidence of distant metastases
	cM0(i+)	No clinical or radiographic evidence of distant metastases in the presence of tumor cells or deposits no larger than 0.2 mm detected microscopically or by molecular techniques in circulating blood, bone marrow, or other nonregional nodal tissues in a patient without symptoms or signs of metastases
cM1		Distant metastases detected by clinical and radiographic means
pM1		Any histologically proven metastases in distant organs; or if in nonregional nodes, metastases greater than 0.2 mm

Note that imaging studies are not required to assign the CMO category

Choice of Therapy

- The treatment of breast cancer is multidisciplinary (see Table 4.6 for key studies leading to current guidelines)
- Address fertility issues and sexual health prior to treatment

Table 4.6 Key studies

	Question	Groups/study design	Inclusion	Outcome	Conclusion
Invasive cancer management					
NSABP B-04 [10]	Determine total mastectomy with or without RT was as effective as radical mastectomy	Randomized 1. Radical mastectomy + ALND 2. Total mastectomy 3. Total mastectomy + RT	Women who are clinically node negative	No difference in overall survival at 25 years.	Total mastectomy is sufficient over RM
Milan I [11]	Compare efficacy in women undergoing radical mastectomy or BCT	Randomized 1. Radical mastectomy 2. Quadrantectomy + ALND + RT	Women with cT1N0 breast cancer	No difference in overall survival at 20 years	BCT sufficient over RM
NSABP B-06 [12]	Compare efficacy in women undergoing total mastectomy or BCT with or without RT	Randomized 1. Modified radical mastectomy 2. Lumpectomy + ALND 3. Lumpectomy + ALND + breast RT	Women Tumor ≤4 cm, node negative (stage I) Tumor ≤4 cm, node positive (stage II)	1. No difference in OS, DFS, and distant DFS 2. Reduction in local recurrence in BCT + RT from 39–14%	BCT is sufficient over MRM
EORTC 1081 [13]	Compare efficacy in women undergoing total mastectomy or BCT with or without RT	1. Modified radical mastectomy 2. Lumpectomy + ALND + WBRT + RT boost to lumpectomy site	Tumor ≤5 cm, node negative (stage I) Tumor ≤5 cm, node positive (stage II) Included some high-risk groups including T2 and positive lymph nodes	No difference in OS, DFS, and distant DFS at 20 years 10 year local recurrence in BCT group 20% vs 12% for MRM	BCT is sufficient over MRM.
CALGB 9343 [7]	Is adjuvant RT after BCT beneficial in women age ≥ 70 with early-stage breast cancer?	Randomized 1. Tamoxifen + RT 2. Tamoxifen	Women age 70+ T1N0M0 ER+ after lumpectomy	No difference in OS, distant DFS at 10 years. IBTR 98% (Tam) vs 90% (TamRT)	Consider omission of RT in age 70+ T1N0M0 ER+ after lumpectomy on tamoxifen.

(continued)

Table 4.6 (continued)

	Question	Groups/study design	Inclusion	Outcome	Conclusion
DCIS management					
NSABP B-17 [14]	Is adjuvant RT required after lumpectomy?	Randomized 1. Lumpectomy 2. Lumpectomy + RT	Women with localized DCIS	No difference in OS DCIS-IBTR from 15.4% to 9.0% Invasive-IBTR from 19.6% to 10.7%	Addition of RT after lumpectomy for DCIS reduces invasive and noninvasive IBTR.
EORTC 10853 [15]	Is adjuvant RT required after lumpectomy?	Randomized 1. Lumpectomy 2. Lumpectomy + RT	Women with DCIS <5 cm	No difference in OS or BCSS at 15 years Reduced local recurrence by 48% (82–69%) at 15 years	Addition of RT after lumpectomy for DCIS reduces local recurrence
ECOG E5194 [16]	What is the risk of developing ipsilateral DCIS after lumpectomy without radiation?	Nonrandomized, prospective 1. Low- or intermediate-grade DCIS, tumor size ≤2.5 cm tumor size 2. High-grade DCIS and tumor size ≤1 cm	Women with DCIS after lumpectomy and no RT	Recurrence at 12 years 1. IBE 14.4% 2. IBE 24.6% ($p = 0.003$) 3. I-IBE 7.5% 4. I-IBE 13.4% ($p = 0.08$) without plateau	Risk of developing IBE or I-IBE is increased in DCIS with more favorable clinical and pathological characteristics treated with lumpectomy but without RT
NSABP B-24 [14]	Does tamoxifen reduce IBTR in DCIS?	Randomized 1. Lumpectomy + RT + placebo 2. Lumpectomy + RT + 5 year Tamoxifen	Women with ER+ DCIS after lumpectomy	8.2% vs 13.4% IBTR (38.8% relative risk reduction)	Consider radiation therapy and tamoxifen-reduced I-IBTR
NSABP B-35 [17]	Tamoxifen or anastrozole for *postmenopausal* DCIS BCT	Randomized 1. Anastrozole 2. Tamoxifen	Women with hormone positive DCIS after lumpectomy and RT	No difference in OS at 10 years Improved BCFI in T (89.1%) vs A (93.1%) also benefit of A in women <60 years.	Anastrozole provided a significant improvement compared to tamoxifen for BCFI, primarily in women <60 years

Neoadjuvant chemotherapy					
NSABP B-18 [5]	Does preop vs postop doxorubicin + cyclophosphamide (AC) improve DFS, OS?	Randomized 1. Preop AC 2. Postop AC	T1–3, N0–1, M0	No difference in DFS, OS. Trends for improved preop DFS and OS in women <50 years.	Neoadjuvant AC equivalent to adjuvant AC
NSABP B-27 [5]	Does preop AC + docetaxel (T), improve tumor response, DFS, OS?	Randomized 1. Preop AC 2. Preop ACT 3. Preop AC, postop T	T1c-T3, N0–1, M0 or T1–3, N1, M0	No change DFS, OS Preop ACT increased pCR compared with AC (26% vs 13%).	Neoadjuvant = adjuvant But preop T improves response
Axillary management					
RAC SNAC [18]	Does ALND confer greater morbidity compared to SLNBx?	Randomized SLNBx pos or neg → ALND SLNBx pos → ALND	Tumor ≤3.0 cm, cN0	RAC increase arm vol in 4.2%, decrease in abduction in 4.4% SNAC increase arm vol in 2.8%, decrease in abduction 2.5%	ALND increases risk for lymphedema. Avoid if able.
NSABP B-32 [19]	Does SLNBx improve survival, regional control, decrease morbidity compared to ALND?	Randomized SLNBx pos or neg → ALND SLNBx pos → ALND	Women with invasive breast cancer, cN0	OS, DFS, regional control equivalent between groups	When cN0 and SLN negative, no ALND required
IBCSG 23–01 [20]	Does ALND required improve DFS if the SLN has micrometastases?	Randomized 1. ALND 2. No ALND	Tumor ≤5 cm, ≥1 SLN with micrometastases without extracapsular extension	DFS equivalent at 10 years Higher rates of lymphedema in ALND group.	Do not perform ALND with micrometastases, as it increases morbidity

(continued)

Table 4.6 (continued)

	Question	Groups/study design	Inclusion	Outcome	Conclusion
ACOSOG Z0011 [21]	Does ALND improve survival or local control compared to observation in invasive breast cancer?	Randomized 1. Completion ALND 2. No ALND	T1–2 breast cancer patients, cN0, with 1 or 2 positive sentinel lymph nodes who undergo BCT	ALND does not improve survival or local control at 10 years	Do not perform routine ALND in T1–2, cN0, with one or two positive lymph nodes
EORTC 10981 AMAROS [22]	Does ALND or RT improve survival or local control in invasive breast cancer?	Randomized 1. ALND 2. RT	cT1–2, cN0 breast cancer and a positive SLNBx	No difference in ARR, OS, or DFS at 10 years ALND was associated with a higher lymphedema rate in updated five-year analyses (24.5% vs 11.9%; $P < 0.001$). A 10-year cumulative incidence of second primary cancers of 12.1% (95% CI, 9.6–14.9) after ART and 8.3% (95% CI, 6.3 to 10.7) after ALND	Axillary RT is preferred over ALND for patients with SN-positive cT1–2 breast cancer
SOUND Trial [23]	Is SLNBx required?	Randomized 1. Omission of axillary surgery 2. SLNBx	Tumor ≤2 cm and neg axillary ultrasound	Distant DFS equivalent at 5 years	Omit SLNBx with negative axillary ultrasound
ACOSOG Z1071 [24]	Is adjuvant RT needed after NACT?	Nonrandomized 1. RT 2. No RT	cT0–4, cN1–2 NAC Lumpectomy or mastectomy SLNBx ALND	Trend toward decreased LRR with adjuvant RT Equivalent OS, BC-specific survival, disease-specific survival	False-negative rate < 10% with ≥3 SLN

4 Breast Cancer

Endocrine therapy				
NSABP P-1 [25]	Does tamoxifen reduce the incidence of breast cancer among women with an increased risk for breast cancer?	Randomized 1. Tamoxifen 5 years 2. Placebo 5 years	Age ≥ 60 years Age 35–59 with a Gail model 5-year risk of breast cancer ≥1.66% Ages 35–59 with a history of LCIS	Tamoxifen reduces the risk of ER-positive breast cancer, but it provides no mortality benefit. Tamoxifen increases the risk of endometrial cancer and pulmonary embolism.	Consider tamoxifen in high-risk women who meet criteria.
ATLAS [26]	Does 10 years of adjuvant tamoxifen compared to 5 years reduce breast cancer recurrence and mortality?	Randomized 1. Continued tamoxifen to 10 years 2. Stop tamoxifen at 5 years	Female Early breast cancer Receiving adjuvant tamoxifen Clinically free of disease	Ten years of adjuvant tamoxifen reduces all-cause mortality and breast cancer recurrence compared to 10 years of therapy, at the expense of marginally increased rates of endometrial cancer and VTE	Consider prolonging adjuvant tamoxifen to 10 years.
STAR P-2 [27]	In postmenopausal women, how does tamoxifen compare to raloxifene in primary breast cancer prevention and side effect profile?	Randomized 1. Tamoxifen 2. Raloxifene	Age ≥ 35 years Gail model 5-year predicted breast cancer risk ≥1.66% or LCIS treated with local excision alone Postmenopausal	Tamoxifen equivalent to raloxifene in reducing the risk of invasive breast cancer Tamoxifen carries a higher incidence of thromboembolic events and cataracts.	Consider raloxifene over tamoxifen

(continued)

Table 4.6 (continued)

	Question	Groups/study design	Inclusion	Outcome	Conclusion
HER2-positive breast cancer					
KATHERINE [28]	Does adjuvant trastuzumab-emtansine (T-DM1) benefit patients after NACT	Open-label, randomized 1. T-DM-1 2. Trastuzumab	HER2-positive early breast cancer with residual invasive disease in breast or axilla at surgery after taxane-based NACT (+/0 anthracycline) and trastuzumab	Invasive DFS higher in T-DM1 88.3% vs trastuzumab 77.0% at 3 years and freedom from distant recurrence	Adjuvant T-DM1 improves DFS and distant recurrence.
EMILIA [29]	Does T-DM1 prolong PFS and OS when compared to lapatanib+capecitabine?	Randomized 1. Lapatinib 1250 mg PO daily and capecitabine 1000 mg PO q12h for 14 days of each 21-day cycle 2. T-DM1 3.6 mg/kg IV every 21 days	Progression of unresectable, locally advanced or metastatic HER2+ breast cancer Previous treatment with a taxane and trastuzumab LVEF ≥50% ECOG 0–1	T-DM1 prolongs PFS and OS when compared to lapatanib+capecitabine	Consider addition of adjuvant T-DM1.

HERA [30]	Does adjuvant trastuzumab improve DFS after adjuvant chemotherapy?	Randomized 1. Trastuzumab for 1 year 2. Trastuzumab for 2 years 3. Observation only	Female Histologically confirmed, early-stage invasive breast cancer after locoregional therapy (surgery ± radiotherapy) HER2 overexpression confirmed on IHC and FISH ≥4 cycles of CT completed prior to randomization LVEF ≥55%	Trastuzumab after adjuvant chemotherapy significantly improves DFS at 1 year among women with HER2-positive breast cancer.	Add adjuvant trastuzumab after CT/RT when HER2 confirmed from surgical pathology
Screening					
Age trial [31]	Does earlier screening with mammograms reduce breast cancer mortality?	Randomized 1. Annual mammogram starting age 40–41 years until the calendar year of the 48th birthday and then routine mammogram starting at ages 50–52 2. Routine mammogram starting at ages 50–52	Women ages 39–41	Mammographic screening at age 40 was reduced compared to screening at age 50, although not statistically significant, at 10 years.	Earlier screening is consistent with improved mortality results of other studies despite not statistically significant in this study.

(continued)

Table 4.6 (continued)

	Question	Groups/study design	Inclusion	Outcome	Conclusion
Swedish Two-County Trial [32]	What is the long-term (29-year) effect of mammographic screening for women ages 40–74 on breast cancer mortality?	Randomized, ITT 1. Offered screening 2. No screening (passive study population)	Women aged 40–74 Residing in one of two counties in Sweden: Dalarna and Östergötland	Mammography screening of women starting at 40 results in a highly significant decrease in breast cancer-specific mortality at 29 years.	Screen women starting at 40
TAILORx [33]	What is the benefit of chemotherapy for patients with a midrange (11–25) Oncotype DX score?	Randomized 1. 11–25: ET 2. 11–25 ET + CT	18–75 years HR positive HER2 negative Axillary node-negative	Improved DFS of women ≤50 years at 9 years Invasive DFS, OS, freedom from disease recurrence at distant site, and freedom from disease at distant or local-regional site equivalent at 9 years	In women ≤50, adjuvant CT + ET provides DFS benefit.

This table is meant to serve as a point of reference for significant conclusions in key landmark papers. Weaknesses, limitations, and criticisms of the studies are not mentioned

ALND axillary lymph node dissection, *ARR* absolute relative risk, *BCFI* breast cancer-free interval, *BCSS* breast cancer-specific survival, *BCT* breast conservation therapy, *CT* chemotherapy, *DCIS* ductal carcinoma in situ, *DFS* disease-free survival, *ECOG* Eastern Cooperative Oncology Group, *ER* estrogen receptor, *ET* endocrine therapy, *HR* hormone receptor, *I-IBE* invasive ipsilateral breast event, *IBE* ipsilateral breast event, *IBTR* ipsilateral breast tumor recurrence, *IDC* invasive ductal carcinoma, *ITT* intention to treat, *LCIS* lobular carcinoma in situ, *LRR* local-regional recurrence, *LVEF* left ventricular ejection fraction, *MRM* modified radical mastectomy, *NACT* neoadjuvant chemotherapy, *OS* overall survival, *PFS* progression-free survival, *RT* radiation therapy, *SLNBx* sentinel lymph node biopsy, *T-DM1* trastuzumab-emtansine

Surgical Therapy

- Breast-conserving therapy (partial mastectomy plus radiation therapy)
- Mastectomy
  - Nipple-sparing mastectomy
  - Skin-sparing mastectomy
  - Simple mastectomy
- Modified Radical Mastectomy
- Axillary Management
  - Sentinel lymph node biopsy
  - Targeted sentinel lymph node biopsy
  - Axillary dissection
- Immediate vs Delayed Reconstruction
  - Implant-based vs autologous tissue transfer
  - Can be influenced by patient preference, comorbidities, tobacco use, breast size and shape, BMI, and tumor factors such as size, depth, and nipple involvement
  - Reconstruction should be delayed in cases of inflammatory breast cancer
- Neoadjuvant Therapy (NAT) [4, 5]
  - Tumor histology, grade, stage, hormone receptors, and HER2 expression guide therapy
  - Candidates
    - Inflammatory breast cancer, unresectable, or locally advanced disease whose disease may be resectable with NAT
    - High-risk HER2-positive or triple-negative breast cancer (TNBC) in whom the finding of residual disease would guide recommendations related to AT
    - Reduce the extent of surgery (BCT or ALND).
    - If delay in surgery is preferable or unavoidable
  - Measuring Response to Treatment
    - Mammography, ultrasound, or MRI
  - A pathologic clinical response (pCR) should guide decision-making
  - Triple-Negative Breast Cancer (TNBC)
  - Clinically node-positive and/or at least T1c disease should be offered an anthracycline- and taxane-containing regimen.
  - Carboplatin may be offered as part of a regimen to increase likelihood of pCR.
  - Insufficient evidence routinely adding immune checkpoint inhibitors in early stages.
  - HR-positive/HER2-negative breast cancer
  - Any patient can be offered NAT instead of AT in whom the chemotherapy decision can be made without surgical pathology data and/or tumor-specific genomic testing.
  - HR-positive/HER2-negative breast cancer—NAET
  - Postmenopausal patients, aromatase inhibitor may be offered to increase locoregional treatment options

- Patients not undergoing surgery, endocrine therapy may be used for disease control
- HER2-positive disease
- Node-positive.
- High-risk node-negative.
- Anthracycline + taxane + trastuzumab.
- Non–anthracycline-based regimen + trastuzumab.
- Pertuzumab may be used with trastuzumab in the neoadjuvant setting.

Adjuvant Therapy

- Hormone receptor positive patients should receive endocrine therapy.
- HER2-positive patients should be offered trastuzumab ± pertuzumab.
- Triple-negative patients are offered pembrolizumab if not given preop or capecitabine.
- BRCA 1/BRCA 2 mutation carriers are offered olaparib times 1 year.

Management of Locally Advanced and Recurrent/Metastatic Disease

- Locally advanced disease (noninflammatory)
  - Preoperative systemic therapy
    - Tumor is operable → mastectomy or partial mastectomy with axillary staging
    - No response and/or tumor remains inoperable → consider additional systemic therapy and/or preop radiation
      - If tumor becomes operable → mastectomy or partial mastectomy with axillary staging
      - Individualized therapy if tumor remains inoperable
- Recurrent/Metastatic Disease
  - Unresectable recurrent disease or stage IV disease should receive systemic therapy according to receptor status as listed above for adjuvant therapy.
    - If bone disease is present, add denosumab, zoledronic acid, or pamidronate.
  - May consider ovarian ablation or suppression in premenopausal women.
  - Biopsy-first recurrence or rebiopsy progression to assess for change in receptor status.
  - Comprehensive germline and somatic profiling to assess potential for additional targeted therapies.
  - If recurrence is localized or isolated to axilla, surgical resection should be performed if possible. Add RT if not initially performed.
  - Supraclavicular or internal mammary nodal recurrence should receive RT if possible.

Radiation Therapy

- Breast [6]
  - Lumpectomy for Invasive Ductal Carcinoma (IDC)
    - Whole breast irradiation is strongly recommended.
    - If adjuvant chemotherapy is indicated after lumpectomy, radiation should be given after chemotherapy is completed.
    - Not always necessary in selected women 70 years of age or older [7].
  - Mastectomy for IDC with Node-Positive Disease
    - Irradiation of chest wall and regional lymph nodes in women with positive ALNs after mastectomy and ALN dissection.
    - Select patients, with clinical stage III disease, and patients with ≥4 positive nodes, receiving preoperative systemic therapy before mastectomy.
  - Node-Negative Disease
    - Features predicting higher risk of local recurrence recommend chest wall irradiation
      - Primary tumors >5 cm.
      - Positive pathologic margin—chest wall irradiation is recommended for these patients.
    - Consider chest wall irradiation in tumors ≤5 cm and negative margins but ≤1 mm
- Chest Wall
  - Recommended for ≥4 positive axillary nodes
  - Strongly consider if 1–3 positive axillary nodes
  - Consider with negative axillary nodes, but tumor >5 cm, margins <1 mm, or for other high-risk features
  - Strongly consider if surgical margins are positive and reexcision is not feasible
- Axilla
  - Inclusion of axilla at the discretion of the radiation oncologist if 1–2 positive axillary nodes with cT1–2 N0 cancers with no preop chemotherapy and whole breast RT is planned
  - Inclusion of axilla is recommended if patient has positive nodes after preop chemotherapy, ≥3 axillary nodes, or ≥cT3

Surveillance

- H&P 1–4 times annually as clinically appropriate for the first 5 years and then annually
- Annual mammogram
- No indication for additional lab work or imaging to check for metastasis unless these are clinical signs and symptoms to suggest recurrent disease
- Cardiotoxicity monitoring for patients who had LEFT-sided radiation therapy, HER2-targeted therapy, or anthracyclines

- Assess adherence to endocrine therapy as appropriate. Some patients cannot tolerate the site effects of commonly prescribed medications
- Encourage low-risk lifestyle (exercise, healthy diet, ideal body weight, low alcohol intake, smoking cessation)

References

1. SEER. Cancer stat facts: cancer of any site. National Cancer Institute Surveillance, Epidemiology, and End Results Program. Published 2023. Accessed September 10, 2023. https://seer.cancer.gov/statfacts/html/all.html
2. Dieci MV, Orvieto E, Dominici M, Conte P, Guarneri V. Rare breast cancer subtypes: histological, molecular, and clinical peculiarities. Oncologist. 2014;19(8):805–13. https://doi.org/10.1634/theoncologist.2014-0108.
3. Kaur M, Tiwana K, Singla N. Rare breast malignancy subtypes: a cytological, histological, and immunohistochemical correlation. Niger J Surg. 2019;25(1):70. https://doi.org/10.4103/njs.NJS_27_18.
4. Korde LA, Somerfield MR, Carey LA, et al. Neoadjuvant chemotherapy, endocrine therapy, and targeted therapy for breast cancer: ASCO guideline. J Clin Oncol. 2021;39(13):1485–505. https://doi.org/10.1200/JCO.20.03399.
5. Rastogi P, Anderson SJ, Bear HD, et al. Preoperative chemotherapy: updates of national surgical adjuvant breast and bowel project protocols B-18 and B-27. J Clin Oncol. 2008;26(5):778–85. https://doi.org/10.1200/JCO.2007.15.0235.
6. Gradishar W, Anderson B, Balassanian R, et al. The NCCN invasive breast cancer: clinical practice guidelines in oncology. JNCCN J Natl Compr Cancer Netw. 2016;5(3):246–312.
7. Hughes KS, Schnaper LA, Bellon JR, et al. Lumpectomy plus tamoxifen with or without irradiation in women age 70 years or older with early breast cancer: long-term follow-up of CALGB 9343. J Clin Oncol. 2013;31(19):2382–7. https://doi.org/10.1200/JCO.2012.45.2615.
8. National Comprehensive Cancer Network. Genetic / familial high-risk assessment: breast, ovarian, and pancreatic. Published online 2024. chrome-extension://efaidnbmnnnibpcajpcglcl efindmkaj/https://www.nccn.org/professionals/physician_gls/pdf/genetics_bop.pdf
9. Hortobagyi GN, Connolly JL, D'Orsi CJ, et al. Breast. In: Amin MB, Edge SB, Green FL, et al., editors. AJCC cancer staging manual. 8th ed. Springer: American Joint Commission on Cancer; 2018. p. 589–634.
10. Fisher B, Jeong JH, Anderson S, Bryant J, Fisher ER, Wolmark N. Twenty-five-year follow-up of a randomized trial comparing radical mastectomy, total mastectomy, and total mastectomy followed by irradiation. N Engl J Med. 2002;347(8):567–75. https://doi.org/10.1056/nejmoa020128.
11. Veronesi U, Cascinelli N, Mariani L, et al. Twenty-year follow-up of a randomized study comparing breast-conserving surgery with radical mastectomy for early breast cancer. N Engl J Med. 2002;347(16):1227–32. https://doi.org/10.1056/NEJMoa020989.
12. Fisher B, Anderson S, Bryant J, et al. Twenty-year follow-up of a randomized trial comparing total mastectomy, lumpectomy, and lumpectomy plus irradiation for the treatment of invasive breast cancer. N Engl J Med. 2002;347(16):1233–41. https://doi.org/10.1056/nejmoa022152.
13. Litière S, Werutsky G, Fentiman IS, et al. Breast conserving therapy versus mastectomy for stage I-II breast cancer: 20 year follow-up of the EORTC 10801 phase 3 randomised trial. Lancet Oncol. 2012;13(4):412–9. https://doi.org/10.1016/S1470-2045(12)70042-6.
14. Wapnir IL, Dignam JJ, Fisher B, et al. Long-term outcomes of invasive ipsilateral breast tumor recurrences after lumpectomy in NSABP B-17 and B-24 randomized clinical trials for DCIS. J Natl Cancer Inst. 2011;103(6):478–88. https://doi.org/10.1093/jnci/djr027.
15. Donker M, Litière S, Werutsky G, et al. Breast-conserving treatment with or without radiotherapy in ductal carcinoma in situ: 15-year recurrence rates and outcome after a recurrence,

from the EORTC 10853 randomized phase III trial. J Clin Oncol. 2013;31(32):4054–9. https://doi.org/10.1200/JCO.2013.49.5077.
16. Solin LJ, Gray R, Hughes LL, et al. Surgical excision without radiation for ductal carcinoma in situ of the breast: 12-year results from the ECOG-ACRIN E5194 study. J Clin Oncol. 2015;33(33):3938–44. https://doi.org/10.1200/JCO.2015.60.8588.
17. Margolese RG, Cecchini RS, Julian TB, et al. Primary results, NRG Oncology/NSABP B-35: a clinical trial of anastrozole (A) versus tamoxifen (tam) in postmenopausal patients with DCIS undergoing lumpectomy plus radiotherapy. J Clin Oncol. 2015;33(18_suppl):LBA500. https://doi.org/10.1200/jco.2015.33.18_suppl.lba500.
18. Gill G. Sentinel-lymph-node-based management or routine axillary clearance? One-year outcomes of sentinel node biopsy versus axillary clearance (SNAC): a randomized controlled surgical trial. Ann Surg Oncol. 2009;16(2):266–75. https://doi.org/10.1245/s10434-008-0229-z.
19. Krag D, Weaver D, Ashikaga T, et al. The sentinel node in breast cancer — a multicenter validation study. N Engl J Med. 1998;339(14):941–6. https://doi.org/10.1056/NEJM199810013391401.
20. Galimberti V, Cole BF, Viale G, et al. Axillary dissection versus no axillary dissection in patients with breast cancer and sentinel-node micrometastases (IBCSG 23-01): 10-year follow-up of a randomised, controlled phase 3 trial. Lancet Oncol. 2018;19(10):1385–93. https://doi.org/10.1016/S1470-2045(18)30380-2.
21. Giuliano AE, Monica Morrow M. Effect of axillary dissection vs no axillary dissection on 10-year overall survival among women with invasive breast cancer and sentinel node metastasis. JAMA J Am Med Assoc. 2017;318(10):918–26. https://doi.org/10.1001/jama.2017.11470.Effect.
22. Bartels SAL, Donker M, Poncet C, et al. Radiotherapy or surgery of the axilla after a positive sentinel node in breast cancer: 10-year results of the randomized controlled EORTC 10981-22023 AMAROS trial. J Clin Oncol. 2023;41(12):2159–65. https://doi.org/10.1200/JCO.22.01565.
23. Gentilini OD, Botteri E, Sangalli C, et al. Sentinel lymph node biopsy vs no axillary surgery in patients with small breast cancer and negative results on ultrasonography of axillary lymph nodes: the SOUND randomized clinical trial. JAMA Oncol. 2023;9:1557. https://doi.org/10.1001/jamaoncol.2023.3759.
24. Haffty BG, McCall LM, Ballman KV, Buchholz TA, Hunt KK, Boughey JC. Impact of radiation on locoregional control in women with node-positive breast cancer treated with neoadjuvant chemotherapy and axillary lymph node dissection: results from ACOSOG Z1071 clinical trial. Int J Radiat Oncol Biol Phys. 2019;105(1):174–82. https://doi.org/10.1016/j.ijrobp.2019.04.038.
25. Vogel VG, Costantino JP, Wickerham DL, Cronin WM. Tamoxifen for prevention of breast cancer: report of the National Surgical Adjuvant Breast and Bowel Project P-1 Study. JNCI J Natl Cancer Inst. 2002;94(19):1504. https://doi.org/10.1093/jnci/94.19.1504.
26. Davies C, Pan H, Godwin J, et al. Long-term effects of continuing adjuvant tamoxifen to 10 years versus stopping at 5 years after diagnosis of oestrogen receptor-positive breast cancer: ATLAS, a randomised trial. Lancet. 2013;381(9869):805–16. https://doi.org/10.1016/S0140-6736(12)61963-1.
27. Corson SL. Effects of tamoxifen vs raloxifene on the risk of developing invasive breast cancer and other disease outcomes. J Minim Invasive Gynecol. 2006;13(5):492–3. https://doi.org/10.1016/j.jmig.2006.06.015.
28. von Minckwitz G, Huang CS, Mano MS, et al. Trastuzumab emtansine for residual invasive HER2-positive breast cancer. N Engl J Med. 2019;380(7):617–28. https://doi.org/10.1056/nejmoa1814017.
29. Diéras V, Miles D, Verma S, et al. Trastuzumab emtansine versus capecitabine plus lapatinib in patients with previously treated HER2-positive advanced breast cancer (EMILIA): a descriptive analysis of final overall survival results from a randomised, open-label, phase 3 trial. Lancet Oncol. 2017;18(6):732–42. https://doi.org/10.1016/S1470-2045(17)30312-1.

30. Cameron D, Piccart-Gebhart MJ, Gelber RD, et al. 11 years' follow-up of trastuzumab after adjuvant chemotherapy in HER2-positive early breast cancer: final analysis of the HERceptin adjuvant (HERA) trial. Lancet. 2017;389(10075):1195–205. https://doi.org/10.1016/S0140-6736(16)32616-2.
31. Moss SM, Wale C, Smith R, Evans A, Cuckle H, Duffy SW. Effect of mammographic screening from age 40 years on breast cancer mortality in the UK Age trial at 17 years' follow-up: a randomised controlled trial. Lancet Oncol. 2015;16(9):1123–32. https://doi.org/10.1016/S1470-2045(15)00128-X.
32. Tabár L, Vitak B, Chen HH, et al. The Swedish Two-County trial twenty years later. Radiol Clin North Am. 2000;38(4):625–51. https://doi.org/10.1016/s0033-8389(05)70191-3.
33. Sparano JA, Gray RJ, Makower DF, et al. Adjuvant chemotherapy guided by a 21-gene expression assay in breast cancer. N Engl J Med. 2018;379(2):111–21. https://doi.org/10.1056/nejmoa1804710.

Esophageal Cancer

Rob Painter and Hari B. Keshava

Introduction

- Eighth most common type of cancer worldwide and sixth leading cause of cancer death (Uhlenhopp)
- Squamous cell carcinoma (SCC) is the most common histological type worldwide
- Adenocarcinoma (AC) is the most common histological type in the United States
  - Fastest-increasing incidence of any solid tumor in the United States (Pera)
- Disproportionately high mortality due to late presentation
- Symptoms: Progressive dysphagia, weight loss, odynophagia, and anorexia
- Risk factors for SCC (Wheeler)
  - Male gender
  - Tobacco use (5–10× risk)
  - Alcohol use (dose-dependent risk)
  - Hot beverages
  - Nitroso-containing foods (pickled vegetables in East Asian cuisine)
  - Caustic injury
  - Low socioeconomic status (Brown)
- Risk factors for AC (Wheeler)
  - Male gender
  - White race
  - GERD/Barrett's esophagus (30× risk)
  - Obesity
  - Smoking

- Nitroso-containing foods
- Familial history of Barrett's esophagus
- Surveillance for patients with risk factors or Barrett's (Spechler)
    - Random endoscopic biopsies in four quadrants every 2 cm with narrow banding imaging
        - No dysplasia: Repeat endoscopy in 3–5 years
        - Low-grade dysplasia: Repeat endoscopy in 6–12 months
        - High-grade dysplasia: Endoscopic eradication therapy
    - Prague Classification (Sharma)
        - Endoscopic method to localize the squamocolumnar junction in BE

Pretreatment Evaluation

- Labs—Full nutritional assessment
- Clinical Staging—Table 5.1
    - SCC and AC
- Endoscopic ultrasound (EUS) for staging (Varghese)
    - Early stage: High-grade dysplasia or T1a
    - Locoregionalized disease: T1b to T4, any N
    - Can include FNA for lymph nodes
- Siewert Classification: Adenocarcinomas involving the GEJ
    - Type I: Epicenter of tumor within 1–5 cm above the anatomic GEJ
    - Type II: Epicenter of tumor within 1 cm above to 2 cm below the anatomic GEJ

Table 5.1 TNM Staging (AJCC 8th edition)

T category	
TX	Tumor cannot be assessed
T0	No evidence of primary tumor
Tis	High-grade dysplasia, defined as malignant cells confined by the basement membrane
T1a	Tumor invades the lamina propria or muscularis mucosae
T1b	Tumor invades the submucosa
T2	Tumor invades the muscularis propria
T3	Tumor invades the adventitia
T4a	Tumor invades the pleura, pericardium, azygos vein, diaphragm, or peritoneum
T4b	Tumor invades any other adjacent structures, such as aorta, vertebral body, or trachea
N category	
NX	Regional lymph nodes cannot be assessed
N0	No regional lymph node metastasis
N1	Metastasis in 1–2 regional lymph nodes
N2	Metastasis in 3–6 regional lymph nodes
N3	Metastasis in seven or more regional lymph nodes
M category	
M0	No distant metastasis
M1	Distant metastasis

- Type III: Epicenter of tumor within 2–5 cm below the anatomic GEJ (NCCN defines as gastric cancer)
- For locoregionalized disease, CT of the chest and abdomen as well as PET for staging (Varghese)
  - NCCN advocates for bronchoscopy for locally advanced upper esophageal tumors
  - No widely accepted use of diagnostic laparoscopy
  - MRI only if suspected metastases to the brain, adrenals, liver, or bone
- Consider further testing in unresectable, recurrent, or metastatic disease (NCCN ESOPH-B)
  - HER2
  - Microsatellite instability
  - PD-L1 testing
  - Next-generation sequencing (NGS)

Management (Ajani)

- Tis or T1a: Consider endoscopic mucosal resection (EMR) + ablation or esophagectomy
- T1b – T2, N0 (low-risk lesions*), N0: upfront Esophagectomy per NCCN, ASCO
  - Role for neoadjuvant in T2N0 is debated
  - Meta-analysis found higher R0 rates after neoadjuvant chemotherapy without a survival advantage (Kidane)
  - Some advocate for neoadjuvant chemotherapy due to inaccuracy of preoperative staging (Samson) (Zhang)
- T2, N0 (high-risk lesion) or T2-T4a, or N + disease: No widely accepted treatment
  - Preoperative chemoradiation
    - No widely accepted regimen
    - Carboplatin + Paclitaxel CROSS trial (van Hagen)
    - Cisplatin + Fluorouracil CALGB 9781 (Tepper)
  - Definitive chemoradiation
    - Persistent local disease, proceed with esophagectomy
    - If complete response can proceed with surveillance
  - Adjuvant therapy: ypT+ and/or N+
    - Nivolumab Checkmate 577 (Kelly)
    - Chemotherapy (Burt) and (Mokdad)
- Unresectable Criteria: Definitive chemoradiation
  - cT4b
  - Bulky, multistation lymphatic involvement is a relative contraindication.
  - Esophagogastric junction or supraclavicular lymph node involvement
  - Any distant metastases
  - <5 cm from the cricopharyngeus

*Low-risk lesions: <3 cm and well differentiated

Surgical Management (NCCN)

- Multidisciplinary tumor board
- Preoperative feeding tube placement
  - Jejunostomy preferred to preserve gastric conduit
- Techniques:
  - Ivor Lewis Esophagogastrectomy: Laparotomy and Right Thoracotomy or Thoracoscopy (Jones)
    - Diagnostic laparoscopy to rule out subclinical metastatic disease
    - Circumferential mobilization of the esophagus at the GEJ
    - Mobilization of greater curvature: Division of the greater omentum and short gastrics while preserving the right gastroepiploic
    - Division of left gastric artery
    - Mobilization of the esophageal hiatus
    - Optional pyloromyotomy
    - Creation of the gastric conduit
    - Feeding jejunostomy (if none preoperatively)
    - Repositioning for right thoracoscopy
    - Subcarinal nodal dissection
    - Mobilization of thoracic esophagus
    - Division of the azygos vein and mobilization of upper esophagus
    - Esophagogastric anastomosis
    - Endoscopy and placement of nasogastric tube
    - Placement of chest tube
  - McKeown Esophagogastrectomy: Laparotomy and Right Thoracotomy or Thoracoscopy with Cervical Anastomosis (Wong)
    - Thoracic phase
      - Anterolateral thoracotomy
      - Division of inferior pulmonary ligament
      - Circumferential mobilization of the lower esophagus
      - Ligation of the thoracic duct
      - Division of the arch of the azygos vein
      - Mediastinal lymphadenectomy with care to preserve the left and right recurrent laryngeal nerves
      - Placement of drain or chest tube
    - Abdominal phase
      - Laparotomy or bilateral subcostal incision
      - Mobilization of the greater curvature of the stomach by division of the short gastrics to the left crus
      - Mobilization of the lesser curvature to the right crus
        - Take care to preserve a replaced left hepatic
    - Cervical phase
      - Left supraclavicular incision

5 Esophageal Cancer

- Division of the middle thyroid vein to expose the carotid sheath
- Apical dissection of the thoracic phase should be present medial to the carotid sheath and lateral to the trachea
- Division of cervical esophagus
- Retrieval of the specimen through the abdomen
- Creation of the gastric conduit
- Optional pyloroplasty or pyloromyotomy
- Cervical anastomosis with nasogastric tube placement
- Transhiatal Esophagogastrectomy: Laparotomy with Cervical Anastomosis (Lin)
  - Abdominal phase
    - Upper midline laparotomy
    - Mobilization of the lesser curvature to the right crus
    - Mobilization of the greater curvature to the left crus
    - Assessment of the esophageal tumor to ensure resectability
    - Opening of the diaphragmatic hiatus to the pericardium
    - Circumferential mobilization of the esophagus to the carina
    - Kocher maneuver to mobilize the pylorus to the hiatus
    - Placement of jejunostomy
  - Cervical phase
    - Left supraclavicular incision
    - Dissection of the prevertebral fascia medial to the carotid sheath
    - Blunt dissection of the superior mediastinum with circumferential mobilization of the esophagus
    - Proximal transection of the esophagus
  - Transhiatal phase
    - Transhiatal blunt dissection of the remaining mediastinal attachments to the esophagus until it can be delivered through the abdomen
    - Evaluation of hemostasis
    - Resection of specimen and creation of conduit
    - Delivery of conduit to cervical incision
    - Cervical anastomosis with nasogastric tube placement
    - Optional pyloromyotomy
    - Suture pexy of the conduit to the hiatus
- Thoracic anastomosis may be associated with lower leak rates (Gooszen) (Biere) although these studies found no difference in mortality
- Some surgeons still choose cervical anastomosis as the complications with cervical leak are less significant
- Gastric conduit most common
  - Can also use colon or jejunum
    - Needs colon cancer screening if colon conduit
- At least 15 lymph nodes should be removed for staging
  - Transthoracic lymphadenectomy has a better yield than transhiatal

Complications After Esophagectomy

- Leak
  - Ivor Lewis—stent and drainage
  - McKeown/Transhiatal—open neck incision
  - Can consider T-tube
  - J tube
  - Newer techniques like endoscopic negative pressure wound therapy
- Necrotic conduit/unstable patient: consider EGD with possible diversion (cervical esophagostomy, removal of conduit, feeding jejunostomy)
- Stricture
  - Upper GI to help with diagnosis
  - EGD and dilation
  - R/O recurrent cancer with biopsies
- Tracheoesophageal Fistula
  - Rare
  - Leak can predispose to this

Palliative Options for Dysphagia

- Brachytherapy
- Endoscopic dilation
- Placement of a metal stent
- External beam radiotherapy
- Palliative/salvage resection reserved for severe refractory dysphagia, stenosis, or strictures

Surveillance (NCCN)

- Tis or T1a treated with EMR
  - EGD every 3 months for the first year, every 6 months for the second year, and then annually
- Tis, T1a, and N0 treated with esophagectomy
  - EGD as needed based on symptoms
  - If incompletely resected BE, serial EGDs
- T1a N+ or T1b or greater treated with esophagectomy ± adjuvant therapy
  - CT chest/abdomen every 6 months for 2 years followed by annually for 5 years
  - EGD as needed based on symptoms
  - If incompletely resected BE, serial EGDs
- Any T, any N treated with neoadjuvant therapy, esophagectomy ±adjuvant therapy
  - CT chest/abdomen every 6 months for 2 years followed by annually for 5 years
- Tumor treated with definitive chemoradiation without surgery

- CT chest/abdomen every 3–6 months for 2 years followed by annually for 5 years
- EGD every 3–6 months for 2 years followed by annually for 3 years

References

1. Ajani JA, D'Amico TA, Bentrem DJ, Cooke D, Corvera C, Das P, et al. Esophageal and esophagogastric junction cancers, version 2.2023, NCCN clinical practice guidelines in oncology. J Natl Compr Cancer Netw. 2023;21(4):393–422.
2. Arnal MJD, Arenas ÁF, Arbeloa ÁL. Esophageal cancer: risk factors, screening and endoscopic treatment in Western and Eastern countries. World J Gastroenterol: WJG. 2015;21(26):7933.
3. Berry MF. Esophageal cancer: staging system and guidelines for staging and treatment. J Thorac Dis. 2014;6(Suppl 3):S289.
4. Biere SSAY, Maas KW, Cuesta MA, Van Der Peet DL. Cervical or thoracic anastomosis after esophagectomy for cancer: a systematic review and meta-analysis. Dig Surg. 2011;28(1):29–35.
5. Brown LM, Devesa SS. Epidemiologic trends in esophageal and gastric cancer in the United States. Surg Oncol Clin. 2002;11(2):235–56.
6. Burt BM, Groth SS, Sada YH, Farjah F, Cornwell L, Sugarbaker DJ, Massarweh NN. Utility of adjuvant chemotherapy after neoadjuvant chemoradiation and esophagectomy for esophageal cancer. Ann Surg. 2017;266(2):297–304.
7. Codipilly DC, Qin Y, Dawsey SM, Kisiel J, Topazian M, Ahlquist D, Iyer PG. Screening for esophageal squamous cell carcinoma: recent advances. Gastrointest Endosc. 2018;88(3):413–26.
8. Gabriel NH, James LC, Carl JD, Stephen BE, Elizabeth AM, Hope SR, et al. AJCC cancer staging manual. 8th ed; 2018. p. 1–50.
9. Gooszen JAH, Goense L, Gisbertz SS, Ruurda JP, Van Hillegersberg R, van Berge Henegouwen MI. Intrathoracic versus cervical anastomosis and predictors of anastomotic leakage after oesophagectomy for cancer. J Br Surg. 2018;105(5):552–60.
10. Jones DR. Minimally invasive Ivor Lewis Esophagectomy. Oper Tech Thorac Cardiovasc Surg. 2013;18(4):254–63.
11. Kelly RJ, Ajani JA, Kuzdzal J, Zander T, Van Cutsem E, Piessen G, et al. Adjuvant nivolumab in resected esophageal or gastroesophageal junction cancer. N Engl J Med. 2021;384(13):1191–203.
12. Kidane B, Korst RJ, Weksler B, Farrell A, Darling GE, Martin LW, et al. Neoadjuvant therapy vs upfront surgery for clinical T2N0 esophageal cancer: a systematic review. Ann Thorac Surg. 2019;108(3):935–44.
13. Lin J, Iannettoni MD. Transhiatal esophagectomy. Surg Clin. 2005;85(3):593–610.
14. Liu CQ, Ma YL, Qin Q, Wang PH, Luo Y, Xu PF, Cui Y. Epidemiology of esophageal cancer in 2020 and projections to 2030 and 2040. Thoracic Cancer. 2023;14(1):3–11.
15. McLaren PJ, Dolan JP. Surgical treatment of high-grade dysplasia and early esophageal cancer. World J Surg. 2017;41:1712–8.
16. Mokdad AA, Yopp AC, Polanco PM, Mansour JC, Reznik SI, Heitjan DF, et al. Adjuvant chemotherapy vs postoperative observation following preoperative chemoradiotherapy and resection in gastroesophageal cancer: a propensity score–matched analysis. JAMA Oncol. 2018;4(1):31–8.
17. Pera M, Manterola C, Vidal O, Grande L. Epidemiology of esophageal adenocarcinoma. J Surg Oncol. 2005;92(3):151–9.
18. Samson P, Puri V, Robinson C, Lockhart C, Carpenter D, Broderick S, et al. Clinical T2N0 esophageal cancer: identifying pretreatment characteristics associated with pathologic upstaging and the potential role for induction therapy. Ann Thorac Surg. 2016;101(6):2102–11.

19. Sharma P, Dent J, Armstrong D, Bergman JJ, Gossner L, Hoshihara Y, et al. The development and validation of an endoscopic grading system for Barrett's esophagus: the Prague C & M criteria. Gastroenterology. 2006;131(5):1392–9.
20. Spechler SJ, Souza RF. Barrett's esophagus. N Engl J Med. 2014;371(9):836–45.
21. Sreedharan A, Harris K, Crellin A, Forman D, Everett SM. Interventions for dysphagia in oesophageal cancer. Cochrane Database Syst Rev. 2009;(4)
22. Tepper J, Krasna MJ, Niedzwiecki D, Hollis D, Reed CE, Goldberg R, et al. Phase III trial of trimodality therapy with cisplatin, fluorouracil, radiotherapy, and surgery compared with surgery alone for esophageal cancer: CALGB 9781. J Clin Oncol Off J Am Soc Clin Oncol. 2008;26(7):1086.
23. Uhlenhopp DJ, Then EO, Sunkara T, Gaduputi V. Epidemiology of esophageal cancer: update in global trends, etiology and risk factors. Clin J Gastroenterol. 2020;13(6):1010–21.
24. van Hagen P, Hulshof MCCM, Van Lanschot JJB, Steyerberg EW, Henegouwen MVB, Wijnhoven BPL, et al. Preoperative chemoradiotherapy for esophageal or junctional cancer. N Engl J Med. 2012;366(22):2074–84.
25. Varghese TK, Hofstetter WL, Rizk NP, Low DE, Darling GE, Watson TJ, et al. The society of thoracic surgeons guidelines on the diagnosis and staging of patients with esophageal cancer. Ann Thorac Surg. 2013;96(1):346–56.
26. Wheeler JB, Reed CE. Epidemiology of esophageal cancer. Surg Clin. 2012;92(5):1077–87.
27. Włodarczyk JR, Kużdżał J. Stenting in palliation of unresectable esophageal cancer. World J Surg. 2018;42:3988–96.
28. Wong I, Law S. McKeown esophagectomy. In: Esophageal cancer: diagnosis and treatment; 2018. p. 99–107.
29. Zhang JQ, Hooker CM, Brock MV, Shin J, Lee S, How R, et al. Neoadjuvant chemoradiation therapy is beneficial for clinical stage T2 N0 esophageal cancer patients due to inaccurate preoperative staging. Ann Thorac Surg. 2012;93(2):429–37.

Gastric Cancer

Carl Schmidt and Mary Garland Kledzik

Introduction

- Most patients in the USA (2/3) present with advanced or incurable disease.
- Diagnosis is made by upper endoscopy.
- Common clinical staging studies include CT, EUS, MRI, and CT/PET.
- Surgical removal with perioperative chemotherapy is the current standard for potentially curable disease.

Diagnosis

- Symptoms may include abdominal pain, weight loss, and anemia.
- Dysphagia may occur with proximal or GEJ tumors (ddx includes esophageal cancer).
- Gastric outlet obstruction may occur with distal tumors (ddx includes peptic ulcer disease).
- Physical exam findings concerning for metastatic disease
    - Virchow's node (palpable left supraclavicular lymph node)
    - Sister Mary Joseph's node (palpable periumbilical mass)
    - Ascites
    - Jaundice
- There are many environmental risk factors [26]:
    - Male sex (x2)
    - *H. pylori* infection (3–5x)
    - Smoking (1.5–2x)

C. Schmidt (✉) · M. G. Kledzik
Department of Surgery, Division of Surgical Oncology, West Virginia University, Morgantown, WV, USA
e-mail: carl.schmidt@hsc.wvu.edu

© The Author(s), under exclusive license to Springer Nature Switzerland AG 2025
C. Schmidt, M. G. Kledzik (eds.), *Complex General Surgical Oncology*,
https://doi.org/10.1007/978-3-031-88954-7_6

- Atrophic gastritis resulting in metaplasia [23]
- Low ferritin, pernicious anemia, and history of distal gastrectomy for peptic ulcer disease [11, 14, 24]
- Unknown if eradicating *H. pylori* reduces incidence [12]
- Red meat consumption [28, 34]
• Countries with high incidence have screening endoscopy programs [33]
  - Japan—EGD every 2 years after age 50
  - Korea—EGD every 2 years after age 40
• Familial risk factors
  - Gastric cancer is familial in approximately 10% [18]
  - Hereditary diffuse gastric cancer (HDGC)
    • Germline mutations of E-cadherin gene (*CDH1*)
    • Autosomal dominant inheritance pattern
    • High penetrance of diffuse subtype gastric cancer [31]
  - Hereditary nonpolyposis colorectal cancer (HNPCC or Lynch syndrome) carries increased risk of colorectal, endometrial, gastric cancers
  - Juvenile polyposis syndrome (JPS), Peutz-Jeghers syndrome (PJS), familial adenomatous polyposis (FAP), ataxia-telengectasia (ATM), Li-Fraumeni (p53), and Cowden (PTEN) syndrome all have increased risk gastric cancer
• Pathologic principles
  - Gastric ulcers discovered by EGD need multiple biopsies
    • Biopsies from edge of ulcer to avoid necrosis
    • Seven biopsies increases sensitivity to detect malignancy [13]
  - Lauren classification system
    • Intestinal type
  - Arises from mucosal glands, defined margins, associated with chronic gastritis
  - Mass or ulcerated mass common
    • Diffuse type
  - Scattered malignant cells, infiltrative margin, submucosal spread, and mucin common
  - May not form discrete mass, thick gastric folds, and difficult to distend on endoscopy
    • Linitis plastic or "leather-bottle-like stomach"
  - Stomach difficult to distend on endoscopy
  - Mucosa may appear normal due to submucosal spread
  - Poor prognosis
  - Reflex pathology for gastric cancer—important pathologic studies
    • *HER2/neu*
  - Overexpressed in 10–38% of gastric cancers
  - Associated with intestinal-type distal cancer
  - Worse prognosis [19]
    • *MMR, PDL1, or TMB* help define prognosis and response to systemic or immunotherapy

Evaluation and Clinical Stage

- Labs—CEA, CA 19-9, and nutrition assessment
- Clinical staging studies—see Table 6.1
- CT scan chest, abdomen, and pelvis
- FDG-PET—18-fluorodeoxyglucose positron emission tomography
  - Consider if indeterminate CT findings for metastatic disease
  - Used to evaluate response to chemotherapy [21]
  - Some diffuse type cancers are not FDG-avid
- Endoscopic ultrasound (EUS)
  - Assess small gastric masses for EMR or ESD
  - Improved accuracy for T and N stage compared to CT scan
- Diagnostic laparoscopy and cytology
  - Staging laparoscopy can avoid unnecessary gastrectomy due to metastatic disease in 24% [6]
  - Positive cytology has a survival similar to macroscopic metastatic disease
- TNM staging—see Table 6.2
  - T stage based on depth penetration into gastric wall
  - N stage defined by number of involved nodes

Table 6.1 Range of sensitivity and specificity for gastric cancer staging modalities

	T1	T2	T3	T4	N
EUS					
Sensitivity	64–92%	54–85%	52–80%	25–78%	17–97%
Specificity	52–98%	80–88%	77–93%	92–99%	49–100%
CT					
Sensitivity	13–94%	29–68%	37–91%	29–86%	63–92%
Specificity	80–100%	78–92%	70–95%	92–99%	42–88%
MRI					
Sensitivity	51–79%	78–90%	78–91%	78–94%	48–100%
Specificity	94–99%	85–93%	83–93%	94–99%	40–100%

Table 6.2 Gastric cancer TNM staging (AJCC 8th edition)

T0	No evidence of tumor
Tis	Intraepithelial tumor without invasion of the lamina propria
T1	Tumor invades the lamina propria, muscularis mucosa, or submucosa
T2	Tumor invades the muscularis propria
T3	Tumor penetrates the subserosal connective tissue without invasion of the visceral peritoneum (serosa) or surrounding structures
T4	Tumor invades the serosa or surrounding structures
N0	No regional lymph nodes involvement*
N1	Metastases in 1–2 regional lymph nodes*
N2	Metastases in 3–6 regional lymph nodes*
N3	Metastases in 7+ regional lymph nodes*
M0	No distant metastases
M1	Distant metastases

Table 6.3 Gastric cancer survival by clinical stage

Clinical	Five-year survival (%)	Postneoadjuvant stage	Five-year survival (%)
I	56.8	I	74.2
IIa	47.4	II	46.3
IIb	33.1		
III	25.9	III	18.6
IV	5.0	IV	7.0

- pTNM stage based on surgical resection
- Regional nodes are perigastric and celiac, splenic, left gastric, and common hepatic arterial nodes
- Paraaortic, retroperitoneal, and other nodes outside regional are classified as distant metastatic disease
- Tumors involving GEJ with tumor epicenter <2 cm into stomach are classified as esophageal cancers
- Table 6.3—estimated survival by TNM stage

Choice of Therapy

- cTNM, clinical stage; pTNM, pathologic stage; and ypTNM, pathologic stage after neoadjuvant therapy
- Palliative intent chemotherapy for patients with distant metastatic disease or cytology positive disease by diagnostic laparoscopy
- T1 and node-negative by clinical stage—evaluate for endoscopic removal or gastrectomy
- T2 and node-negative—evaluate for neoadjuvant therapy or gastrectomy
- T3–4 or node-positive by clinical stage—evaluate for neoadjuvant therapy
- See Fig. 6.2

Endoscopic Therapy

- Endoscopic mucosal resection (EMR) and endoscopic submucosal dissection (ESD)
- Indicated if risk of lymph node metastases <1% [1]
  - T1a (mucosal invasion) LNM risk = 1–3%
  - T1b (submucosal invasion) LNM risk = 15%
- classic indications—nonulcerated, differentiated, T1a, and diameter ≤ 2 cm
- ESD expanded criteria [25]
  - Ulcerated, differentiated, T1a, and diameter ≤ 3 cm
  - Nonulcerated, undifferentiated, T1a, and diameter ≤ 2 cm

Surgical Therapy

- Surgical removal of primary gastric cancer is required for potential cure
- Determination of resectability
  - Contraindications to resection for potential cure include distant metastatic disease, encasement of aorta, and celiac or hepatic artery occlusion (rare)
  - En bloc removal of left lateral liver segment, distal pancreas and spleen, or partial colectomy are not contraindications to resection
  - Linitis plastica, patients needing a Whipple operation or other contiguous organ resection should prompt strong consideration of neoadjuvant therapy
- Total gastrectomy
  - For tumors of GEJ, gastric cardia and upper one-third of stomach
  - Siewert's classification for GEJ tumors
    - Type I: distal esophagus -may infiltrate the GEJ from above; typically treated surgically with esophagogastrectomy
    - Type II: carcinoma of cardia arising at GEJ within 1 cm above/2 cm below
    - Type III: arising below cardia infiltrating GEJ and distal esophagus from below
  - Reconstruction with Roux-en-Y esophagojejunostomy [see Fig. 6.1]
- Subtotal and distal gastrectomy
  - For tumors in distal two-thirds of stomach
  - Improved QOL compared to total gastrectomy [4, 5, 9]
  - Reconstruction with either Roux-en-Y gastrojejunostomy or Billroth II gastrojejunostomy [see Fig. 6.2]

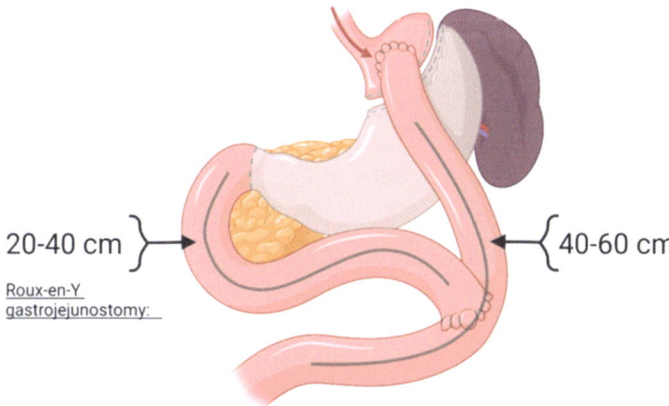

Fig. 6.1 Roux-en-Y gastrojejunostomy reconstruction after total gastrectomy or distal subtotal gastrectomy; the Roux limb is typically made 40–60 cm in length

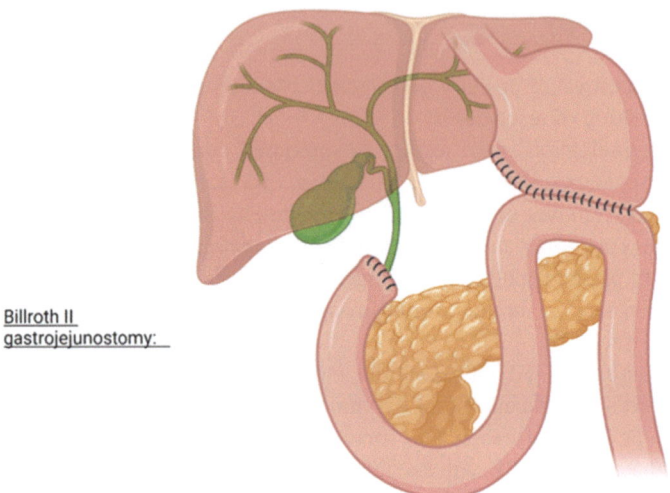

Fig. 6.2 Billroth II gastrojejunostomy reconstruction after distal gastrectomy

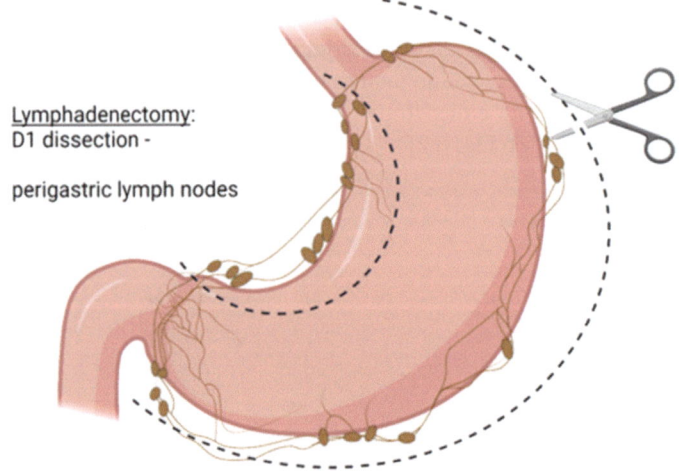

Fig. 6.3 Lymph node regions removed for D1 (perigastric) lymphadenectomy

- Extent of Lymphadenectomy
  - Minimum of 16 lymph nodes required for adequate staging
  - D1 dissection includes perigastric lymph nodes [see Fig. 6.3]
  - D2 dissection includes hepatic, left gastric, celiac, and splenic artery nodes and spleen [see Fig. 6.4]
  - Modified D2 includes hepatic, left gastric, celiac, and splenic artery nodes

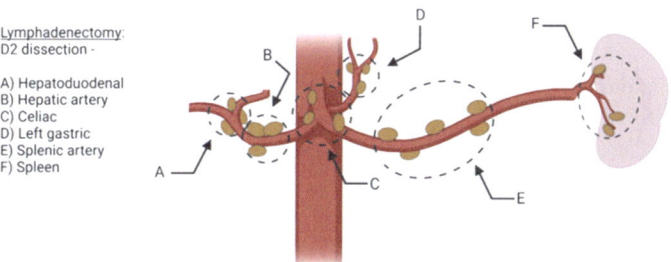

Fig. 6.4 Lymph node regions removed for D2 (extended) lymphadenectomy

- D3 dissection includes porta hepatis and retropancreatic and periaortic nodes
- Dutch D1D2 lymphadenectomy trial [3]
  - Operative morbidity and mortality higher in D2 versus D1 group (43%/10% vs 25%/4%, respectively)
  - D2 lymphadenectomy—higher DSS and lower local (12% vs 22%) and regional (13% vs 19%) recurrence [15, 29]
- Italian Gastric Cancer Study Group—organ-preserving D2 lymphadenectomy [10]
  - Morbidity and mortality—12% and 3% for D1 and 18% and 2% for D2
  - A five-year DSS 71% and 73% for D1 and D2 groups for all comers
  - If node-positive disease—A five-year DSS 61% for D2 group vs 46% D1
- Extent of resection
  - Traditional necessity of wide >5 cm proximal margin for distal cancers may not be necessary [30]
  - Multivisceral resection is indicated when required to achieve R0 resection
  - Frozen section margins of can be considered, but surgical clearance of a microscopic positive esophageal or duodenal margin may not be beneficial if increased operative morbidity; other factors such as number of positive nodes may outweigh prognostic impact of margin
- Minimally invasive gastrectomy [7]
  - Laparoscopic distal gastrectomy not inferior to open for stage I GC
    - KLASS-01 trial (Korea)
    - JCOG0912 trial (Japan)
  - Laparoscopic distal gastrectomy not inferior to open for advanced GC
    - KLASS-02 trial (Korea)
    - CLASS-01 trial (China)
- Cytoreduction and heated intraperitoneal chemotherapy (CRS/HIPEC)
  - Currently under evaluation for patients with limited peritoneal disease
  - GASTRIPEC-1 trial awaiting publication, 105 patients; RCT comparing CRS +/− HIPEC with mitomycin C + cisplatin for gastric adenocarcinoma with peritoneal metastases, OS 14.9 months for both groups (PFS 7.1 v 3.5 months), 55 pts. progressed prior to operation

Adjuvant therapy (Table 6.4)

- McDonald trial / INT-0116 (2001)—Macdonald et al. [22]
  - Most patients T3/T4
  - 5FU/LV for five days and then chemoradiation 4500 cGy compared to surgery alone
- MAGIC trial (2006)—Cunningham et al. [8]
  - $\geq$ T1b GC
  - Three cycles ECF pre- and postoperative compared to surgery alone
  - 42% patients completed all therapies in ECF arm
- FLOT 4 trial (2019)—Al-Batran et al. [2]
  - $\geq$ T2 GC
  - Three cycles ECF or ECX pre- and postoperative compared to four cycles FLOT pre- and post
  - 50% completed all therapies in FLOT arm

Table 6.4 Randomized trials evaluating adjuvant therapy for gastric cancer

Trial	Patients	Results
INT-0116 (MacDonald)	556 patients, RCT Resectable gastric adenocarcinoma Surgery + adjuvant 5-FU + leucovorin × 5 days and then 4500 cGy vs surgery alone	OS 36 vs 27 months RFS 30 vs 19 months 3-year OS 50% vs 41% Only 10% received D2 lymphadenectomy
MAGIC trial	503 patients, RCT StageII+ gastric/EGJ adenocarcinoma ECFx3 + surgery+ ECFx3 v surgery alone	5 yr. OS 36% vs 23% PFS Complication rates 46% vs 45% Only 41% received D2 lymphadenectomy Only 42% in the perioperative chemotherapy group completed all of therapy
CLASSIC trial (Noh et al. Lancet 2014)	1035 patients, RCT Stage II–IIIB gastric adenocarcinoma in Asia All received D2 lymphadenectomy Surgery + adjuvant CAPEOX vs surgery alone	Five-year DFS 68% vs 53% Five-year OS 78% vs 69%
FLOT4	716 patients, RCT Stage T2+ or N+, M0 resectable gastric/GEJ adenocarcinoma FLOT4 + surgery + FLOT4 v ECF/ECX × 3 + surgery + ECF/ECX × 3	OS 50 vs 35 months DFS 30 vs 18 months Toxicities were equal

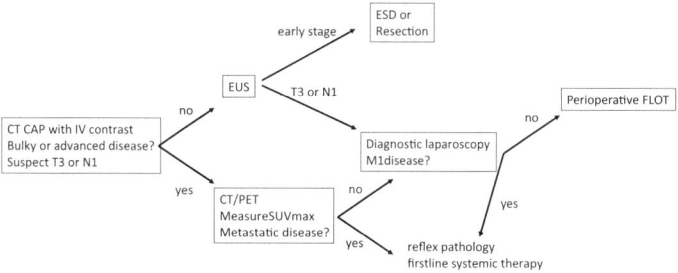

Fig. 6.5 A diagnostic and treatment algorithm for gastric cancer

- Algorithm for multidisciplinary evaluation and management of gastric cancer [see Fig. 6.5]
    - Initial staging with contrast-enhanced CT scan chest, abdomen, and pelvis
    - Consider CT/PET scan if concern for metastatic disease or to measure primary tumor SUV response with neoadjuvant therapy
    - Consider EUS especially if early-stage cancer amenable to ESD
    - Consider diagnostic laparoscopy with cytologic washings for any patient prior to neoadjuvant chemotherapy or radical resection
    - A perioperative chemotherapy strategy is preferred for most patients with T2/T3/T4 or node-positive gastric cancer s

Management of Locally Advanced and Metastatic Disease

- First-line therapy
    - ECF—response rate 46%, median survival nine months [32]
    - ECX, EOF, EOX, and FOLFIRI also options
    - Trastuzumab combined with chemotherapy if HER2/neu-expressing tumors
- Second-line therapies
    - Irinotecan or docetaxel and median survival <6 months
    - Paclitaxel and ramucirumab, median survival nine months
- Immunotherapy/targeted therapy—see Table 6.5

Table 6.5 Immunotherapy and biologic therapy trials for gastric cancer

Trial	Patients	Results
Checkmate-649 [16]	790 patients; RCT Nivolumab + FOLFOX/CAPEOX v FOLFOX/CAPEOX	PD-L1 CPS $\geq$ 5%: PFS 7.7 vs 6.1 months OS 14.4 vs 11.1 months PD-L1 CPS $\geq$ 1% PFS 7.5 vs 6.9 months OS 14.0 vs 11.2 months
CheckMate-577 [17]	794 patients; RCT Stage II/stage III esophageal/GEJ s/p neoadjuvant CRT Nivolumab vs placebo for one year	DFS 22.4 vs 11.0 months
Keynote-811 Chung HC et al. First-line pembrolizumab/placebo plus trastuzumab and chemotherapy in HER2-positive advanced gastric cancer: KEYNOTE-811 Future Oncol 2021;17:491–501	434 patients; RCT Unresectable or metastatic gastric/GEJ adenocarcinoma HER2—Positive Platinum-based chemotherapy+ trastuzumab +/− pembrolizumab	Response on imaging Objective response 74.4 v 51.9% Disease control 96.2 vs 89.3% CR 11.3 vs 3.1% PR 63.2 vs 48.9% Stable 21.8 vs 37.4%
Destiny-Gastric01 (https://www.annalsofoncology.org/article/S0923-7534(20)39363-7/fulltext)	187 patients; RCT phase II Advanced gastric/GEJ adenocarcinoma HER2-positive Third line; all patients had prior HER2 therapy Trastuzumab deruxtecan vs irinotecan or paclitaxel	ORR 51.3 vs 14.3% DOR 11.3 vs 3.9 months PFS 5.6 vs 3.5 months OS 12.5 vs 8.4 months
Destiny-Gastric01 (https://www.annalsofoncology.org/article/S0923-7534(20)39363-7/fulltext)	187 patients; RCT phase II Advanced gastric/GEJ adenocarcinoma HER2-positive Third line; all patients had prior HER2 therapy Trastuzumab deruxtecan vs irinotecan or paclitaxel	ORR 51.3 vs 14.3% DOR 11.3 vs 3.9 months PFS 5.6 vs 3.5 months OS 12.5 vs 8.4 months

Radiation Therapy

- Adjuvant radiation considered for microscopically positive margins if risk higher for locoregional versus systemic recurrence
- ARTIST trial (Korea)—no difference in survival between adjuvant chemoradiation and chemotherapy alone [20]
- CRITICS trial—no difference between adjuvant chemotherapy versus adjuvant chemoradiation [27]

Key Numbers

Here are some key general numbers to remember

Question	Answer
% of gastric cancers that are familial	10%
% of CT-occult metastatic dz. detected by PET	20%
Prognostic change in SUVmax by PET	35%
% patients positive by cytology for M1 disease	10–15%
% yield occult peritoneal disease by laparoscopy	20–25%
Survival benefit with D2 LND in node-positive cancer	15%
FLOT chemotherapy response rate	40–60%

Bibliography

1. Abe N, Watanabe T, Suzuki K, Machida H, Toda H, Nakaya Y, Masaki T, Mori T, Sugiyama M, Atomi Y. Risk factors predictive of lymph node metastasis in depressed early gastric cancer. Am J Surg. 2002;183:168–72.
2. Al-Batran SE, Homann N, Pauligk C, Goetze TO, Meiler J, Kasper S, Kopp HG, Mayer F, Haag GM, Luley K, Lindig U, Schmiegel W, Pohl M, Stoehlmacher J, Folprecht G, Probst S, Prasnikar N, Fischbach W, Mahlberg R, Trojan J, Koenigsmann M, Martens UM, Thuss-Patience P, Egger M, Block A, Heinemann V, Illerhaus G, Moehler M, Schenk M, Kullmann F, Behringer DM, Heike M, Pink D, Teschendorf C, Löhr C, Bernhard H, Schuch G, Rethwisch V, von Weikersthal LF, Hartmann JT, Kneba M, Daum S, Schulmann K, Weniger J, Belle S, Gaiser T, Oduncu FS, Güntner M, Hozaeel W, Reichart A, Jäger E, Kraus T, Mönig S, Bechstein WO, Schuler M, Schmalenberg H, Hofheinz RD. Perioperative chemotherapy with fluorouracil plus leucovorin, oxaliplatin, and docetaxel versus fluorouracil or capecitabine plus cisplatin and epirubicin for locally advanced, resectable gastric or gastro-oesophageal junction adenocarcinoma (FLOT4): a randomised, phase 2/3 trial. Lancet. 2019;393:1948–57.
3. Bonenkamp JJ, Hermans J, Sasako M, van de Velde CJ. Extended lymph-node dissection for gastric cancer. Dutch gastric cancer group. N Engl J Med. 1999;340:908–14.
4. Bozzetti F. Total versus subtotal gastrectomy in cancer of the distal stomach: facts and fantasy. Eur J Surg Oncol. 1992;18:572–9.
5. Bozzetti F, Marubini E, Bonfanti G, Miceli R, Piano C, Gennari L. Subtotal versus total gastrectomy for gastric cancer. Five year survival rates in a multicenter randomized Italian trial. Ann Surg. 1999;230:170–8.
6. Burke EC, Karpeh MS, Conlon KC, Brennan MF. Laparoscopy in the management of gastric adenocarcinoma. Ann Surg. 1997;225:262–7.
7. Choi S, Hyung WJ. Modern surgical therapy for gastric cancer-robotics and beyond. J Surg Oncol. 2022;125:1142–50.
8. Cunningham D, Allum WH, Stenning SP, Thompson JN, Van de Velde CJ, Nicolson M, Scarffe JH, Lofts FJ, Falk SJ, Iveson TJ, Smith DB, Langley RE, Verma M, Weeden S, Chua YJ, Participants MT. Perioperative chemotherapy versus surgery alone for resectable gastroesophageal cancer. N Engl J Med. 2006;355:11–20.
9. Davies J, Johnston D, Sue-Ling H, Young S, May J, Griffith J, Miller G, Martin I. Total or subtotal gastrectomy for gastric carcinoma? A study of quality of life. World J Surg. 1998;22:1048–55.
10. Degiuli M, Sasako M, Ponti A, Vendrame A, Tomatis M, Mazza C, Borasi A, Capussotti L, Fronda G, Morino M. Randomized clinical trial comparing survival after D1 or D2 gastrectomy for gastric cancer. Br J Surg. 2014;101:23–31.

11. Dubrow R. Gastric cancer following peptic ulcer surgery [editorial; comment]. J Natl Cancer Inst. 1993;85:1268–70.
12. Ford AC, Forman D, Hunt RH, Yuan Y, Moayyedi P. Helicobacter pylori eradication therapy to prevent gastric cancer in healthy asymptomatic infected individuals: systematic review and meta-analysis of randomised controlled trials. BMJ (Clinical research ed.). 2014;348:g3174.
13. Graham DY, Schwartz JT, Cain GD, Gyorkey F. Prospective evaluation of biopsy number in the diagnosis of esophageal and gastric carcinoma. Gastroenterology. 1982;82:228–31.
14. Guiraldes E, Pena A, Duarte I, Trivino X, Schultz M, Larrain F, Espinosa MN, Harris P. Nature and extent of gastric lesions in symptomatic Chilean children with helicobacter pylori-associated gastritis. Acta Paediatr. 2002;91:39–44.
15. Hartgrink HH, van de Velde CJ, Putter H, Bonenkamp JJ, Klein Kranenbarg E, Songun I, Welvaart K, van Krieken JH, Meijer S, Plukker JT, van Elk PJ, Obertop H, Gouma DJ, van Lanschot JJ, Taat CW, de Graaf PW, von Meyenfeldt MF, Tilanus H, Sasako M. Extended lymph node dissection for gastric cancer: who may benefit? Final results of the randomized Dutch gastric cancer group trial. J Clin Oncol. 2004;22:2069–77.
16. Janjigian YY, Shitara K, Moehler M, Garrido M, Salman P, Shen L, Wyrwicz L, Yamaguchi K, Skoczylas T, Campos Bragagnoli A, Liu T, Schenker M, Yanez P, Tehfe M, Kowalyszyn R, Karamouzis MV, Bruges R, Zander T, Pazo-Cid R, Hitre E, Feeney K, Cleary JM, Poulart V, Cullen D, Lei M, Xiao H, Kondo K, Li M, Ajani JA. First-line nivolumab plus chemotherapy versus chemotherapy alone for advanced gastric, gastro-oesophageal junction, and oesophageal adenocarcinoma (CheckMate 649): a randomised, open-label, phase 3 trial. Lancet. 2021;398:27–40.
17. Kelly RJ, Ajani JA, Kuzdzal J, Zander T, Van Cutsem E, Piessen G, Mendez G, Feliciano J, Motoyama S, Lièvre A, Uronis H, Elimova E, Grootscholten C, Geboes K, Zafar S, Snow S, Ko AH, Feeney K, Schenker M, Kocon P, Zhang J, Zhu L, Lei M, Singh P, Kondo K, Cleary JM, Moehler M. Adjuvant Nivolumab in resected esophageal or gastroesophageal junction cancer. N Engl J Med. 2021;384:1191–203.
18. La Vecchia C, Negri E, Franceschi S, Gentile A. Family history and the risk of stomach and colorectal cancer. Cancer. 1992;70:50–5.
19. Lee EY, Cibull ML, Strodel WE, Haley JV. Expression of HER-2/neu oncoprotein and epidermal growth factor receptor and prognosis in gastric carcinoma. Arch Pathol Lab Med. 1994;118:235–9.
20. Lee J, Lim DH, Kim S, Park SH, Park JO, Park YS, Lim HY, Choi MG, Sohn TS, Noh JH, Bae JM, Ahn YC, Sohn I, Jung SH, Park CK, Kim KM, Kang WK. Phase III trial comparing capecitabine plus cisplatin versus capecitabine plus cisplatin with concurrent capecitabine radiotherapy in completely resected gastric cancer with D2 lymph node dissection: the ARTIST trial. J Clin Oncol. 2012;30:268–73.
21. Lordick F, Ott K, Krause BJ, Weber WA, Becker K, Stein HJ, Lorenzen S, Schuster T, Wieder H, Herrmann K, Bredenkamp R, Hofler H, Fink U, Peschel C, Schwaiger M, Siewert JR. PET to assess early metabolic response and to guide treatment of adenocarcinoma of the oesophagogastric junction: the MUNICON phase II trial. Lancet Oncol. 2007;8:797–805.
22. Macdonald JS, Smalley SR, Benedetti J, Hundahl SA, Estes NC, Stemmermann GN, Haller DG, Ajani JA, Gunderson LL, Jessup JM, Martenson JA. Chemoradiotherapy after surgery compared with surgery alone for adenocarcinoma of the stomach or gastroesophageal junction. N Engl J Med. 2001;345:725–30.
23. Morson B. Carcinoma arising from areas of intestinal metaplasia in the gastric mucosa. Br J Cancer. 1955;9:377–85.
24. Nomura A, Chyou PH, Stemmermann GN. Association of serum ferritin levels with the risk of stomach cancer. Cancer Epidemiol Biomarkers Prev. 1992;1:547–50.
25. Ortigão R, Libânio D, Dinis-Ribeiro M. The future of endoscopic resection for early gastric cancer. J Surg Oncol. 2022;125:1110–22.
26. Shah D, Bentrem D. Environmental and genetic risk factors for gastric cancer. J Surg Oncol. 2022;125:1096–103.

27. Slagter AE, Jansen EPM, van Laarhoven HWM, van Sandick JW, van Grieken NCT, Sikorska K, Cats A, Muller-Timmermans P, Hulshof M, Boot H, Los M, Beerepoot LV, Peters FPJ, Hospers GAP, van Etten B, Hartgrink HH, van Berge Henegouwen MI, Nieuwenhuijzen GAP, van Hillegersberg R, van der Peet DL, Grabsch HI, Verheij M. CRITICS-II: a multicentre randomised phase II trial of neo-adjuvant chemotherapy followed by surgery versus neo-adjuvant chemotherapy and subsequent chemoradiotherapy followed by surgery versus neo-adjuvant chemoradiotherapy followed by surgery in resectable gastric cancer. BMC Cancer. 2018;18:877.
28. Song P, Lu M, Yin Q, Wu L, Zhang D, Fu B, Wang B, Zhao Q. Red meat consumption and stomach cancer risk: a meta-analysis. J Cancer Res Clin Oncol. 2014;140:979–92.
29. Songun I, Putter H, Kranenbarg EM, Sasako M, van de Velde CJ. Surgical treatment of gastric cancer: 15-year follow-up results of the randomised nationwide Dutch D1D2 trial. Lancet Oncol. 2010;11:439–49.
30. Squires MH 3rd, Kooby DA, Pawlik TM, Weber SM, Poultsides G, Schmidt C, Votanopoulos K, Fields RC, Ejaz A, Acher AW, Worhunsky DJ, Saunders N, Jin LX, Levine E, Cho CS, Bloomston M, Winslow E, Cardona K, Staley CA 3rd, Maithel SK. Utility of the proximal margin frozen section for resection of gastric adenocarcinoma: a 7-institution study of the US gastric cancer collaborative. Ann Surg Oncol. 2014;21:4202.
31. van der Post RS, Vogelaar IP, Carneiro F, Guilford P, Huntsman D, Hoogerbrugge N, Caldas C, Schreiber KE, Hardwick RH, Ausems MG, Bardram L, Benusiglio PR, Bisseling TM, Blair V, Bleiker E, Boussioutas A, Cats A, Coit D, DeGregorio L, Figueiredo J, Ford JM, Heijkoop E, Hermens R, Humar B, Kaurah P, Keller G, Lai J, Ligtenberg MJ, O'Donovan M, Oliveira C, Pinheiro H, Ragunath K, Rasenberg E, Richardson S, Roviello F, Schackert H, Seruca R, Taylor A, Ter Huurne A, Tischkowitz M, Joe ST, van Dijck B, van Grieken NC, van Hillegersberg R, van Sandick JW, Vehof R, van Krieken JH, Fitzgerald RC. Hereditary diffuse gastric cancer: updated clinical guidelines with an emphasis on germline CDH1 mutation carriers. J Med Genet. 2015;52:361–74.
32. Waters JS, Norman A, Cunningham D, Scarffe JH, Webb A, Harper P, Joffe JK, Mackean M, Mansi J, Leahy M, Hill A, Oates J, Rao S, Nicolson M, Hickish T. Long-term survival after epirubicin, cisplatin and fluorouracil for gastric cancer: results of a randomized trial. Br J Cancer. 1999;80:269–72.
33. Xia JY, Aadam AA. Advances in screening and detection of gastric cancer. J Surg Oncol. 2022;125:1104–9.
34. Zhu H, Yang X, Zhang C, Zhu C, Tao G, Zhao L, Tang S, Shu Z, Cai J, Dai S, Qin Q, Xu L, Cheng H, Sun X. Red and processed meat intake is associated with higher gastric cancer risk: a meta-analysis of epidemiological observational studies. PLoS One. 2013;8:e70955.

Gastrointestinal Stromal Tumor

Nicholas W. Miller, Dane C. Olevian, and Alan A. Thomay

Introduction

Background

- Gastrointestinal stromal tumors (GISTs) are the most common mesenchymal neoplasms identified in the gastrointestinal (GI) tract [1].
  - Despite this, they are still relatively rare, representing less than 1% of all GI tumors [2].
- The American Cancer Society estimates that there are 4000–6000 cases of GISTs diagnosed in the USA each year [3].
- The location of these tumors may vary, but they are most commonly found in the stomach (60–70%), small bowel (20–25%), colon (5%), rectum (5%), and esophagus (5%) [4].
  - Very rare reports described GISTs in the appendix on surgical pathology from appendectomy [5].
  - They have also been discovered in the retroperitoneum, omentum, and mesentery [1, 4].

N. W. Miller
West Virginia University, School of Medicine, Morgantown, WV, USA
e-mail: nwm0006@mix.wvu.edu

D. C. Olevian
West Virginia University, Department of Pathology, Morgantown, WV, USA
e-mail: dane.olevian@hsc.wvu.edu

A. A. Thomay (✉)
West Virginia University, Department of Surgery, Morgantown, WV, USA
e-mail: aathomay@hsc.wvu.edu

© The Author(s), under exclusive license to Springer Nature Switzerland AG 2025
C. Schmidt, M. G. Kledzik (eds.), *Complex General Surgical Oncology*,
https://doi.org/10.1007/978-3-031-88954-7_7

- These tumors can range in size from several millimeters to many centimeters with the average size being about 6 cm, and they most often originate within the muscularis propria layer of the GI wall [2, 6].
  - Some smaller lesions may originate from the muscularis mucosa layer [7].
- It is common for these tumors to grow intramurally or in an exophytic pattern to invade other structures [8].
- Those smaller than 1 cm can be designated as microGISTs, and those 1–2 cm can be called miniGISTs [9].
- The largest GIST documented in the literature was measured to be 55 × 45 × 20 cm [10].

Epidemiology

- It is estimated that there are upward of 20 cases of GISTs per million people each year worldwide [1, 2, 9].
- Diagnostic rates have been increasing in recent years with more widespread use of advanced imaging technology [4].
- While all ages can be affected, the mean age at diagnosis is within the sixth decade of life, and males and females tend to be affected equally [1, 4].
  - About 0.02 GIST cases per million people per year occur in individuals under 14 years of age and are more often clinically malignant [11, 12].
- Studies have not identified associations related to geography, race, ethnicity, or occupation [2].
- Most cases develop sporadically (97%), but there are descriptions of germline mutations and associations with systemic diseases such as primary familial GIST syndrome, neurofibromatosis type 1, Carney-Stratakis syndrome, and Carney triad (Table 7.1) [2, 6, 13].

Table 7.1 GIST genetic syndromes. Genes involved and other clinical manifestations of various genetic syndromes presenting with GISTs

Syndrome	Gene involved	Clinical manifestations
Primary familial GIST syndrome [62]	KIT PDGFRA	GISTs, cutaneous hyperpigmentation, mastocytosis, dysphagia
Neurofibromatosis type 1 [63]	NF1	Neurofibromas, optic pathway gliomas, malignant peripheral nerve sheath tumors, GISTs, pheochromocytomas, juvenile monomyelocytic leukemia, café-au-lait macules, skinfold freckling, Lisch nodules
Carney-Stratakis syndrome, Carney Triad [64, 65]	SDH	Paragangliomas, GISTs, (also pulmonary chondromas in Carney Triad)

Pathophysiology

- Within the myenteric (Auerbach's) plexus, interstitial cells of Cajal (ICCs), the pacemaker cells of the GI tract, appear to be the origination of neoplasia in GIST [1, 14].
    - These ICCs direct peristalsis of the GI tract by providing autonomic innervation, and their location and function coincide with GISTs, which can be of smooth muscle and/or neuronal differentiation [2, 11].
- Affected cells have been found to have oncogenic gain-of-function mutations in *c-KIT* (75%) and/or *platelet-derived growth factor receptor alpha* (*PDGFRA*) (10%), which encode for the receptor tyrosine kinases (RTKs) KIT and PDGFRA, respectively [1, 4, 15].
    - The most common *c-KIT* mutations are within exon 11, which encodes for the juxtamembrane domain of the RTK.
    - The second most common *c-KIT* mutation is within exon 9, encoding for the extracellular domain.
- While these mutations may represent the initial genetic alterations leading to neoplasia, they appear to only be the first events among a series of additional genotypic changes necessary for malignancy [4].
- Additional documented mutations in malignant GISTs affected tumor suppressor genes on chromosomes 14q, 22q, 1p, and 15q [16].
- A smaller subset of GISTs do not possess changes in KIT or PDGFRA.
    - Rather, these cases tend to have defects in *SDH* (14%), *BRAF* (0.5%), *NF1* (0.5%), *RAS* (<0.5%), or *ETV1* (<0.5%) [4, 6, 15].
- Investigations into targeted therapies for GISTs associated with these genes are ongoing [17, 18].

Diagnosis

Symptoms

- Because GISTs can arise anywhere along the GI tract and even in extraintestinal sites, clinical symptoms can vary widely.
- Up to 30% of GISTs are asymptomatic and discovered incidentally on diagnostic imaging or in abdominal surgery for another reason [1, 19].
- When symptoms do present, they may include melena, hematemesis, anemia, weakness, abdominal pain, perforation, bowel obstruction, and/or distention [1, 5].
- There have been unusual case reports where GISTs have presented with suspected appendicitis and inguinal hernias [5, 20].

Endoscopy

- Endoscopy is one of the most common imaging modalities aiding in diagnosing GISTs.
- Typically, GISTs will appear as a subepithelial lesion completely covered by normal mucosa.
    - This is a nonspecific finding associated with a wide array of differential diagnoses including GIST, lipoma, schwannoma, leiomyoma, ectopic pancreas, or varices (Table 7.2).
- Those GISTs found to have malignant courses may have irregular borders, ulceration, and/or growth of the lesion on follow-up endoscopy.
- The subepithelial lesion associated with GIST is generally firm and has a negative cushion (pillow) sign or formation of indentation in surface of lesion on contact with forceps [1, 21].
- Standard endoscopy alone is unable to narrow the differential diagnoses after identification of a subepithelial lesion.

Table 7.2 Differential diagnoses of subepithelial lesion (SEL). Endoscopic descriptions, endoscopic ultrasound (EUS) descriptions, and immunohistochemical (IHC) findings of various pathologies presenting as SEL

Differential diagnosis	Endoscopic description	EUS description	IHC findings
GIST [7, 66, 67]	Submucosal mass, smooth margins, normal overlying mucosa, may protrude into lumen, negative cushion sign	Hypoechoic, homogeneous, well-defined margins, arising from muscularis propria or muscularis mucosa	CD117, DOG-1, PKC-theta
Lipoma [68]	Isolated solid bulge, smooth margins, normal overlying mucosa, yellow hue, positive cushion sign	Hyperechoic, homogeneous, well-defined margins, arising from submucosa	
Leiomyoma [69]	Submucosal mass, smooth margins, normal overlying mucosa, may protrude into lumen	Hypoechoic, homogeneous, well-defined margins, arising from muscularis propria or muscularis mucosa	Smooth muscle actin, desmin
Neuroendocrine tumor [70]	Small, round, sessile or polypoid, normal overlying mucosa	Hypoechoic or isoechoic, homogenous, arising from mucosa	Synaptophysin, chromogranin
Schwannoma [71]	Small, isolated, nodular or polypoid, normal overlying mucosa, yellow hue	Hypoechoic, homogeneous, well-defined margins, arising from mucosa or submucosa	S-100
Ectopic pancreas [72]	Submucosal nodule, central umbilication	Hypoechoic or isoechoic, heterogeneous, indistinct margins, arise from submucosa or muscularis mucosa	
Varices [73]	Enlarged tortuous vessels, easily compressed with instrument, blue hue	Anechoic, round, arising from muscularis propria or submucosa, Color Doppler	

7 Gastrointestinal Stromal Tumor

- Therefore, endoscopic ultrasound (EUS) is often utilized to provide more details about GI wall layer of origin, consistency of lesion, and size.
  - Due to characteristic EUS findings, some pathologies, including lipomas, cysts, and varices, can be diagnosed with these images alone.
  - However, if these results are inconclusive (such as in the case of GIST), the differential diagnosis list may remain broad.
  - Lesions less than 1 cm are typically followed with periodic EUS every six months to one year (Fig. 7.1) [1].
- GISTs will typically appear as hypoechoic, homogeneous, solid masses on EUS [1, 4].
  - These findings may be seen in other GI tumors, including leiomyomas, so obtaining sample for biopsy is helpful.
- The most effective method for diagnosing lesions found with EUS is to perform an EUS-guided fine needle aspiration.

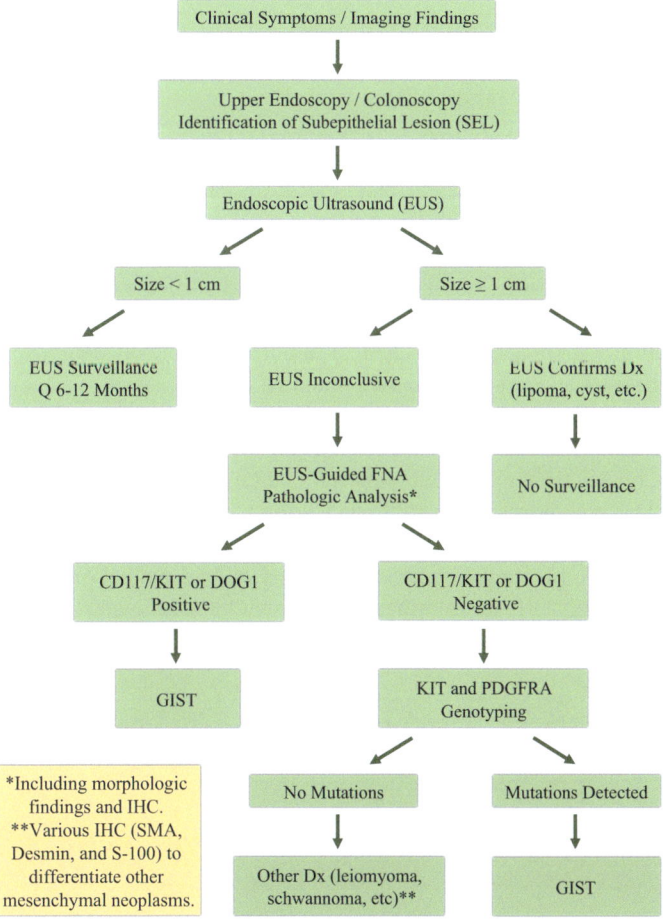

Fig. 7.1 GIST diagnostic tree. An overview of diagnostic studies characterizing GIST and other subepithelial lesion differential diagnoses

- This has been found to have an accuracy of up to 93% [1, 22].
- Performed in lesions greater than 1 cm, diagnostic accuracy increases with tumor size.
- Alternative biopsy methods, including endoscopic forceps biopsy, endoscopic submucosal dissection, or endoscopic snare resection are not preferred for obtaining samples for pathology [1].
- Further, tunnel biopsies can sometimes be collected safely and efficiently on initial endoscopy, preventing the need for follow-up EUS-FNA [23].

Histology

- GISTs are notorious for their broad and variable morphologic spectrum, though three principal types are recognized: spindled, epithelioid, and mixed [1].
- All tend to be well-circumscribed lesions often surrounded by a pseudocapsule [2].
- Spindle-cell GISTs are the most common and represent 70% of all cases.
  - These tumors feature uniform fusiform cells arranged in sheets, fascicles, bundles, or whorls (Fig. 7.2).
  - They have relatively monomorphic nuclei with fine chromatin and inconspicuous nucleoli.
  - The cytoplasm is typically pale and eosinophilic and often has a fibrillary appearance.
  - Paranuclear vacuoles are common, particularly in gastric tumors.
  - There may be a fibrocollagenous or myxoid stroma, while other cases may show prominent stromal hyalinization or sclerosis.
- Epithelioid GISTs account for 20% of tumors and typically demonstrate a markedly different appearance than their spindled counterparts.
  - These tumors have uniform, rounded cells arranged in sheets, nests, or clusters with a fibrous or myxoid stroma (Fig. 7.3).
  - The nuclei are typically monomorphic, though a subset may show significant nuclear pleomorphism or multinucleation.
  - Cytoplasmic vacuolization may be present and is occasionally prominent.
- Roughly 10% of tumors show mixed spindled and epithelioid morphology or cytologic characteristics intermediate between these extremes.

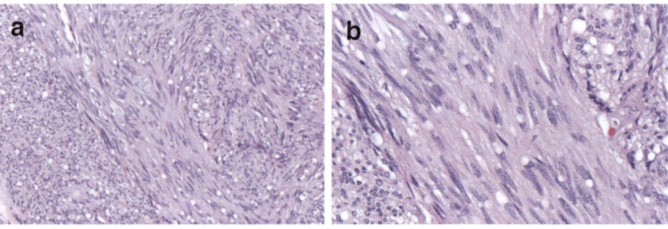

Fig. 7.2 Spindle cell GIST. (**a**, left) 20× magnification. (**b**, right) 40× magnification

7 Gastrointestinal Stromal Tumor

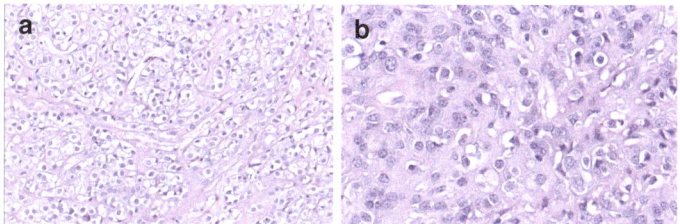

Fig. 7.3 Epithelioid GIST. (**a**, left) 20× magnification. (**b**, right) 40× magnification

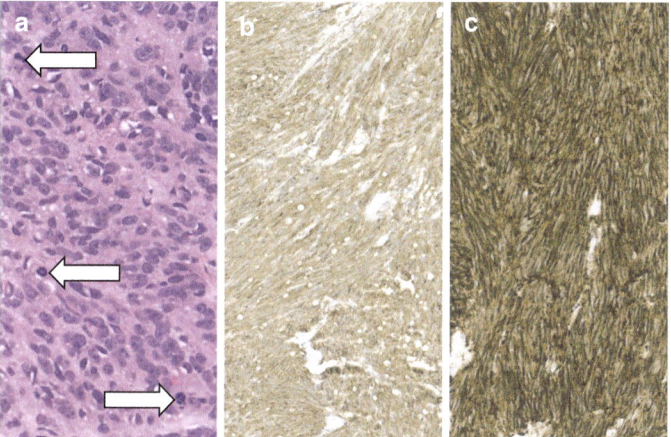

Fig. 7.4 Mitotic figures and immunohistochemical analysis. (**a**, left) Mitotic figures at 40× magnification. (**b**, center) CD117 immunostain at 20× magnification. (**c**, right) DOG-1 immunostain at 20× magnification

- Regardless of the morphology, tumors tend to have inconspicuous stromal vasculature and may show a brisk stromal lymphocytic infiltrate.
- Coagulative tumor necrosis is uncommon and is associated with more aggressive cases.
- GISTs may also undergo therapy-associated morphologic changes, manifest by hypocellularity, fibrosis, hyalinization, myxoid change, necrosis, and increased nuclear pleomorphism.
- SDH-deficient GISTs may show characteristic multinodular and plexiform growth within the muscularis propria and typically feature predominately epithelioid morphology [24–26].
- In rare cases, GISTs have been known to dedifferentiate, in which case a conventional GIST shows an abrupt transition to a high-grade, pleomorphic (dedifferentiated) area with abundant mitosis and necrosis.
- GIST grading is based entirely on mitotic count, expressed as the number of mitoses per 5 mm^2 (Fig. 7.4).

Immunohistochemistry

- Immunohistochemistry is an important ancillary tool for the diagnosis of GIST and is necessary to distinguish GISTs from their histologic mimics—most notably leiomyomas, schwannomas, and desmoid fibromatosis.
- A basic initial panel comprising CD117 (KIT), DOG-1, desmin, S100, and CD34 is recommended.
  - Approximately 95% of GISTs are immunoreactive to CD117, while DOG-1 has been shown to have over 99% sensitivity (Fig. 7.4).
  - Approximately 70% of GISTs are also positive for CD34, 30–40% for smooth muscle actin, 5–10% for desmin, 5% for S100, and 1–2% for keratin.
  - Staining for these less common markers is usually weak or focal—strong or diffuse CD117 and DOG-1 staining should provide diagnostic clarification.
- Notably, the expression of CD117 on IHC evaluation does not necessarily imply mutation in c-KIT, with one study finding that only about 73% of CD117-positive GISTs actually carried a mutation in c-KIT [26].
- Given that succinate dehydrogenase (SDH)-deficient GISTs have specific clinical implications, some authors recommend screening all gastric GISTs for SDH deficiency by immunohistochemistry, which can be accomplished by staining for SDH-B specifically, as this subunit is lost in all forms of SDH-deficient GISTs [24–28].

Molecular Analysis

- Genotyping can also be utilized in GIST diagnosis and is particularly recommended if tyrosine kinase inhibitors are a possible treatment modality.
- Approximately 75% of GISTs have activating mutations in the KIT gene (exon 11 is most common), whereas another 10% have mutations in the PDGFRA gene [1].
  - Mutations in KIT and PDGRFA are mutually exclusive.
- Approximately 10–15% of tumors harbor neither KIT nor PDGFRA mutations.
  - The majority of these so-called wild-type GISTs are SDH-deficient, which harbor mutations in SDH subunit genes.
  - Rare tumors are also associated with mutations in NF1, BRAF, KRAS, and other genes.
- Interestingly, more than 90% of metastatic GISTs have inactivation of the DMD gene on chromosome Xp21.1 encoding for dystrophin [17].
- Despite the increased relevance of genotypic analysis, this is not universally performed for all patients [10].
  - In fact, a team of researchers found that among cases of GIST from 2000 to 2018, only 47% of cases had mutational analysis despite its known benefit in guiding directed medical therapy.

- As a result, this team recommended two phases of mutational analysis—basic testing solely to assess c-KIT and PDGFRA followed by advanced testing for various other potential genes implicated in pathogenesis if preliminary testing is inconclusive [27].

Imaging

- Cross-sectional imaging studies, most frequently by computed tomography (CT), can provide information into tumor size, location, and organ involvement.
- Further, positron emission tomography (PET) can be utilized to assess tumor metabolic activity [4].
- Other imaging modalities including magnetic resonance imaging (MRI) and ultrasound may also be useful [6].
- When GISTs are suspected in rarer sites, such as the esophagus or rectum, modified CT scans can be performed with sufflated carbon dioxide to distend the GI wall for better visualization [29].
- In an initial diagnosis, it is possible for the tumor to be so large that it is difficult to identify the originating location.
    - However, imaging will show a heterogeneous mass often with necrosis and patchy uptake of contrast.
- Size can usually be estimated easily on imaging, and metastatic spread can be assessed.
- CT and PET imaging is particularly useful in regularly assessing the response to medical therapy [30].

Evaluation and Clinical Stage

Pathologic Stage Classification

- The 8th edition of the AJCC considers tumor size, lymph node involvement, and distant metastasis to establish the pathologic stage of all GISTs, regardless of site.
- The T stage is based solely on tumor size.
    - A GIST measuring 2 cm or less is considered T1, while those measuring 2 cm to 5 cm are classified as T2.
    - T3 tumors are greater than 5 cm and up to 10 cm, while any tumor greater than 10 cm is classified as T4.
- No regional lymph node metastasis receives the N0 stage, while any number of positive lymph nodes is designated N1.
- Similarly, M0 represents no spread to distant sites, whereas M1 indicates spread to remote sites of the body.

- Most GISTs metastasize to intraabdominal soft tissues, liver, or both if they metastasize at all.
• Although T, N, and M definitions are identical for all GISTs, the AJCC provides separate stage groupings for gastric/omental GISTs versus those arising in the small intestine, esophagus, colon, rectum, or peritoneum.
    - This reflects the lower rates of metastasis of gastric and omental GISTs than those originating elsewhere.
    - Therefore, the criteria is more liberal in assigning a higher stage to a tumor in the small intestine, esophagus, colon, rectum, or peritoneum.
        • For example, a 6 cm GIST originating from the small intestine with low mitotic rate and no nodal involvement or distant metastasis would be assigned to AJCC stage II, whereas a tumor of the same characteristics located in the stomach would only be stage IB (Tables 7.3 and 7.4) [30].
• Regarding histologic grading of GIST, the College of American Pathologists make assignments based solely on mitotic activity of the tumor and highlight that histologic grading is not well suited to GISTs.
    - This is because, in comparison to other soft tissue tumors, GISTs already have lower mitotic rates but tend to have more aggressive features.

Table 7.3 GIST AJCC staging system. AJCC 8th edition staging system for GISTS originating in the stomach or omentum [74]

AJCC stage	TMN	Mitotic rate
IA	T1 or T2, N0, M0	Low
IB	T3, N0, M0	Low
II	T1, N0, M0	High
	T2, N0, M0	High
	T4, N0, M0	Low
IIIA	T3, N0, M0	High
IIIB	T4, N0, M0	High
IV	Any T, N1, M0	Any
	Any T, any N, M1	Any

Table 7.4 GIST AJCC taging system. AJCC 8th edition staging system for GISTS originating in the small intestine, esophagus, colon, rectum, or peritoneum [74]

AJCC stage	TMN	Mitotic rate
I	T1 or T2, N0, M0	Low
II	T3, N0, M0	Low
IIIA	T1, N0, M0	High
	T4, N0, M0	Low
IIIB	T2, N0, M0	High
	T3, N0, M0	High
	T4, N0, M0	High
IV	Any T, N1, M0	Any
	Any T, any N, M1	Any

Table 7.5 Histologic Ggrade of GIST. College of American Pathologists grading system for GIST based solely on mitotic activity. Note that 5 mm² is equivalent to 50 high power fields (HPF)

Histologic grade	Mitotic activity
GX (grade cannot be assessed)	Unable to assess
G1 (low grade)	≤5 mitoses per 5 mm²
G2 (high grade)	>5 mitoses per 5 mm²

- The classification system used for histologic grade is broken down into three categories: GX, G1, and G2.
  - GX is assigned when a grade cannot be assessed.
  - G1 is considered low grade and is assigned when mitotic rates are less than or equal to 5 mitoses per 5 mm².
  - G2 is considered high grade and is assigned when mitotic rates are greater than 5 mitoses per 5 mm² (Table 7.5) [31].

Risk Stratification

- The biological behavior of GISTs exists on a continuum such that traditional concepts of benign and malignant are difficult to apply.
  - Furthermore, most GISTs are regarded as having some potential for distant metastasis.
- Consequently, a stratification scheme for risk of progressive disease is advocated by the College of American Pathologists based on the classification set forth by Miettinen and Lasota [32].
  - This scheme stratifies risk of progressive disease based on anatomic site, mitotic rate, and tumor size (Table 7.6).
    - Smaller tumors with lower mitotic rates and those arising in the stomach are considered lower risk than larger tumors with high mitotic rates arising in the jejunum/ileum.
    - For tumor sites not listed in the table, such as esophagus, peritoneum, and mesentery, the risk criteria for jejunum/ileum is recommended.

Prognosis

- The same factors used in establishing malignancy risk can aid in determining disease prognosis.
- Metastasis of GISTs is typically to the liver (65%) or peritoneum (21%) [1, 33].
  - It is rare for GISTs to metastasize to lymph nodes (6%), bone (6%), or lung (2%) [33].

Table 7.6 Guidelines for risk assessment of primary GIST

Tumor parameters		Risk of progressive disease#(%)			
Mitotic rate	Size	Gastric	Duodenum	Jejunum/ileum	Rectum
≤5 per 5 mm²	≤2 cm	None (0%)	None (0%)	None (0%)	None (0%)
	>2–≤5 cm	Very low (1.9%)	Low (8.3%)	Low (4.3%)	Low (8.5%)
	>5–≤10 cm	Low (3.6%)	(Insufficient data##)	Moderate (24%)	(Insufficient data##)
	>10 cm	Moderate (12%)	High (34%)	High (52%)	High (57%)
>5 per 5 mm²	≤2 cm	None	(Insufficient data##)	High	High (54%)
	>2–≤5 cm	Moderate (16%)	High (50%)	High (73%)	High (52%)
	>5–≤10 cm	High (55%)	(Insufficient data##)	High (85%)	(Insufficient data##)
	>10 cm	High (86%)	High (86%)	High (90%)	High (71%)

Adapted from Miettinen and Lasota. # defined as metastasis or tumor-related death. ## denotes small number of cases

Table 7.7 Differentiating GIST prognosis based on location

GIST location	Percentage of cases [4]	Five-year survival with surgical resection [34]	Symptoms [75]
Stomach	60–70%	88%	GI bleeding, abdominal pain, asymptomatic
Small intestine	20–25%	84%	GI bleeding, abdominal pain
Colon	5%	92%	GI bleeding
Rectum	5%	90%	GI bleeding
Esophagus	5%	80%	Abdominal pain

Survival data derived from large population-based study using the surveillance, epidemiology, and end results (SEER) database from the National Cancer Institute

- The strongest indicator of metastasis to the liver is angioinvasion [14].
- The risk of GIST metastasis has been correlated with size regardless of mitotic index [1].
- One of the largest studies of GIST assessed over 10,000 cases from 2000 to 2018 and found the following factors to impact survival most negatively: tumor size greater than 5 cm and poorly differentiated or undifferentiated histology [34].
- According to SEER, the five-year survival rate for GIST is 85% for all stages combined.
  - Localized disease has a five-year survival rate of 95%, regional disease is 84%, and distant disease is 52% [34].
  - Survival rates also vary based on the organ the GIST originated (Table 7.7).

Follow-Up

- Follow-up after GIST treatment focuses on assessing local recurrence and metastasis.
- Abdominal CT scanning can allow visualization from the diaphragm to the inguinal region and is widely used [1].
- For intermediate and high-risk GISTs, imaging is recommended every 3–6 months for three years and then every 6 months for an additional two years and annually thereafter.
- Low-risk GISTs can be followed with imaging every 6–12 months for 5 years and annually thereafter.
- Very low-risk GISTs do not have recommended follow-up guidelines established [4].

Treatment

Surgical

- Treatment of GISTs requires multidisciplinary teams that include surgeons, medical oncologists, pathologists, and radiologists [13].
- Preoperative planning with imaging studies is necessary to understand affected organs and assess for metastasis [10].
- Following appropriate diagnosis, surgical resection is the widely accepted first choice of therapy for localized GISTs that are larger than 2 cm [1, 4, 5].
- The goal of surgical intervention is an R0 complete resection with negative microscopic margins with intent to cure [1, 4].
- Depending on the location, wedge or segmental resections may be performed to preserve organs to the greatest extent; this is generally indicated for tumors that are smaller than 10 cm [1, 13].
- When tumors are adherent to contiguous organs, en bloc resection is utilized.
- Partial resections are only considered with very large tumors or palliative purposes [35].
- Laparoscopic techniques have even been found to benefit resection of smaller gastric GISTs less than 2 cm and have the benefits of decreasing blood loss and length of hospital stay [1, 2, 13].
- It is critical to prevent rupture of the pseudocapsule surrounding the GIST to avoid implanted recurrence to the peritoneum [4].
- Notably, lymph node metastasis is rare in GISTs, so lymphadenectomy is not standard of care during resection [1].
- In cases of metastatic GIST, surgery may be utilized for debulking [9].
  - It is estimated that up to 30% of presenting patients with GIST have already developed metastatic disease [13].

- Reducing tumor burden may prevent the development of additional mutations that influence effectiveness of medical therapies [9].
- The goal for surgical intervention in metastatic disease is to remove all gross disease; this may require specialized techniques including multivisceral resection, omentectomy, and peritoneal stripping.
- Due to the multifocal presentation of liver metastasis in GIST, traditional hepatectomy techniques are usually not indicated, but radiofrequency ablation or hepatic embolization may provide some benefit [13].
- Interventional radiologists can be particularly helpful in radiofrequency ablation and hepatic artery embolization and chemoembolization in cases of metastatic disease to the liver refractory to traditional surgical or medical approaches [36].

Endoscopic

- Though not the usual standard of care, studies into the efficacy and safety of endoscopic treatment approaches for GIST are ongoing [1, 37].
- A systemic review assessed the utility of various approaches, including endoscopic band ligation, endoscopic submucosal dissection, endoscopic submucosal excavation, endoscopic full-thickness resection, and submucosal tunneling endoscopic resection in the treatment of gastric GIST.
  - While the authors believed these approaches to be an option for smaller GIST confined to the gastric muscularis propria, the study found the most common complications associated with endoscopic approaches to be bowel perforation and rupture of the tumor pseudocapsule [37].
- Overall, long-term disease control with endoscopic approaches remains unknown.

Medical

- Originally approved in 2001 for treatment of certain leukemias, imatinib revolutionized the approach to treating cancer.
  - This small molecular inhibitor directly acts on tyrosine kinase, one of the receptors transmitting growth signals to certain cancer cells and is hypothesized to be effective in cancers with high proliferation through tyrosine kinase-mediated signaling [38].
  - Further trials found it to be useful in the treatment of advanced GIST by inhibiting KIT [39].
  - Imatinib is now the now most widely used medical treatment for GIST, often used in the adjuvant setting.
  - It is even used as sole therapy for unresectable, metastatic, or recurrent cases of GIST [1, 5].

- Deciding who qualifies for adjuvant imatinib therapy requires assessing the risk of disease recurrence, discussed previously, which requires consideration of tumor location, size, mitotes, and rupture.
  - Several risk stratification models have been studied including an original National Institutes of Health (NIH) consensus criteria, a modified version of this NIH criteria, and the Armed Forces Institute of Pathology (AFIP) prognostic model.
    - In the USA, the AFIP model appears to be most widely used (Table 7.6).
    - There does not appear to be data supporting that one of these models outperforms the other in assessing risk [40].
  - Overarching factors increasing risk of disease recurrence include increased size, increased mitoses, site of origin outside stomach, and presence of rupture [32].
  - Imatinib is usually considered in patients whose classification of disease recurrence falls into moderate or high risk [41, 42].
- Three notably large Phase III clinical trials assessed the use of adjuvant imatinib for GIST: ACOSOG Z9001, SSG trial XVIII, and EORTC trial 62026 [42].
  - ACOSOG Z9001 compared 400 mg/day of adjuvant imatinib for one year with a placebo group receiving surgery alone and found one-year RFS to be 98% in adjuvant imatinib group compared with 83% in placebo group [43].
  - The SSG XVIII trial compared 400 mg/day imatinib duration between two groups: one receiving adjuvant treatment for one year and the other receiving for three years.
    - They found five-year RFS to be 65.6% in three-year group compared to 47.9% in one-year group [44].
  - The EORTC trial 62026 compared 400 mg/day of adjuvant imatinib for two years with placebo group receiving surgery alone and found RFS to be 69% in imatinib group and 63% in placebo group [45].
- While originally considered for three years, adjuvant treatment with imatinib for GIST may show benefit with extension to five years based on the Postresection Evaluation of Recurrence-free Survival for Gastrointestinal Stromal Tumors With 5 Years of Adjuvant Imatinib (PERSIST-5) clinical trial.
  - This study found that no patients had recurrence during therapy when receiving five years of adjuvant imatinib after resection of primary GIST with imatinib-sensitive mutations.
  - Inclusion criteria for this study included adults with primary GIST expressing KIT who had complete resection within 12 weeks before starting the adjuvant imatinib; Eastern Cooperative Oncology Group performance status of 0 or 1, which is an assessment of functional status; adequate liver, kidney, and bone marrow function; and intermediate or high risk of GIST recurrence based on the Miettinen and Lasota risk classification (meaning having primary GIST at any site that is 2 cm or larger with ≥ 5 mitoses per 50 high-power field or having a nongastric primary GIST that is 5 cm or larger).
  - Overall, the study found a five-year estimated recurrence-free survival (RFS) to be 90% and the overall survival rate to be 95%.

- Notably, this study had about half of the participants discontinue therapy early and noted some recurrences after discontinuation, highlighting the need for improved support in maintaining patient compliance to therapy [46].
- Other studies have shown imatinib therapy for at least three years has shown promising results, significantly improving recurrence-free survival, and further studies are underway comparing outcomes in varying durations of adjuvant therapy [47].
- In cases where imatinib is unsuccessful, newer TKIs, including sunitinib, sorafenib, nilotinib, dasatinib, avapritinib, regorafenib, larotrectinib, and entrectinib, may provide benefit [1, 4, 9].
  - Notably, these drugs have varying targets and many studies are underway to assess their utility in GIST with differing mutations.
  - Specifically, sunitinib, often the second-line to imatinib, may target multiple receptor tyrosine kinases including VEGFR, PDGFR, KIT, FLT3, RET, and CSF1R [48].
  - Sorafenib can target VEGFR, KIT, and PDGFR [49].
  - Nilotinib has been shown to target KIT, PDGFR, and BCR-ABL [50].
  - Dasatinib can inhibit KIT, PDGFR, and SRC kinases [51].
  - Avapritinib notably targets KIT and PDGFR and may show particular benefit in GISTs with PDGFRA exon 18 D824V mutations [52].
  - Regorafenib can also inhibit KIT, PDGFR, and VEGFR [51].
  - Larotrectinib and entrectinib can both target tropomyosin receptor kinases, which results from *NTRK* fusions that are present in some wild-type GISTs [53].
- There has also been investigation into using TKIs in the neoadjuvant setting.
  - It is believed that this can provide reduction in tumor sizes to allow greater feasibility in obtaining appropriate surgical margins; it may also have benefits in sparing organs and decreasing rates of bleeding and tumor rupture [4].
  - Specifically, since rectal GIST resections tend to be more difficult, imatinib is recommended in the neoadjuvant setting as it has been shown to aid in tumor shrinkage for R0 resection and improve overall survival compared to upfront surgery [9, 54].
  - When used as neoadjuvant treatment, surgery should ideally be scheduled within 6–12 months [4].
  - After one month from initiation of neoadjuvant therapy, imaging exams are usually repeated to assess for response [55].
  - A systematic review found that neoadjuvant imatinib in cases of localized GIST demonstrated progression in 0–2% of cases with the eventual R0 resection occurring in 77–91% of cases.
    - This same study found that when the case was metastatic and neoadjuvant imatinib was administered, 4.5% of cases progressed with eventual R0 resection occurring in 58% of cases [47].
- Unfortunately, not all GISTs show similar responsiveness to TKI therapy.
  - It has been demonstrated that different locations of mutation in *c-KIT* may predict success.

- Specifically, when the *c-KIT* mutation is within exon 11, imatinib therapy has its best response; however, when located within exon 9, imatinib is less beneficial [2].
- A meta-analysis of data from the US-CDN and EU-AUS trials comparing imatinib dosing for treatment of unresectable or metastatic GIST showed that 800 mg imatinib daily did not have much advantage over 400 mg daily with less toxicity for most patients and recommended the 400 mg daily dosing.
  - They found an exception for patients with the exon 9 KIT mutations who may benefit from treatment at 800 mg, though this higher dose has not been extensively studied in adjuvant setting [42, 56].
- GISTs with mutations in *PDGFRA* on exons 12, 14, and 18 tend to be less responsive to imatinib with the exon 18 D824V mutation being imatinib-resistant [6, 16].
- Some studies have found sunitinib and other newer TKIs to be useful in imatinib-resistant GIST; avapritinib is recommended for the *PDGFRA* D824V mutation [2, 9].
- Because of these differences in treatment response dependent on tumor genetics, mutational analysis is recommended in all patients being considered for medical therapy [9].
- It is hypothesized that secondary mutations may develop with imatinib therapy in *c-KIT* exons 13, 14, and 17 contributing to medical therapy resistance [57].
- Current recommendations for adjuvant imatinib remains 400 mg/day for most patients, particularly for patients with high risk of relapse based on the ACOSOG, SSG, and EORTC trials [42].
- In the neoadjuvant setting, mutational analysis before initiating treatment is critical as certain mutations (PDGFRA D842V) will not respond to imatinib and would not be used.
- Some evidence suggests the KIT exon 11 mutations responds better to neoadjuvant imatinib compared to other mutations [58].
- Metastatic GIST makes surgical resection difficult as tumors appear multifocal and have usually spread to liver and peritoneum [4].
  - In these cases, imatinib may be initiated and has been shown to extend median overall survival from 1.5 to 5 years in metastatic disease [6].
  - Importantly, in cases of metastatic disease, there can be different mutations in various tumor foci within the same patient.
    - This means that some of these foci could be capable of responding to imatinib, while others are resistant.
    - Therefore, in such cases, a combination of surgical treatment for imatinib-resistant lesions and imatinib medical therapy may be required.
- In addition to TKI therapy, there have been investigations into the use of immunotherapy in GIST treatment.
  - There are ongoing studies regarding the utility of cytokine-based therapy, immune checkpoint inhibitors, anti-KIT monoclonal antibodies, bispecific monoclonal antibodies, and therapy with CAR T cells [59].

- While these investigations expand the potential for GIST therapy, they are not currently standard of care [9].
- Further, there are ongoing investigations to understand the potential role of microRNAs in diagnosis and treatment since the genetic aberrations associated with GIST are well described.
  - These microRNAs are thought to play a role in carcinogenesis by affecting posttranscriptional gene expression.
  - Implications for clinical practice could include future therapy directed at these or even their use as biomarkers with advanced technologies in detecting RNA [58, 60, 61].

Summary

- While GISTs are rarer tumors of the GI tract, they represent the most common GI tract mesenchymal neoplasm.
- Diagnostic rates are increasing with greater widespread use of more advanced imaging technology.
- Most are associated with mutations in *c-KIT* and/or *PDGFRA*, and there is high potential and increasing investigations into targeted molecular medical therapy.
- Currently, endoscopic ultrasound-guided fine needle aspiration typically provides a tissue sample that is assessed for morphology, mitoses, and immunohistochemical staining (KIT, CD34, DOG1, etc.) to diagnose GIST.
- All GISTs are considered potentially malignant with factors including size, mitoses, rupture, and location being beneficial in determining risk (very low, low, intermediate, high) of malignancy.
- The most widely accepted initial therapy is complete R0 surgical resection of the GIST with techniques varying based on size and location of the disease.
- Imatinib and other newer TKI therapies have shown promise in both neoadjuvant and adjuvant settings and even in cases of metastatic disease.

General Numbers to Remember

- Percent of All GI Tumors: <1%
- Percent of Sarcomas: 30–45%
- Percent By Location:
  - Stomach: 60–70%
  - Small Bowel: 20–25%
  - Colon: 5%
  - Rectum: 5%
  - Esophagus: 5%
- Percent Malignant: 30%
- Percent Sporadic: 97%
- Percent Asymptomatic: 30%

- Percent By Mutation:
  - *c-KIT*: 80%
  - *PDGFRA*: 5%
- Percent By Morphology:
  - Spindle-Shaped: 70%
  - Epithelioid: 20%
  - Mixed: 10%
- Percent By Immunohistochemistry
  - KIT: 95%
  - CD34: 60–70%
  - SMA: 30–40%
  - Desmin: 5–10%
  - S-100: 5%
- Percent Having Mutational Analysis: 47%
- Total 5-Year Survival: 85%
  - Localized Disease Five-Year Survival: 95%
  - Regional Disease Five-Year Survival: 84%
  - Distant Disease Five-Year Survival: 52%

Bibliography

1. Akahoshi K, Oya M, Koga T, Shiratsuchi Y. Current clinical management of gastrointestinal stromal tumor. World J Gastroenterol. 2018;24(26):2806–17. https://doi.org/10.3748/wjg.v24.i26.2806.
2. Gupta P, Tewari M, Shukla HS. Gastrointestinal stromal tumor. Surg Oncol. 2008;17(2):129–38. https://doi.org/10.1016/j.suronc.2007.12.002.
3. Key Statistics for Gastrointestinal Stromal Tumors. American Cancer Society.
4. Eisenberg BL, Pipas JM. Gastrointestinal stromal tumor--background, pathology, treatment. Hematol Oncol Clin North Am. 2012;26(6):1239–59. https://doi.org/10.1016/j.hoc.2012.08.003.
5. Nasasra A, Hershkovitz Y, Zager Y, Lavy R. Gastrointestinal stromal tumor of the appendix. Isr Med Assoc J. 2022;24(10):677–8.
6. Mantese G. Gastrointestinal stromal tumor: epidemiology, diagnosis, and treatment. Curr Opin Gastroenterol. 2019;35(6):555–9. https://doi.org/10.1097/mog.0000000000000584.
7. Chak A, Canto MI, Rösch T, et al. Endosonographic differentiation of benign and malignant stromal cell tumors. Gastrointest Endosc. 1997;45(6):468–73. https://doi.org/10.1016/s0016-5107(97)70175-5.
8. Kang HC, Menias CO, Gaballah AH, et al. Beyond the GIST: mesenchymal tumors of the stomach. Radiographics. 2013;33(6):1673–90. https://doi.org/10.1148/rg.336135507.
9. Sharma AK, Kim TS, Bauer S, Sicklick JK. Gastrointestinal stromal tumor: New insights for a multimodal approach. Surg Oncol Clin N Am. 2022;31(3):431–46. https://doi.org/10.1016/j.soc.2022.03.007.
10. Nemec HM, Smith AM, Benjamin CD. Giant gastrointestinal stromal tumor of the stomach. Am Surg. 2022;88(2):303–5. https://doi.org/10.1177/0003134820942137.
11. Rosai J. Gastrointestinal stromal tumor and its mimics. Int J Surg Pathol. 2010;18(3 Suppl):79s–87s. https://doi.org/10.1177/1066896910369928.
12. Kotb M, Abdelaziz M, Beyaly M, Mekawy M, Rashwan H, Mashali N. Neonatal gastrointestinal stromal tumor of the sigmoid colon: a case report and review of literature. Fetal Pediatr Pathol. 2020;39(2):172–8. https://doi.org/10.1080/15513815.2019.1641861.

13. Grignol VP, Termuhlen PM. Gastrointestinal stromal tumor surgery and adjuvant therapy. Surg Clin North Am. 2011;91(5):1079–87. https://doi.org/10.1016/j.suc.2011.06.007.
14. Yamamoto H, Oda Y. Gastrointestinal stromal tumor: recent advances in pathology and genetics. Pathol Int. 2015;65(1):9–18. https://doi.org/10.1111/pin.12230.
15. Schaefer IM, DeMatteo RP, Serrano C. The GIST of advances in treatment of advanced gastrointestinal stromal tumor. Am Soc Clin Oncol Educ Book. 2022;42:1–15. https://doi.org/10.1200/edbk_351231.
16. Schaefer IM, Mariño-Enríquez A, Fletcher JA. What is new in gastrointestinal stromal tumor? Adv Anat Pathol. 2017;24(5):259–67. https://doi.org/10.1097/pap.0000000000000158.
17. Nannini M, Rizzo A, Indio V, Schipani A, Astolfi A, Pantaleo MA. Targeted therapy in SDH-deficient GIST. Ther Adv Med Oncol. 2021;13:17588359211023278. https://doi.org/10.1177/17588359211023278.
18. Blay JY, Kang YK, Nishida T, von Mehren M. Gastrointestinal stromal tumours. Nat Rev Dis Primers. 2021;7(1):22. https://doi.org/10.1038/s41572-021-00254-5.
19. Chan CH, Cools-Lartigue J, Marcus VA, Feldman LS, Ferri LE. The impact of incidental gastrointestinal stromal tumours on patients undergoing resection of upper gastrointestinal neoplasms. Can J Surg. 2012;55(6):366–70. https://doi.org/10.1503/cjs.009111.
20. Yuan Y, Ding L, Tan M, Han AJ, Zhang X. A concealed inguinal presentation of a gastrointestinal stromal tumor (GIST): a case report and literature review. BMC Surg. 2021;21(1):111. https://doi.org/10.1186/s12893-021-01088-4.
21. Mummadi R, Raju GS. New endoscopic approaches to removing colonic lipomas. Gastroenterol Hepatol (N Y). 2007;3(11):882–3.
22. Larghi A, Fuccio L, Chiarello G, et al. Fine-needle tissue acquisition from subepithelial lesions using a forward-viewing linear echoendoscope. Endoscopy. 2014;46(1):39–45. https://doi.org/10.1055/s-0033-1344895.
23. Koutsoumpas A, Perera R, Melton A, Kuker J, Ghosh T, Braden B. Tunneled biopsy is an underutilised, simple, safe and efficient method for tissue acquisition from subepithelial tumours. World J Clin Cases. 2021;9(21):5822–9. https://doi.org/10.12998/wjcc.v9.i21.5822.
24. Ibrahim A, Chopra S. Succinate Dehydrogenase-Deficient Gastrointestinal Stromal Tumors. Arch Pathol Lab Med. 2020;144(5):655–60. https://doi.org/10.5858/arpa.2018-0370-RS.
25. Doyle LA, Nelson D, Heinrich MC, Corless CL, Hornick JL. Loss of succinate dehydrogenase subunit B (SDHB) expression is limited to a distinctive subset of gastric wild-type gastrointestinal stromal tumours: a comprehensive genotype–phenotype correlation study. Histopathology. 2012;61(5):801–9. https://doi.org/10.1111/j.1365-2559.2012.04300.x.
26. Wagner AJ, Remillard SP, Zhang YX, Doyle LA, George S, Hornick JL. Loss of expression of SDHA predicts SDHA mutations in gastrointestinal stromal tumors. Mod Pathol. 2013;26(2):289–94. https://doi.org/10.1038/modpathol.2012.153.
27. Sarlomo-Rikala M, Kovatich AJ, Barusevicius A, Miettinen M. CD117: a sensitive marker for gastrointestinal stromal tumors that is more specific than CD34. Mod Pathol. 1998;11(8):728–34.
28. Espinosa I, Lee CH, Kim MK, et al. A novel monoclonal antibody against DOG1 is a sensitive and specific marker for gastrointestinal stromal tumors. Am J Surg Pathol. 2008;32(2):210–8. https://doi.org/10.1097/PAS.0b013e3181238cec.
29. Han XF, Liang Y, Ma L. Disabled fingers due to infantile digital fibromatosis: A report of two cases with residual functional joint deformity. Dermatol Ther. 2022;35(3):e14335. https://doi.org/10.1111/dth.14335.
30. King DM. The radiology of gastrointestinal stromal tumours (GIST). Cancer Imaging. 2005;5(1):150–6. https://doi.org/10.1102/1470-7330.2005.0109.
31. Rivera AKU, Jabiles AG, Passiuri IC, et al. Gastrointestinal stromal tumour of the rectum and intestinal obstruction: case report. Ecancermedicalscience. 2020;14:1139. https://doi.org/10.3332/ecancer.2020.1139.
32. Miettinen M, Lasota J. Gastrointestinal stromal tumors: pathology and prognosis at different sites. Semin Diagn Pathol. 2006;23(2):70–83. https://doi.org/10.1053/j.semdp.2006.09.001.

33. Abuzakhm SM, Acre-Lara CE, Zhao W, et al. Unusual metastases of gastrointestinal stromal tumor and genotypic correlates: Case report and review of the literature. J Gastrointest Oncol. 2011;2(1):45–9. https://doi.org/10.3978/j.issn.2078-6891.2011.006.
34. Khan J, Ullah A, Waheed A, et al. Gastrointestinal stromal tumors (GIST): a population-based study using the SEER database, including management and recent advances in targeted therapy. Cancers (Basel). 2022;14(15) https://doi.org/10.3390/cancers14153689.
35. Stamatakos M, Douzinas E, Stefanaki C, et al. Gastrointestinal stromal tumor. World J Surg Oncol. 2009;7:61. https://doi.org/10.1186/1477-7819-7-61.
36. Avritscher R, Gupta S. Gastrointestinal stromal tumor: role of interventional radiology in diagnosis and treatment. Hematol Oncol Clin North Am. 2009;23(1):129–37., ix. https://doi.org/10.1016/j.hoc.2008.11.002.
37. Tan Y, Tan L, Lu J, Huo J, Liu D. Endoscopic resection of gastric gastrointestinal stromal tumors. Transl Gastroenterol Hepatol. 2017;2:115. https://doi.org/10.21037/tgh.2017.12.03.
38. Lemonick MD, Park A. New hope for cancer. San Francisco: Time; 2001.
39. Demetri GD, von Mehren M, Blanke CD, et al. Efficacy and safety of imatinib mesylate in advanced gastrointestinal stromal tumors. N Engl J Med. 2002;347(7):472–80. https://doi.org/10.1056/NEJMoa020461.
40. Joensuu H, Vehtari A, Riihimäki J, et al. Risk of recurrence of gastrointestinal stromal tumour after surgery: an analysis of pooled population-based cohorts. Lancet Oncol. 2012;13(3):265–74. https://doi.org/10.1016/s1470-2045(11)70299-6.
41. Balachandran VP, DeMatteo RP. Gastrointestinal stromal tumors: who should get imatinib and for how long? Adv Surg. 2014;48(1):165–83. https://doi.org/10.1016/j.yasu.2014.05.014.
42. Laurent M, Brahmi M, Dufresne A, et al. Adjuvant therapy with imatinib in gastrointestinal stromal tumors (GISTs)-review and perspectives. Transl Gastroenterol Hepatol. 2019;4:24. https://doi.org/10.21037/tgh.2019.03.07.
43. Dematteo RP, Ballman KV, Antonescu CR, et al. Adjuvant imatinib mesylate after resection of localised, primary gastrointestinal stromal tumour: a randomised, double-blind, placebo-controlled trial. Lancet. 2009;373(9669):1097–104. https://doi.org/10.1016/s0140-6736(09)60500-6.
44. Joensuu H, Eriksson M, Sundby Hall K, et al. One vs three years of adjuvant imatinib for operable gastrointestinal stromal tumor: a randomized trial. JAMA. 2012;307(12):1265–72. https://doi.org/10.1001/jama.2012.347.
45. Casali PG, Le Cesne A, Poveda Velasco A, et al. Time to definitive failure to the first tyrosine kinase inhibitor in localized gastrointestinal stromal tumors (GIST) treated with imatinib as an adjuvant: Final results of the EORTC STBSG, AGITG, UNICANCER, FSG, ISG, and GEIS randomized trial. J Clin Oncol. 2015;33(36):4276–83. https://doi.org/10.1200/jco.2015.62.4304.
46. Raut CP, Espat NJ, Maki RG, et al. Efficacy and tolerability of 5-year adjuvant imatinib treatment for patients with resected intermediate-or high-risk primary gastrointestinal stromal tumor: the PERSIST-5 clinical trial. JAMA Oncol. 2018;4(12):e184060. https://doi.org/10.1001/jamaoncol.2018.4060.
47. Brinch CM, Aggerholm-Pedersen N, Hogdall E, Krarup-Hansen A. Medical oncological treatment for patients with Gastrointestinal Stromal Tumor (GIST) - A systematic review. Crit Rev Oncol Hematol. 2022;172:103650. https://doi.org/10.1016/j.critrevonc.2022.103650.
48. Mulet-Margalef N, Garcia-Del-Muro X. Sunitinib in the treatment of gastrointestinal stromal tumor: patient selection and perspectives. Onco Targets Ther. 2016;9:7573–82. https://doi.org/10.2147/ott.S101385.
49. Heinrich MC, Marino-Enriquez A, Presnell A, et al. Sorafenib inhibits many kinase mutations associated with drug-resistant gastrointestinal stromal tumors. Mol Cancer Ther. 2012;11(8):1770–80. https://doi.org/10.1158/1535-7163.Mct-12-0223.
50. Reichardt P, Blay JY, Gelderblom H, et al. Phase III study of nilotinib versus best supportive care with or without a TKI in patients with gastrointestinal stromal tumors resistant to or intolerant of imatinib and sunitinib. Ann Oncol. 2012;23(7):1680–7. https://doi.org/10.1093/annonc/mdr598.

51. Schuetze SM, Bolejack V, Thomas DG, et al. Association of dasatinib with progression-free survival among patients with advanced gastrointestinal stromal tumors resistant to imatinib. JAMA Oncol. 2018;4(6):814–20. https://doi.org/10.1001/jamaoncol.2018.0601.
52. George S, Jones RL, Bauer S, et al. Avapritinib in patients with advanced gastrointestinal stromal tumors following at least three prior lines of therapy. Oncologist. 2021;26(4):e639–49. https://doi.org/10.1002/onco.13674.
53. Cao Z, Li J, Sun L, et al. GISTs with NTRK gene fusions: A clinicopathological, immunophenotypic, and molecular study. Cancers (Basel). 2022;15(1) https://doi.org/10.3390/cancers15010105.
54. Liu Z, Zhang Z, Sun J, et al. Comparison of prognosis between neoadjuvant imatinib and upfront surgery for GIST: A systematic review and meta-analysis. Front Pharmacol. 2022;13:966486. https://doi.org/10.3389/fphar.2022.966486.
55. Rodrigues J, Campanati RG, Nolasco F, Bernardes AM, Sanches SRA, Savassi-Rocha PR. Preoperative gastric gist downsizing: the importance of neoadjuvant therapy. Arq Bras Cir Dig. 2019;32(1):e1427. https://doi.org/10.1590/0102-672020180001e1427.
56. Comparison of two doses of imatinib for the treatment of unresectable or metastatic gastrointestinal stromal tumors: a meta-analysis of 1,640 patients. J Clin Oncol. 2010;28(7):1247–53. https://doi.org/10.1200/jco.2009.24.2099.
57. Joensuu H. Gastrointestinal stromal tumor (GIST). Ann Oncol. 2006;17(Suppl 10):x280–6. https://doi.org/10.1093/annonc/mdl274.
58. Liu X, Chu KM. Molecular biomarkers for prognosis of gastrointestinal stromal tumor. Clin Transl Oncol. 2019;21(2):145–51. https://doi.org/10.1007/s12094-018-1914-4.
59. Arshad J, Costa PA, Barreto-Coelho P, Valdes BN, Trent JC. Immunotherapy strategies for gastrointestinal stromal tumor. Cancers (Basel). 2021;13(14) https://doi.org/10.3390/cancers13143525.
60. Kim WK, Yang HK, Kim H. MicroRNA involvement in gastrointestinal stromal tumor tumorigenesis. Curr Pharm Des. 2013;19(7):1227–35. https://doi.org/10.2174/138161213804805748.
61. Kupcinskas J. Small molecules in rare tumors: emerging role of microRNAs in GIST. Int J Mol Sci. 2018;19(2) https://doi.org/10.3390/ijms19020397.
62. Miettinen M, Lasota J. Gastrointestinal stromal tumors: review on morphology, molecular pathology, prognosis, and differential diagnosis. Arch Pathol Lab Med. 2006;130(10):1466–78. https://doi.org/10.5858/2006-130-1466-gstrom.
63. Ly KI, Blakeley JO. The diagnosis and management of neurofibromatosis type 1. Med Clin North Am. 2019;103(6):1035–54. https://doi.org/10.1016/j.mcna.2019.07.004.
64. Stratakis CA, Carney JA. The triad of paragangliomas, gastric stromal tumours and pulmonary chondromas (Carney triad), and the dyad of paragangliomas and gastric stromal sarcomas (Carney-Stratakis syndrome): molecular genetics and clinical implications. J Intern Med. 2009;266(1):43–52. https://doi.org/10.1111/j.1365-2796.2009.02110.x.
65. McWhinney SR, Pasini B, Stratakis CA. Familial gastrointestinal stromal tumors and germline mutations. N Engl J Med. 2007;357(10):1054–6. https://doi.org/10.1056/NEJMc071191.
66. Rodriguez SA, Faigel DO. Endoscopic diagnosis of gastrointestinal stromal cell tumors. Curr Opin Gastroenterol. 2007;23(5):539–43. https://doi.org/10.1097/MOG.0b013e32829fb39f.
67. Miettinen M, Lasota J. Gastrointestinal stromal tumors--definition, clinical, histological, immunohistochemical, and molecular genetic features and differential diagnosis. Virchows Arch. 2001;438(1):1–12. https://doi.org/10.1007/s004280000338.
68. Hwang JH, Saunders MD, Rulyak SJ, Shaw S, Nietsch H, Kimmey MB. A prospective study comparing endoscopy and EUS in the evaluation of GI subepithelial masses. Gastroint Endosc. 2005;62(2):202–8. https://doi.org/10.1016/s0016-5107(05)01567-1.
69. Xu GQ, Zhang BL, Li YM, et al. Diagnostic value of endoscopic ultrasonography for gastrointestinal leiomyoma. World J Gastroenterol. 2003;9(9):2088–91. https://doi.org/10.3748/wjg.v9.i9.2088.
70. Nakamura S, Iida M, Yao T, Fujishima M. Endoscopic features of gastric carcinoids. Gastrointest Endosc. 1991;37(5):535–8. https://doi.org/10.1016/s0016-5107(91)70823-7.

71. Palazzo L, Landi B, Cellier C, et al. Endosonographic features of esophageal granular cell tumors. Endoscopy. 1997;29(9):850–3. https://doi.org/10.1055/s-2007-1004320.
72. Matsushita M, Hajiro K, Okazaki K, Takakuwa H. Gastric aberrant pancreas: EUS analysis in comparison with the histology. Gastrointest Endosc. 1999;49(4 Pt 1):493–7. https://doi.org/10.1016/s0016-5107(99)70049-0.
73. Boyce GA, Sivak MV Jr, Rösch T, et al. Evaluation of submucosal upper gastrointestinal tract lesions by endoscopic ultrasound. Gastrointest Endosc. 1991;37(4):449–54. https://doi.org/10.1016/s0016-5107(91)70778-5.
74. Amin MB, Edge SB, Greene FL, et al. AJCC cancer staging manual. Springer International Publishing; 2018.
75. Aghdassi A, Christoph A, Dombrowski F, et al. Gastrointestinal stromal tumors: clinical symptoms, location, metastasis formation, and associated malignancies in a single center retrospective study. Dig Dis. 2018;36(5):337–45. https://doi.org/10.1159/000489556.

Genetic Syndromes

8

Jacob Swords, Carly Likar, and Mary Garland Kledzik

Breast Guidelines to Test

Mutations	National Comprehensive Cancer Network® (NCCN®) [1]	ASBS [2]

BRCA 1
BRCA 2
PALB2
ATM
PTEN
CHD1
Neurofibromatosis
PTEN
	Age ≤ 50 years at diagnosis
	All patients:
	  Ashkenazi Jewish ancestry
	  Male breast cancer
	  To aid in systemic treatment decisions using PARP inhibitors for breast cancer in the metastatic setting
	  Triple-negative breast cancer
	  Multiple primary breast cancers (synchronous or metachronous)
	  Lobular breast cancer with personal or family history of diffuse gastric cancer
	  Family history of >1 close blood relative with ANY breast cancer at age ≤ 50, male breast cancer, ovarian cancer, pancreatic cancer, and prostate cancer with metastatic or high grade
	  Family history of ≥3 total diagnoses of breast cancer in patient and/or close blood relatives
	  Family history ≥2 close blood relatives with either breast or prostate cancer (any grade)
		All breast cancer patients are eligible for genetic screening.

J. Swords · C. Likar (✉)
West Virginia University, Department of Surgery, Morgantown, WV, USA
e-mail: cnszmyd@hsc.wvu.edu

M. G. Kledzik
Department of Surgery, Division of Surgical Oncology West Virginia Universityy, Morgantown, WV, USA

Colon Guidelines for Testing

Mutations	NCCN [3]	Bethesda Criteria [4] (Lynch syndrome / HNPCC)	Further testing [3]
Lynch FAP STK11 MUTYH SMAD4 Juvenile Polyposis CHEK2 PTEN	Age ≤ 50 years at diagnosis All patients: Personal or family history of ≥10 cumulative adenomas (polyposis syndrome) ≥2 hamartomas or polyps ≥20 serrated lesions throughout the colon ≥5 serrated polyps proximal to the rectum greater than 5 mm with 2 greater than 10 mm dMMR tumor	At least three relatives with a Lynch syndrome-associated cancer (see below) 1 is first-degree relative 2 successive generations At least 1 at age ≤ 50 years HNPCC-associated tumors include colon, endometrial, ovarian, renal, bladder, gastric, small bowel, pancreas, biliary, prostate, breast, and skin. Risk of each is dependent on exact gene mutation and further explained in gene-specific recommendations.	All tumors should be sent for mismatch repair deficiency (MLH1, MSH2, MSH6, PMS2, and EPCAM). This is immunohistochemistry If MLH1 deficient, they need further testing with BRAF for MLH1 promoter hypermethylation (implies somatic mutation rather than germline mutation) Microsatellite instability needs to be assessed by PCR testing.

Pancreas Guidelines for Genetic Testing

Mutations	NCCN [1]
BRCA 1 ATM CDKN2A TP3 PRSS1 Lynch PALB2 STK11	All patients with exocrine pancreatic cancer and/or all patients with first-degree relatives with exocrine pancreatic cancer should have genetic testing

Gastric Guidelines for Genetic Testing

Mutations	NCCN [5]
CDH1 FAP MEN2 SMAD4 Peutz Jeghers Syndrome	Known mutation in gene related to gastric cancer in the family or young patients with a family member meeting below criteria: Age ≤ 40 year with gastric cancer Gastric cancer ≤50 years old with a first- or second-degree relative with gastric cancer Anyone with gastric cancer with 2+ first- or second-degree relatives with gastric cancer Gastric and breast cancer diagnosed ≤50 years old Gastric cancer with a family history of Lynch or polyposis syndrome Gastric cancer in patient with Maori ancestry Gastric cancer in patient with history of cleft lip

Sarcoma Guidelines for Genetic Testing

Mutations	Classic Li-Fraumeni [1]	Chompret [1]
LiFraumeni (LFS) Neurofibromatosis Lynch syndrome (see colon guidelines)	Known TP53 mutation in family Age ≤ 45 sarcoma diagnosis and first- or second-degree family member with cancer <45 years	LFS tumor diagnosed age ≤ 45 years old and at least a first- or second-degree relative with LFS-related cancers diagnosed age ≤ 55 years or multiple primaries at any age or individual with multiple LFS tumors diagnosed ≤45 years old or adrenal cortical carcinoma, choroid plexus carcinoma, or rhabdomyosarcoma of embryonal anaplastic subtype at any age or breast cancer ≤30 years old LFS-associated tumors include adrenocortical carcinoma, breast cancer, osteosarcoma, soft tissue sarcoma, and CNS tumor

Endocrine Guidelines for Genetic Testing

Mutations	
VHL SDHA/B/C/D MEN1 MEN2	All patients with medullary thyroid cancer [6]

Guidelines Once Positive:

APC—familial adenomatous polyposis [3]
- Colon adenocarcinoma
- 100% lifetime risk of colorectal cancer
- Annual colonoscopy starting at 10–15
- Proctocolectomy at 18, if delaying recommend annual colonoscopy
- Post colectomy—care depends on type of colectomy
  - Ileorectal anastomosis—Lifetime risk 10–30% risk of colorectal cancer
    - Rectal endoscopy every 6–12 months
    - If endoscopy shows dense polyposis or high-grade dysplasia in any individual, then a completion proctocolectomy is recommended.
  - Ileal pouch—anal anastomosis. Lifetime risk 1–3% of colorectal cancer
    - Endoscopic evaluation of pouch and anastomosis every year
- Duodenal adenocarcinoma [14]
  - 1–10% absolute risk
  - Screening
    - Upper endoscopy starting at 20–25 years old with follow-up depending on Spigelman score

Spigelman score [14]			
Criteria	1 point	2 point	3 points
Polyp number	1–4	5–20	>20
Polyp size (mm)	1–4	5–10	>10
Histology	Tubular	Tubulovillous	Villous
Dysplasia	Mild	Moderate	Severe

- Stage 0–0 pts
  - Repeat upper endoscopy and duodenoscopy in four years
- Stage 1–1–4 pts
  - Repeat upper endoscopy and duodenoscopy in three years
- stage 2–5–6 pts.
  - Repeat upper endoscopy and duodenoscopy in 1–3 years
- stage 3–7–8 pts.
  - Repeat upper endoscopy and duodenoscopy in 6–12 months
- Stage 4–9–12 pts
  - Surgical evaluation
- Gastric adenocarcinoma
  - 0.1–7.1% absolute risk
  - Screening—during endoscopy for duodenal adenocarcinoma
- Thyroid carcinoma
  - 1–12% absolute risk
  - Screening—baseline thyroid ultrasound starting in late teenage years, if normal repeat every 2–5 years
- Desmoids
  - 10–24% absolute risk
  - Higher risk with mutations at 3' end of APC gene
  - If patient develops abdominal symptoms, then CT abdomen/pelvis
  - If patient develops symptomatic desmoids, recommend annual CT or MRI

ATM [1]

- Breast cancer 20–30% absolute risk, ovarian cancer 2–3% absolute risk, and pancreatic adenocarcinoma 5–10% absolute risk
- Risk reduction—insufficient evidence for prophylactic mastectomy, bilateral salpingo-oophorectomy (BSO) not recommended
- Screening
  - Annual mammogram starting at 40
  - Consider annual MRI at 30–35 (Note: MRI is often recommended at younger ages due to increased breast density)
  - Pancreatic cancer screening in patients with family history of exocrine pancreatic cancer (MRCP or EUS at age 50 or 10 years prior to earliest first-degree relative)

BARD1 [1]

- Breast cancer 20–40% absolute risk, no associated cancers
- Risk reduction—insufficient evidence for prophylactic mastectomy

8 Genetic Syndromes

- Screening
  - Annual mammogram starting at 40
  - Consider annual MRI at 40 (Note: MRI is often recommended at younger ages due to increased breast density)

BRCA1 [1]
- Absolute lifetime risk >60% breast cancer in females; 0.2–1.2% absolute risk of male breast cancer prior to age 70, 39–58% absolute risk of ovarian cancer, <5% absolute risk of pancreatic adenocarcinoma, and 7–26% absolute risk of prostate cancer
- Breast screening (females)
  - Clinical exam every 6–12 months starting at 25
  - 25–29 annual MRI (Note: MRI is often recommended at younger ages due to increased breast density)
  - 30–75 annual mammogram and MRI
  - >75 screening on individual basis
  - Discuss prophylactic mastectomy
- Breast screening (males)
  - Annual clinical exam starting at 35
  - Consider annual mammogram starting at 50
- Ovarian
  - Recommend risk reduction bilateral salpingo-oophorectomy at 35–40 (after done with childbearing)
    - However, data has started to show higher rates of cancer originating from the fallopian tubes in the premenopausal age group. There are ongoing trials looking at salpingectomy followed by delayed oophorectomy after menopause vs bilateral salpingo-oophorectomy in this patient subset. Recommend discussion with an ovarian cancer expert in this patient subset.
- Prostate
  - Consider screening starting at age 40

BRCA 2 [1]
- Absolute lifetime risk >60% breast cancer in females, 1.8–7.1% absolute risk of male breast cancer, 13–29% absolute risk of ovarian cancer, 5–10% absolute risk of pancreatic adenocarcinoma, and 19–61% absolute risk prostate cancer
- Breast screening (females)
  - Clinical exam every 6–12 months starting at 25
  - 25–29 annual MRI (Note: MRI is often recommended at younger ages due to increased breast density)
  - 30–75 annual mammogram and MRI
  - >75 screening on individual basis
  - Discuss risk reduction mastectomy
- Breast Screening (males)
  - Annual clinical exam starting at 35
  - Annual mammogram starting at 50

- Ovarian
  - Recommend risk reduction bilateral salpingo-oophorectomy at 40–45 (after done with childbearing)
- Prostate
  - Screening starting at age 40
- Pancreas
  - For patients with first-degree family member with exocrine pancreatic cancer recommend MRCP or EUS starting at 50 or 10 years prior to age at diagnosis of earliest family member

CDH1 [1]
- Absolute lifetime risk 41–60% for breast cancer, 70% lifetime risk of gastric adenocarcinoma in men, and 56% lifetime risk in women$_7$. Gastric penetrance however is dependent on whether the patient has family members with history of gastric cancer with patients with positive family history at higher risk. [1, 7]
- Screening
  - Annual mammogram, consider breast MRI starting at 30 (Note: MRI is often recommended at younger ages due to increased breast density)
- Gastric cancer
  - Recommend prophylactic total gastrectomy from 18–40 with preop endoscopy$_1$
  - If deferring gastrectomy recommend endoscopies every 6–12 months

CDKN2A [1]
- Pancreatic adenocarcinoma—absolute risk >15%
- Screening—EUS or MRCP at 50 or 10 years before age at diagnosis of earliest family member if applicable
- Melanoma—absolute risk 28–76%
  - Screening—comprehensive skin exam every six months
- P14ARF mutation specifically also at risk for nerve sheath tumors and sarcoma

CHEK2 [1]
- Breast—absolute risk 20–40%
- Screening—annual mammogram starting at 40, consider MRI starting at 30
- Risk reduction—not enough data supporting prophylactic mastectomy
- Colorectal—absolute risk 5–10%
  - Screening—colonoscopy every 5 years starting at 40 or 10 years prior to age at diagnosis of earliest family member

MEN1 [8]
- Initial evaluation
- Serum calcium
- CT abdomen/pelvis with multiphase contrast or MRI
- CT chest with contrast
- Pituitary MRI

- Parathyroid adenoma
  - >90% lifetime risk
  - Surveillance—annual calcium
- Pancreatic or duodenal neuroendocrine tumor
  - 20–80% lifetime risk
    - Gastrinoma—20–60%
    - Insulinoma—7–31%
    - Glucagonoma—1–5%
    - VIPoma—<2%
  - CT abdomen/pelvis or MRI abdomen every 1–3 years
  - Consider serial EUS
- Pituitary adenomas
  - 30–40% lifetime risk
  - Pituitary MRI every 3–5 years
  - Prolactin, IGF-1, and other previously abnormal pituitary hormones every 3–5 years
- Gastric carcinoid
  - 7–35% lifetime risk
- Bronchial/thymic carcinoid
  - <8% lifetime risk
  - Consider MRI or CT chest every 1–3 years
- Adrenal adenoma
  - 27–36% lifetime risk

MEN2A [6, 8]
- Medullary thyroid cancer
- >98% lifetime risk
- Basal serum calcitonin level
- Central and lateral neck compartment ultrasound
- Consider neck CT with contrast if ultrasound is unclear
- Total thyroidectomy prior to age five or at diagnosis
- Therapeutic neck dissection as indicated; would consider prophylactic bilateral central neck dissection (level VI) depending on disease burden on presentation and during operation
- Pheochromocytoma
  - 50% lifetime risk
  - Surveillance starting at ages 10–15
    - Blood pressure monitoring annually
    - Annual plasma free or 24 hour fractionated metanephrines
- Parathyroid adenoma
  - 25% lifetime risk
  - Surveillance—annual calcium
- Cutaneous lichens amyloidosis
- Hirschsprung disease

MEN2B [6, 8]
- Medullary thyroid cancer
- >98% lifetime risk
- Basal serum calcitonin level
- Central and lateral neck compartments ultrasound
- Consider CT neck with contrast
- Total thyroidectomy during the first year of life or at diagnosis
- Recommend referral to facilities with experience in pediatric thyroid surgery
- RET918 oncogene highest risk, recommend prophylactic central node dissection as well [6]
- Therapeutic neck dissection as indicated; consider prophylactic bilateral central neck dissection (level VI)
- Pheochromocytoma
  - 50% lifetime risk
- Surveillance starting at ages 6–10
  - BP monitoring annually
  - Annual plasma free or 24-hour fractionated metanephrines
- Intestinal ganglioneuromas
- Mucosal neuromas
- Marfanoid habitus

MUTYH [3]
- Screening—colonoscopy every 1–2 years starting at 20–25 years old
- If adenoma burden is too high (>20 adenomas <1 cm or any polyps with high-grade dysplasia) recommend total colectomy with ileorectal anastomosis or proctocolectomy with ileal pouch-anal anastomosis if there is a high rectal polyp burden
- Ileal rectal anastomosis screening—endoscopy every 6–12 months
- Duodenal screening—baseline endoscopy at 30–35 years old and further management based on Spigelman score (see APC recommendations)

Neurofibromatosis (NF1) [1]
- Breast
- 20–40% absolute risk
- Screening—Annual mammogram with tomosynthesis starting at age 30 and consider breast MRI with contrast from ages 30–50 (Note: MRI is often recommended at younger ages due to increased breast density)
- Risk reduction—Evidence insufficient for risk reduction mastectomy, manage based on family history
- Malignant peripheral nerve sheath tumors and GIST
  - Refer to NF1 specialist

PALB2 [1]
- Breast
- Absolute risks of breast cancer 40–60%, 1% risk of male breast cancer

- Screening: MRI/mammography with tomosynthesis every 6 months starting at 30 years old.
- Consider risk reduction mastectomy
- Ovarian
  - Absolute risk of ovarian cancer 10%
  - Consider risk reduction bilateral salpingo-oophorectomy
- Pancreatic
  - Absolute risk of 5–10%
  - Screening—EUS/MRCP at age 50 if family history of pancreatic cancer

PTEN (Cowdens) [1, 3]
- Breast
- Absolute risk 40–60%
- Screening—Clinical exam every 6–12 months starting at 25
- Screening—Annual mammography and breast MRI screening with contrast starting at age 35 years or 10 years before the earliest known breast cancer in the family (Note: MRI is often recommended at younger ages due to increased breast density)
- Discuss risk reduction mastectomy in patients with known mutation
- Colon
  - Absolute risk 11–20%
  - Colonoscopy starting at age 35 or 10 yrs. prior to earliest relative
  - At least every 5 years
- Endometrial
  - Consider endometrial biopsy every 1–2 years
  - Consider hysterectomy once done with childbearing years
- Renal
  - Consider renal ultrasound every 1–2 years starting at age 40
- Thyroid
  - Annual exam starting at age 7

Lynch [3]
- Most Lynch cancers (60–80%) come from mutations in MLH1 or MSH2. MSH6 and PMS2 have much lower penetrance for cancer. Lynch-related cancers are rarely related to EpCAM MSH6 carriers are much more common and are more related to extracolonic cancers, particularly endometrial cancer.
- Total colectomy in Lynch syndrome when a new cancer is diagnosed is often debated. The risk of a metachronous second colon cancers is less than 20% at 10 years but up to 60% at 30 years. Especially in older patients with less than 20 years of life expectancy, the risk/benefit ratio of total colectomy should be carefully weighed in reliable patients willing to be screened.

MLH1 [3]
- Colorectal
- Absolute risk 46–61%

- Screening—colonoscopy starting at age 20–25 or 2–5 years prior to age at diagnosis of earliest family member and every 1–2 years after
- No indication for prophylactic total proctocolectomy
- Pancreatic
  - Absolute risk 6.2%
  - Screening—For patients with first-degree family member with exocrine pancreatic cancer MRCP or EUS Start at age 50 or 10 years prior to earliest family member
- Endometrial
  - Absolute risk 34–54%
  - Screening can consider endometrial biopsy every 1–2 years starting at ages 30–35
  - Consider prophylactic hysterectomy—decreases incidence but has not been shown to improve overall mortality
- Ovarian
  - Absolute risk 4–20%
  - Screening—none
  - No evidence for prophylactic BILATERAL SALPINGO-OOPHORECTOMY
- Gastric—(5–7% absolute risk) /small bowel—0.4–11% absolute risk
  - Recommend EGD starting at age 30–35 with repeat every 2–4 years in conjunction with colonoscopy
- Other high cancer risks
  - Prostate 4.4–13.8% absolute risk

MSH2 [3]
- Colorectal
- Absolute risk 33–52%
- Screening—colonoscopy starting at age 20–25 and every 1–2 years after
- No indication for prophylactic total proctocolectomy
- Pancreatic
  - Absolute risk 0.5–1.6%
  - Screening—For patients with first-degree family member with exocrine pancreatic cancer, consider MRCP or EUS at age 50 or 10 years prior to earliest family member
- Endometrial
  - Absolute risk 21–57%
  - Screening—can consider endometrial biopsy every 1–2 years starting at ages 30–35
  - Consider prophylactic hysterectomy—decreases incidence but has not been shown to improve overall mortality
- Gastric (0.2–9% absolute risk)/small bowel (1.1–10% absolute risk)
  - Recommend EGD starting at ages 30–35 with repeat every 2–4 years in conjunction with colonoscopy

- Ovarian
  - Absolute risk 8–38%
  - Screening—none
  - Can consider prophylactic *bilateral salpingo-oophorectomy*
- Other high-risk cancers
  - Renal/ureter—2.2–28% absolute risk
  - Bladder—4.4–12.8% absolute risk
  - Prostate—3.9–23.8% absolute risk

MSH6 [3]
- Colorectal
- Absolute risk 10–44%
- Screening—colonoscopy starting at ages 30–35 and every 1–3 years after
- No indication for prophylactic total proctocolectomy
- Pancreatic
  - Absolute risk 1.4–1.6%
  - Screening—none
- Endometrial
  - Absolute risk 16–49%
  - Screening—can consider endometrial biopsy every 1–2 years starting at age 30–35
  - Consider prophylactic hysterectomy—decreases incidence but has not been shown to improve overall mortality
- Gastric (1–8% absolute risk)/small bowel (1–4% absolute risk)
  - Recommend EGD starting at ages 30–40 with repeat every 2–4 years in conjunction with colonoscopy
- Ovarian
  - Absolute risk 1–13%
  - Screening—none
  - Can consider prophylactic bilateral salpingo-oophorectomy
- Other high-risk cancers
  - Renal/ureter—0.7–5.5% absolute risk
  - Bladder—4.4–12.8% absolute risk
  - Prostate—2–11% absolute risk

PMS2 [3]
- Colorectal
- Absolute risk—8–20%
- Screening—colonoscopy starting at 30–35 years old and every 1–2 years after
- No indication for prophylactic total proctocolectomy
- Pancreatic
  - Absolute risk 0.5–1.6—not increased from general population
- Endometrial
  - Absolute risk 13–26%

- Screening—can consider endometrial biopsy every 1–2 years starting at ages 30–35
- Consider prophylactic hysterectomy—decreases incidence but has not been shown to improve overall mortality
- Gastric/small bowel—minimal data for increased risk from general population
- Ovarian
  - Absolute risk 1–3%
  - Screening—none
  - No evidence for prophylactic bilateral salpingo-oophorectomy
- Other high-risk cancers
  - Renal/ureter—not increased
  - Bladder—not increased
  - Prostate—4–11% absolute risk

RAD51C/D [1]
- Breast
- 17–30% absolute risk
- Screening—Annual mammogram and consider breast MRI with contrast starting at age 40
- Ovarian
  - C—10–15% absolute risk; D—10–20% absolute risk
  - Recommend—consider risk reduction bilateral salpingo-oophorectomy at 45–50

SDHA/B/C/D [8]
- Hereditary paraganglioma
- Pheochromocytoma
- Surveillance starting at ages 6–10 (B) or 10–15 (others)
  - BP monitoring annually
  - Annual plasma free or 24 hour fractionated metanephrines

SMAD4- Juvenile Polyposis [3]
- Diagnosed by >5 juvenile colon polyps or multiple juvenile polyps throughout GI tract or any juvenile polyps

Colon adenocarcinoma
  - Absolute risk 50%
  - Colonoscopy at ages 12–15 if no polyps repeat every 2–3 years starting at 18 years old, if polyps found repeat every 2–3 years

Stomach adenocarcinoma
  - Absolute risk 21%
  - Endoscopy at 12–15 if no polyps repeat every 2–3 years starting at 18 years old, if polyps found repeat every 2–3 years

STK11—Peutz-Jeghers Syndrome [1, 3]
- Breast cancer

- 32–54% absolute risk
- Screening—mammogram and breast MRI with contrast starting at age 30
- Discuss risk reduction mastectomy
- Pancreatic adenocarcinoma
  - Around 15% absolute risk
  - Screening EUS/MRCP starting at 30–35 years old or 10 years younger than earliest family member
- Colon and stomach adenocarcinoma
  - 39% absolute risk (colon) 29% (stomach)
  - Screening—endoscopy and colonoscopy starting at 8–10 years, repeat every 2–3 years if polyps are found, shorter intervals depending on polyp findings
- Small intestine
  - 13% absolute risk
  - Screening—capsule endoscopy or CT/MR enterography every 2–3 years starting at age 18
- Cervix
  - 10% absolute risk
  - Annual pelvic exam and pap smear starting at age 18–20
  - Consider total hysterectomy once done with childbearing
- Endometrial carcinoma
  - 9% absolute risk
  - Annual pelvic exam and endometrial biopsy if abnormal bleeding starting at age 18–20
- Ovary—sex cord stromal tumors
  - 20% absolute risk
  - Annual pelvic exam and pelvic ultrasound starting at ages 18–20
  - Physical exams for signs of precocious puberty starting at age 8

TP53—LiFraumeni [1, 3]
- Breast
- >60% absolute risk
- Screening
- Age 20–25—annual breast MRI
- Age 30–75—annual breast MRI and mammogram
- >75—screening on individual basis
- Discuss risk reducing mastectomy
- Pancreatic
  - 5–10% absolute risk
  - Consider EUS/MRCP at age 50 or 10 years younger than earliest family member with pancreatic cancer
- Colon
  - >20% absolute risk
  - Screening
    - Colonoscopy every 2–5 years starting at age 25 or 5 years before earliest first-degree family member

- Stomach
  - Upper endoscopy every 2–5 years starting at age 25 or 5 years before earliest first-degree family member
- Consider annual whole body MRI

Von Hippel Lindau [8, 9]
- Pheochromocytoma
- 10–20% lifetime risk
- Blood pressure monitoring at all medical visits starting at age two years.
- Abdominal MRI or CT with/without contrast every 2–3 years starting at 15 years.
- Paraganglioma
  - 10–20% lifetime risk
- Pancreatic neuroendocrine tumors
  - 5–17% lifetime risk
- Clear cell renal cell carcinoma
  - Abdominal MRI or CT with/without contrast to assess kidneys, pancreas, and adrenal glands every two years starting at age 15
- Also associated with hemangioblastoma

Disclaimers

Single nucleotide polymorphisms (SNPs) [10–13]
- SNPs are variations within the human genome that can be germline or sporadic.
- Many SNPs do not alter function and are thus labeled as "silent."
- SNPs alone may not confer a biological affect but together may influence gene expression.
- There is currently testing to assess breast cancer risk using SNPs. As SNPs between family members are extremely variable, family history should not be a criteria for this testing, although it is not well defined.
- Patients considered high risk based on SNPs should be considered for increased screening practices.
- There is similar data in colorectal cancer, although newer, that can potentially guide screening and treatment.

Risk reduction
- It is important to note that some risk-reducing surgeries such as breast still leave a 5–10% risk of breast cancer, but patients are no longer screened with mammograms or MRIs. This means that any cancers found would be clinically palpable and thus invasive.
- The benefit of risk reduction surgery diminishes as a patient passes their peak risk age (e.g., a 70-year-old woman found to have BRCA1 mutation will get little benefit from a prophylactic mastectomy and a hysterectomy with bilateral salpingo-oophorectomy as her risk of either after age 70 is <5%).

Variants of Undetermined Significance (VUS)
- VUS is a change, or variant, in a gene that has never been seen before or because of conflicting or incomplete information in the medical literature. Its association with cancer risk is unknown.
- Therefore, it cannot be determined yet whether this genetic variant is associated with an increased risk of cancer (pathogenic) or is a harmless, normal genetic variant (benign). At this time, predictive testing for variants of unknown significance is not recommended for at-risk family members. In the absence of a definitive mutation, the patient's risk of future cancers and medical management recommendations must be based on personal and family history of cancer.

References

NCCN

1. Referenced with permission from the NCCN Clinical Practice Guidelines in Oncology (NCCN Guidelines®) for NCCN Genetic/Familial High Risk Assessment: Breast, Ovarian and Pancreatic Version 2.2024. © National Comprehensive Cancer Network, Inc. 2023. All rights reserved. Accessed 11/28/23. To view the most recent and complete version of the guideline, go online to NCCN.org.
2. American Society of Breast Surgeons: Consensus Guideline on Genetic Testing for Hereditary Breast Cancer
3. Referenced with permission from the NCCN Clinical Practice Guidelines in Oncology (NCCN Guidelines®) for NCCN Genetic/Familial High Risk Assessment: Colorectal Version 2.2023© National Comprehensive Cancer Network, Inc. 2023. All rights reserved. Accessed 11/28/23. To view the most recent and complete version of the guideline, go online to NCCN.org.
4. Umar A, Boland CR, Terdiman JP, Syngal S, de la Chapelle A, Rüschoff J, Fishel R, Lindor NM, Burgart LJ, Hamelin R, Hamilton SR, Hiatt RA, Jass J, Lindblom A, Lynch HT, Peltomaki P, Ramsey SD, Rodriguez-Bigas MA, Vasen HF, Hawk ET, Barrett JC, Freedman AN, Srivastava S. Revised Bethesda Guidelines for hereditary nonpolyposis colorectal cancer (Lynch syndrome) and microsatellite instability. J Natl Cancer Inst. 2004;96(4):261–8. https://doi.org/10.1093/jnci/djh034. PMID: 14970275; PMCID: PMC2933058.
5. Referenced with permission from the NCCN Clinical Practice Guidelines in Oncology (NCCN Guidelines®) for Gastric Cancer Version 1.2023© National Comprehensive Cancer Network, Inc. 2023. All rights reserved. Accessed 11/28/23. To view the most recent and complete version of the guideline, go online to NCCN.org.
6. Referenced with permission from the NCCN Clinical Practice Guidelines in Oncology (NCCN Guidelines®) for Thyroid Cancer Version 3.2023 National Comprehensive Cancer Network, Inc. 2023. All rights reserved. Accessed 11/28/23. To view the most recent and complete version of the guideline, go online to NCCN.org.
7. Hansford S, Kaurah P, Li-Chang H, et al. Hereditary diffuse gastric cancer syndrome: CDH1 mutations and beyond. JAMA Oncol. 2015;1(1):23–32. https://doi.org/10.1001/jamaoncol.2014.168.
8. Referenced with permission from the NCCN Clinical Practice Guidelines in Oncology (NCCN Guidelines®) for Neuroendocrine and adrenal tumors Version 1.2023 National Comprehensive Cancer Network, Inc. 2023. All rights reserved. Accessed 11/28/23. To view the most recent and complete version of the guideline, go online to NCCN.org.
9. Referenced with permission from the NCCN Clinical Practice Guidelines in Oncology (NCCN Guidelines®) for Kidney cancer Version 1.2024National Comprehensive Cancer Network,

Inc. 2023. All rights reserved. Accessed 11/28/23. To view the most recent and complete version of the guideline, go online to NCCN.org.
10. Erichsen H, Chanock S. SNPs in cancer research and treatment. Br J Cancer. 2004;90:747–51. https://doi.org/10.1038/sj.bjc.6601574.
11. van Veen EM, Brentnall AR, Byers H, Harkness EF, Astley SM, Sampson S, Howell A, Newman WG, Cuzick J, Evans DGR. Use of single-nucleotide polymorphisms and mammographic density plus classic risk factors for breast cancer risk prediction. JAMA Oncol. 2018;4(4):476–82. https://doi.org/10.1001/jamaoncol.2017.4881. PMID: 29346471; PMCID: PMC5885189.
12. Cuzick J, Brentnall A, Dowsett M. SNPs for breast cancer risk assessment. Oncotarget. 2017;8(59):99211–2. https://doi.org/10.18632/oncotarget.22278. PMID: 29245890; PMCID: PMC5725081.
13. Jenkins MA, Makalic E, Dowty JG, Schmidt DF, Dite GS, MacInnis RJ, et al. Quantifying the utility of single nucleotide polymorphisms to guide colorectal cancer screening. Future Oncol. 2016;12:503–13.
14. Syngal S, Brand RE, Church JM, Giardiello FM, Hampel HL, Burt RW; American College of Gastroenterology. ACG clinical guideline: Genetic testing and management of hereditary gastrointestinal cancer syndromes. Am J Gastroenterol. 2015;110(2):223–62; quiz 263. https://doi.org/10.1038/ajg.2014.435. Epub 2015 Feb 3. PMID: 25645574; PMCID: PMC4695986.

Hepatocellular Carcinoma

Brian Sparkman, Kyeong Ri Yu, Apara Sai Jella, Leopoldo Fernandez, Jose Trevino, and Adam Khader

Introduction

- Cirrhosis is present in 90% of patients who develop HCC.
- About 40% of HCC patients do not secrete AFP.
- Diagnosis is primarily made by CT, MRI, and contrast-enhanced US on LI-RADS criteria in patients with known cirrhosis or hepatitis B (Fig. 9.1). All others require a biopsy for pathologic diagnosis.
- Consider screening with ultrasound (US) and alpha fetoprotein (AFP) in at-risk populations.
- AFP > 400 mg/mL, tumor size >5 cm, and vascular invasion are associated with metastasis.
- Several staging systems for HCC are available, but none are universally adopted; the severity of the liver disease, the size and extent of the tumor, and the presence of metastases are important factors to consider.

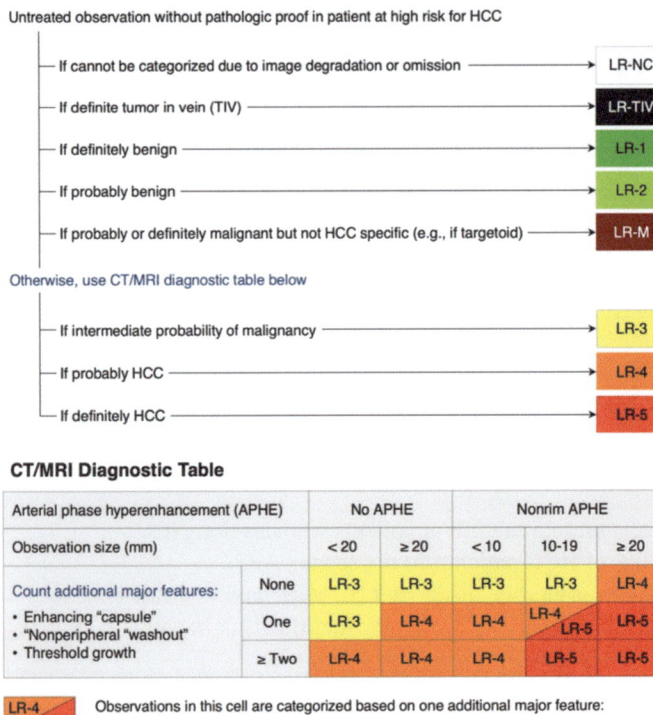

Fig. 9.1 Li-RADS v2018 diagnostic algorithm for CT and MRI ((LI- RADS) v2018 ACR.org. [29]). (Reproduced under CC BY-NC-ND 4.0)

- Curative treatments include resection and transplantation; locoregional and systemic therapies are available for nonsurgical candidates and as adjunct therapy in postoperative patients.

Epidemiology

- Most common cause HBV worldwide and HCV in the USA
- A third of cases not associated with a virus
    - NAFLD affects up to one-third of HCC patients and is associated with obesity and metabolic syndrome
- Other risk factors
    - Male sex (2–8× higher than women)
    - Older age: typically presents in 50–60 s
    - Smoking
    - Alcohol use
        - Synergistic effect with HBV and HCV

- Chemical exposure: aflatoxin (B1), nitrites, hydrocarbons, pesticide, anabolic steroid use
- Less common risk factors
  - Hemochromatosis
  - Alpha-1-antitrypsin deficiency
  - Primary sclerosing cholangitis
  - History of hepatic adenoma
  - Primary biliary cirrhosis
  - Wilson's disease

Diagnosis

- Symptoms
  - May include RUQ abdominal pain, weight loss, and palpable mass
  - Advanced malignant disease may present with nonspecific symptoms such as anorexia, nausea, and lethargy
  - If cirrhotic, may have hepatic decompensation
  - Can be asymptomatic
  - Rarely present with paraneoplastic syndrome (usually poor prognosis)
    - Hypercalcemia, hypoglycemia, erythrocytosis, and diarrhea
- Imaging
  - Critical for diagnosis of HCC
  - Abdominal US
    - Screening and surveillance in patients with cirrhosis
    - Masses with poorly defined margins
  - Multiphase contrast CT abdomen or MRI abdomen
    - Confirmatory study
    - A focal nodule with early enhancement in the arterial phase and rapid contrast washout in the delayed portal venous phase
    - Enhancing capsule appearance
    - Growth of $\geq 50\%$ in size (threshold >5 mm) in ≤ 6 months on previous CT or MRI
  - LI-RADS [Liver Imaging Reporting And Data System] criteria (Fig. 9.1)
    - Comprehensive system to standardize the terminology, technique, interpretation, reporting, and data collection of liver imaging
    - Applies to high-risk patients with the following:
      - Cirrhosis from noncongenital causes
      - Chronic HBV infection
      - History of HCC
      - Listed for or after liver transplant
      - Over age 18
    - Used to estimate likelihood of HCC and malignancy associated with each category and guide subsequent work up and management, including repeat imaging and biopsy

- Biopsy
  - Diagnosis should be as noninvasive as possible
    - Not recommended for LRs 1, 2, 3, and 5
  - May be pursued for LR-4 and LR-M lesions
    - Patient's risk of HCC is not high (e.g., no cirrhosis)
    - Imaging studies are inconclusive for HCC
    - Lesion is <1 cm
    - Not candidate for curative resection and needs diagnosis for systemic therapy or transplant
  - Risks include bleeding, pneumothorax, and biliary peritonitis
    - Overall risk for needle tract seeding 2.7% [16]
  - Histopathology
    - Most widely used grading system is 4-scale Edmondson and Steiner system.
    - Graded well, moderately, poorly differentiated, or undifferentiated.
    - Central necrosis of large tumors is common.
    - Bile globules and acidophilic inclusions may be present.
    - Growth patterns can vary
      - Can be attached to the liver via a vascular stalk
      - A demarcated mass often surrounded by a fibrous capsule, displacing vascular structures without invasion
      - Infiltrative into vascular structure
- Serum markers
  - AFP (alpha-fetoprotein)
    - Usual threshold for HCC evaluation is at AFP level > 20 ng/mL
    - Not used as primary surveillance test due to low sensitivity and specificity [31]
    - However, serum level AFP >400 ng/mL in high-risk patients is diagnostic for HCC
    - Used as adjunctive test for diagnosis and for monitoring patients after treatment (tumor marker)
  - Other labs to obtain in patient with liver mass suspicious for HCC
    - CBC + platelet count
    - Liver function tests including albumin
    - Renal function tests
    - Coagulation panel
    - CA 19–9, CEA
- Staging
  - Tumor, node, and metastasis (TNM) staging (Table 9.1)
    - T stage based on number and size of the primary tumor and presence of vascular invasion
    - N stage defined by presence of regional lymph node metastasis
      - Regional lymph nodes are hilar, hepatoduodenal ligament, inferior phrenic, and caval lymph nodes
    - M stage defined by presence of distant metastasis

Table 9.1 AJCC 8th edition T, N, and M for HCC [26]

Primary tumor (T)		Regional lymph nodes (N)		Distant metastases (M)	
T1a	Solitary tumor ≤2 cm with/without vascular invasion	Nx	Regional lymph nodes cannot be assessed	M0	No distant metastasis
T1b	Solitary tumor >2 cm without vascular invasion	N0	No regional lymph node metastasis	M1	Distant metastasis
T2	Solitary tumor >2 cm with vascular invasion or multifocal tumors, none >5 cm	N1	Regional lymph node metastasis		
T3	Multifocal tumors of at least one of which is >5 cm				
T4	Single tumor or multifocal tumors of any size involving a major branch of the portal vein or hepatic vein or tumor(s) with direct invasion of adjacent organs other than the gallbladder or with perforation of visceral peritoneum				

Table 9.2 AJCC 8th edition for staging for HCC [26]

Stage	Tumor	Node	Distant metastasis
Stage IA	T1a	N0	M0
Stage IB	T1b	N0	M0
Stage II	T2	N0	M0
Stage IIIA	T3	N0	M0
Stage IIIB	T4	N0	M0
Stage IVA	Any T	N1	M0
Stage IVB	Any T	Any N	M1

- Common extrahepatic metastases include lungs (most common), bones, brains, and adrenal glands
    - Anatomic stage/prognostic group dependent on TNM classification (Table 9.2)
- Barcelona Clinic Liver Cancer (BCLC) staging classification
    - Integrates assessment of extent of the primary tumor, liver function, vascular invasion, and distant metastases
    - Guides surgical vs nonsurgical management (Fig. 9.2)
    - Currently most used in the Western countries
    - If radiologic progression, change management
- Okuda system
    - Includes size and volume of the tumor and measures of liver function such as albumin, bilirubin, and presence of ascites
    - Identifies and distinguishes patients with poor prognosis who are not candidates for resection
- Cancer of Liver Italian Program (CLIP)

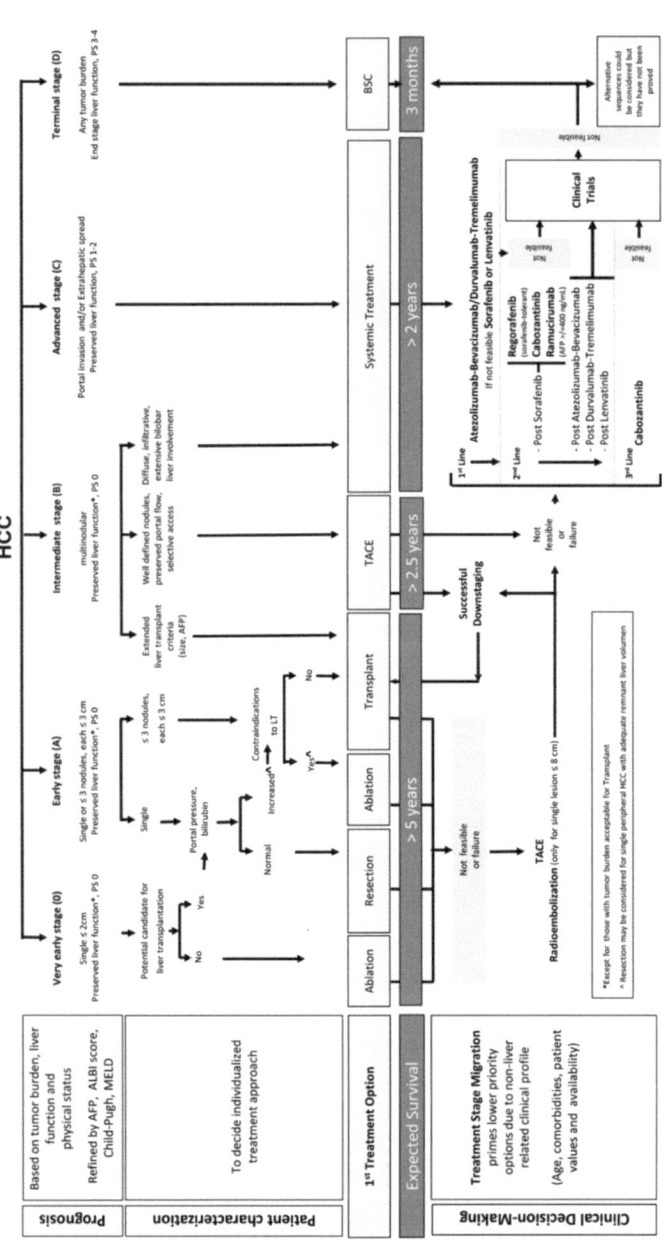

Fig. 9.2 The BCLC system establishes a prognosis in accordance with the five stages that are linked to first-line treatment recommendation. The expected outcome is expressed as median survival of each tumor stage according to the available scientific evidence. Individualized clinical decision-making, according to the available data on September 15, 2021, is defined by teams responsible for integrating all available data with the individual patient's medical profile. Note that liver function should be evaluated beyond the conventional Child-Pugh staging.++Full availability of the data from the trial testing the combination of tremelimumab and durvalumab may lead to these agents being incorporated as a first-line alternative. AFP alpha-fetoprotein; ALBI albumin-bilirubin; BCLC Barcelona Clinic Liver Cancer; BSC best supportive care; ECOG PS Eastern Cooperative Oncology Group-performance status; LT liver transplantation; MELD model of end-stage liver disease; TACE transarterial chemoembolization. (Source: Reig et al. [25])

- Considers tumor morphology, AFP level, presence of portal vein thrombosis, and the severity of cirrhosis per Child-Pugh score
  - Shown to be more reliable in predicting survival than other systems
- Others less frequently used include GRETCH score, Tokyo score, and CUPI

Choice of Therapy

- Surgical Resection
  - Selection criteria for safe and effective resection for potential cure is highly subjective; these are some general guidelines:
    - Solitary mass without major vascular invasion and adequate liver function
    - Future liver remnant—20% in healthy individuals; >30% if status post neoadjuvant therapy; >40% in patients with cirrhosis
    - 1 cm margins needed
    - About 10–20% of patients considered to have resectable disease at the time of presentation
  - Contraindications: For major hepatectomy, FLR <40% in cirrhosis, portal hypertension (platelet count <100), Child-Pugh class B or C
- Transplant
  - Potentially curative for patients with early-stage HCC and cirrhosis
  - Candidate patients with HCC granted extra MELD points
  - Criteria:
    - At least T2 and AFP <1000 ng/ml
    - BCLC stage 0/A or B
    - Milan criteria
      - Single tumor <5 cm or no more than three tumors with none >3 cm
      - Other expanded criteria exist such as UCSF
      - No significant difference between the two in overall survival rate (de Sousa)
  - Contraindications: severe cardiopulmonary disease, extrahepatic malignancy, active alcohol/substance use, active infection/sepsis, and lack of psychosocial support
- Locoregional therapies
  - Ablation
    - For one or few small lesions <3–4 cm
    - Radiofrequency, microwave, and cryotherapy
    - Contraindications: proximity to bowel/gallbladder, injury; blood vessels, heat sink effect, size >4 cm
  - Transarterial chemoembolization (TACE)
    - For larger, unresectable lesions ≥5 cm
    - Can be combined with ablation, including for patients with portal vein tumor thrombus

- Intraarterial chemotherapy (IACT)
  - For those not eligible for ablation or refractory to other regional therapies
  - Typically multiagent approach without embolization
- Intraarterial radiotherapy
  - Administers yttrium-90 microspheres into hepatic artery
  - Risk of microspheres shunting into lungs or GI tract
  - Pretreatment study to measure the lung shunt fraction (LSF)—need LSF <20% to minimize risk of radiation pneumonitis. Larger tumors (>5 cm) correlate with higher LSF.
  - Other contraindications: severe cardiopulmonary disease, total bilirubin >2 mg/dL, albumin <2.8 g/dL, AST or ALT >5x upper limit of normal, and presence of ascites
- External beam radiotherapy (EBRT)
  - Selection criteria: unresectable HCC ineligible for transplant or locoregional therapies as above
  - Contraindications: extrahepatic disease and advanced cirrhosis
  - Difficult to deliver effective dose without causing toxicity in the past, improving with development of 3D-CRT and SBRT
  - SBRT utilizes larger fractional doses in fewer fractions
- High-intensity-focused ultrasound ablation (HIFU)
  - Does not puncture tumor, less risk of bleeding or needle tract seeding
  - Limited by cost, availability, and need for general or epidural anesthesia
- Histotripsy
  - Noninvasive, nonthermal, and nonionizing focused ultrasound
  - Phase 1 study, THERESA trial [27]
  - First-in-man study
  - Correlated well with planned histotripsy volume with high safety profile
- Systemic Therapy
  - For patients with advanced unresectable disease inappropriate for surgical therapy nor liver directed therapy listed above
  - Must have adequate liver function and performance status to tolerate systemic therapy
  - Advanced Liver Cancer Prognostic System (ALCPS), the ALBI (albumin and bilirubin) score
  - Considering ongoing clinical trials
  - First line therapy
    - Preferred regimens
      - Atezolizumab plus bevacizumab
      - Tremelimumab plus durvalumab
    - Sorafenib
    - Lenvatinib
    - Durvalumab
    - Pembrolizumab
    - Nivolumab

- Subsequent-line systemic therapy with disease progression
  - Child-Pugh Class A only
    - Regorafenib
    - Cabozantinib
    - Lenvatinib
    - Sorafenib
    - Nivolumab plus ipilimumab
    - Pembrolizumab
  - Ramucirumab (Child-Pugh class A and AFP ≥400 ng/ml)
  - Nivolumab (Child-Pugh class B)
  - Dostarlimab-gxly (For MSI-H/dMMR tumors)
  - Selpercatinib (for RET gene fusion-positive tumors)
  - Nivolumab plus ipilimumab (for TMB-H tumors)
- Hospice
  - Patients with poor liver function (Child B and C) may be ineligible for local, regional, and systemic treatment options
  - Patients with poor performance status
- Adjuvant therapy
  - Recurrence common after surgical resection
  - Antiviral therapy against HBV and/or HCV
  - Systemic therapy—no standard adjuvant therapy after resection
    - STORM trial, evaluation of sorafenib as adjuvant therapy [28]
    - Potential role of capecitabine for intrahepatic cholangiocarcinoma or mixed tumors
- Clinical trials for HCC
  - Table 9.3 lists recent studies that have led to changes by the FDA.
  - Various recently reported
  - Phase 1
    - Histotripsy, see THERESA trial [27] above
  - Phase 2 trials
    - IMMUTACE
      - 49 patients received at least one dose of nivolumab
      - Transarterial chemoembolization (TACE) in combination with nivolumab for patients with intermediate-stage HCC
      - No new safety signals in enrolled patients
    - Hepatic artery infusion chemotherapy combined with sintilimab and bevacizumab biosimilar in unresectable hepatocellular carcinoma.
      - Single arm, phase II study
      - 30 patients enrolled
        - 20 patients had partial response and were eligible for surgical resection
        - 14 patients underwent resection
          - pCR rate 52%
      - Manageable safety profile for initially unresectable HCC.

Table 9.3 Past clinical trials on systemic treatments in HCC resulted in regulatory approval by the US FDA

Trial name/ID	Arms	Line of therapy	Primary end-point	ORR	PFS	OS
SHARP	Sorafenib vs placebo	First	OS	2 vs 1%	5.5 vs 2.8 months	10.7 vs 7.9 months (HR 0.69)
REFLECT	Lenvatinib vs sorafenib	First	OS	24.1 vs 9.2%	7.4 vs 3.7 months	13.6 vs 12.3 months (HR 0.92)
IMbrave150	Atezolizumab+bevacizumab vs sorafenib	First	OS and PFS	29.8 vs 11.3%	6.8 vs 4.3 months	19.2 vs 13.4 months (HR 0.66)
RESORCE	Regorafenib vs placebo	Second	OS	11 vs 4%	3.1 vs 1.5 months	10.6 vs 7.8 months (HR 0.63)
CELESTIAL	Cabozantinib vs placebo	Second and third	OS	4 vs 1%	5.2 vs 1.9 months	10.2 vs 8.0 months (HR 0.76)
REACH-2	Ramucirumab vs placebo (AFP >400 ng/mL)	Second	OS	5 vs 1%	2.8 vs 1.6 months	8.5 vs 7.3 months (HR 0.71)
CHECKMATE 040	Nivolumab single arm	Second	ORR	15%	N/A	N/A
KEYNOTE 224	Pembrolizumab single arm	Second	ORR	17%	N/A	N/A
CHECKMATE 040	Nivolumab + ipilimumab single arm	Second	ORR	32%	N/A	N/A

Source: Foerster et al. [23]

- Phase 3 trials
  - STORM trial
    - Sorafenib versus placebo for adjuvant therapy for advanced HCC
    - Did not achieve primary endpoint (RFS)
    - BIOSTORM
      - Added targeted exome sequencing, immunohistochemistry, FISH, and immunome.
      - Some improvement with highly selected, by gene signature, sorafenib RFS responders

Bibliography

1. Marrero JA, Kulik LM, Sirlin CB, Zhu AX, Finn RS, Abecassis MM, Roberts LR, Heimbach JK. Diagnosis, staging, and management of hepatocellular carcinoma: 2018 practice guidance by the American Association for the Study of Liver Diseases. Hepatology. 2018;68(2):723–50. https://doi.org/10.1002/hep.29913. PMID: 29624699.
2. Siegel RL, Miller KD, Wagle NS, Jemal A. Cancer statistics, 2023. CA Cancer J Clin. 2023;73(1):17–48. https://doi.org/10.3322/caac.21763. PMID: 36633525.
3. Anstee QM, Reeves HL, Kotsiliti E, et al. From NASH to HCC: current concepts and future challenges. Nat Rev Gastroenterol Hepatol. 2019;16:411–28. https://doi.org/10.1038/s41575-019-0145-7.
4. Stickel F, Schuppan D, Hahn EG, Seitz HK. Cocarcinogenic effects of alcohol in hepatocarcinogenesis. Gut. 2002;51(1):132–9. https://doi.org/10.1136/gut.51.1.132. PMID: 12077107; PMCID: PMC1773267.
5. Schlageter M, Terracciano LM, D'Angelo S, Sorrentino P. Histopathology of hepatocellular carcinoma. World J Gastroenterol. 2014;20(43):15955–64. https://doi.org/10.3748/wjg.v20.i43.15955.
6. Zhao YJ, Ju Q, Li GC. Tumor markers for hepatocellular carcinoma. Mol Clin Oncol. 2013;1(4):593–598. https://doi.org/10.3892/mco.2013.119. Epub 2013 May 13. PMID: 24649215; PMCID: PMC3915636.
7. Russo FP, Imondi A, Lynch EN, Farinati F. When and how should we perform a biopsy for HCC in patients with liver cirrhosis in 2018? A review. Dig Liver Dis. 2018;50(7):640–6. https://doi.org/10.1016/j.dld.2018.03.014. Epub 2018 Mar 20. PMID: 29636240.
8. Di Tommaso L, Spadaccini M, Donadon M, et al. Role of liver biopsy in hepatocellular carcinoma. World J Gastroenterol. 2019;25(40):6041–52. https://doi.org/10.3748/wjg.v25.i40.6041.
9. Wu W, He X, Andayani D, et al. Pattern of distant extrahepatic metastases in primary liver cancer: a SEER based study. J Cancer. 2017;8(12):2312–2318. Published 2017 Jul 21. https://doi.org/10.7150/jca.19056.
10. Maida M, Orlando E, Cammà C, Cabibbo G. Staging systems of hepatocellular carcinoma: a review of literature. World J Gastroenterol. 2014;20(15):4141–50. https://doi.org/10.3748/wjg.v20.i15.4141. PMID: 24764652; PMCID: PMC3989950.
11. Bento de Sousa JH, Calil IL, Tustumi F, et al. Comparison between Milan and UCSF criteria for liver transplantation in patients with hepatocellular carcinoma: a systematic review and meta-analysis. Transl Gastroenterol Hepatol. 2021;6:11. Published 2021 Jan 5. https://doi.org/10.21037/tgh.2020.01.06.
12. Varma V, Mehta N, Kumaran V, Nundy S. Indications and contraindications for liver transplantation. Int J Hepatol. 2011;2011:121862. https://doi.org/10.4061/2011/121862.

13. Refaat R, Hassan M. The relationship between the percentage of lung shunting on Tc-99m macroaggregated albumin (Tc-99m MAA) scan and the grade of hepatocellular carcinoma vascularity. Egyptian J Radiol Nucl Med. 2014;45 https://doi.org/10.1016/j.ejrnm.2014.01.001.
14. Zavaglia C, Mancuso A, Foschi A, Rampoldi A. High-intensity focused ultrasound (HIFU) for the treatment of hepatocellular carcinoma: is it time to abandon standard ablative percutaneous treatments? Hepatobiliary Surg Nutr. 2013;2(4):184–7. https://doi.org/10.3978/j.issn.2304-3881.2013.05.02.
15. Matsuo Y. Stereotactic body radiotherapy for hepatocellular carcinoma: A brief overview. Curr Oncol. 2023;30(2):2493–500. Published 2023 Feb 18. https://doi.org/10.3390/curroncol30020190.
16. Silva MA, Hegab B, Hyde C, Guo B, Buckels JA, Mirza DF. Needle track seeding following biopsy of liver lesions in the diagnosis of hepatocellular cancer: a systematic review and meta-analysis. Gut. 2008;57(11):1592–6. https://doi.org/10.1136/gut.2008.149062. Epub 2008 Jul 31. PMID: 18669577.
17. Ma MC, Chen YY, Li SH, et al. Intra-arterial chemotherapy with doxorubicin and cisplatin is effective for advanced hepatocellular cell carcinoma. ScientificWorldJournal. 2014;2014:160138. https://doi.org/10.1155/2014/160138.
18. Okusaka T, Kasugai H, Shioyama Y, Tanaka K, Kudo M, Saisho H, Osaki Y, Sata M, Fujiyama S, Kumada T, Sato K, Yamamoto S, Hinotsu S, Sato T. Transarterial chemotherapy alone versus transarterial chemoembolization for hepatocellular carcinoma: a randomized phase III trial. J Hepatol. 2009;51(6):1030–6. https://doi.org/10.1016/j.jhep.2009.09.004. Epub 2009 Oct 1. PMID: 19864035.
19. Lewandowski RJ, Salem R. Yttrium-90 radioembolization of hepatocellular carcinoma and metastatic disease to the liver. Semin Intervent Radiol. 2006;23(1):64–72. https://doi.org/10.1055/s-2006-939842.
20. Murthy R, Kamat P, Nuñez R, Salem R. Radioembolization of yttrium-90 microspheres for hepatic malignancy. Semin Intervent Radiol. 2008;25(1):48–57. https://doi.org/10.1055/s-2008-1052306.
21. Akateh C, Black SM, Conteh L, et al. Neoadjuvant and adjuvant treatment strategies for hepatocellular carcinoma. World J Gastroenterol. 2019;25(28):3704–21. https://doi.org/10.3748/wjg.v25.i28.3704.
22. Li SH, Mei J, Cheng Y, Li Q, Wang QX, Fang CK, Lei QC, Huang HK, Cao MR, Luo R, Deng JD, Jiang YC, Zhao RC, Lu LH, Zou JW, Deng M, Lin WP, Guan RG, Wen YH, Li JB, Zheng L, Guo ZX, Ling YH, Chen HW, Zhong C, Wei W, Guo RP. Postoperative adjuvant hepatic arterial infusion chemotherapy with FOLFOX in hepatocellular carcinoma with microvascular invasion: a multicenter, phase III, randomized study. J Clin Oncol. 2023;41(10):1898–908. https://doi.org/10.1200/JCO.22.01142. Epub 2022 Dec 16. PMID: 36525610; PMCID: PMC10082249.
23. Foerster F, Galle PR. The current landscape of clinical trials for systemic treatment of HCC. Cancers (Basel). 2021;13(8):1962. https://doi.org/10.3390/cancers13081962. PMID: 33921731; PMCID: PMC8073471.
24. Shi C, Li Y, Geng L, Shen W, Sui C, Dai B, Lu J, Pan M, Yang J. Adjuvant stereotactic body radiotherapy after marginal resection for hepatocellular carcinoma with microvascular invasion: A randomised controlled trial. Eur J Cancer. 2022;166:176–84. https://doi.org/10.1016/j.ejca.2022.02.012. Epub 2022 Mar 15. PMID: 35303509.
25. Reig M, Forner A, Rimola J, Ferrer-Fàbrega J, Burrel M, Garcia-Criado Á, Kelley RK, Galle PR, Mazzaferro V, Salem R, Sangro B, Singal AG, Vogel A, Fuster J, Ayuso C, Bruix J. BCLC strategy for prognosis prediction and treatment recommendation: The 2022 update. J Hepatol. 2022;76(3):681–93. https://doi.org/10.1016/j.jhep.2021.11.018. Epub 2021 Nov 19. PMID: 34801630; PMCID: PMC8866082.

26. Kamarajah SK, Frankel TL, Sonnenday C, Cho CS, Nathan H. Critical evaluation of the American Joint Commission on Cancer (AJCC) 8th edition staging system for patients with Hepatocellular Carcinoma (HCC): A Surveillance, Epidemiology, End Results (SEER) analysis. J Surg Oncol. 2018;117(4):644–50. https://doi.org/10.1002/jso.24908. Epub 2017 Nov 11. PMID: 29127719.
27. Vidal-Jove J, Serres X, Vlaisavljevich E, Cannata J, Duryea A, Miller R, Merino X, Velat M, Kam Y, Bolduan R, Amaral J, Hall T, Xu Z, Lee FT Jr, Ziemlewicz TJ. First-in-man histotripsy of hepatic tumors: the THERESA trial, a feasibility study. Int J Hyperth. 2022;39(1):1115–23. https://doi.org/10.1080/02656736.2022.2112309. PMID: 36002243.
28. Pinyol R, Montal R, Bassaganyas L, Sia D, Takayama T, Chau GY, Mazzaferro V, Roayaie S, Lee HC, Kokudo N, Zhang Z, Torrecilla S, Moeini A, Rodriguez-Carunchio L, Gane E, Verslype C, Croitoru AE, Cillo U, de la Mata M, Lupo L, Strasser S, Park JW, Camps J, Solé M, Thung SN, Villanueva A, Pena C, Meinhardt G, Bruix J, Llovet JM. Molecular predictors of prevention of recurrence in HCC with sorafenib as adjuvant treatment and prognostic factors in the phase 3 STORM trial. Gut. 2019;68(6):1065–75. https://doi.org/10.1136/gutjnl-2018-316408. Epub 2018 Aug 14. PMID: 30108162; PMCID: PMC6580745.
29. Elmohr M, Elsayes KM, Chernyak V. LI-RADS: review and updates. Clin Liver Dis (Hoboken). 2021;17(3):108–12. https://doi.org/10.1002/cld.991. PMID: 33868648; PMCID: PMC8043699.
30. American College of Radiology. Liver Imaging Reporting and Data System (LI- RADS) v2018 ACR.org: ACR. Available at: https://www.acr.org/-/media/CR/Files/RADS/LI-RADS/LI-RADS-2018-Core.pdf?la=en. Published 2018.
31. Hanif H, Ali MJ, Susheela AT, Khan IW, Luna-Cuadros MA, Khan MM, Lau DT. Update on the applications and limitations of alpha-fetoprotein for hepatocellular carcinoma. World J Gastroenterol. 2022;28(2):216–29.

Large Intestine Cancers

10

Abhineet Uppal

Introduction

- Colorectal cancer (CRC): 150 k cases per year in the USA, third most common for both sexes
  - 20% diagnosed before age 55, median age is 66, and 70% nonmetastatic at diagnosis
  - Colonoscopy for diagnosis, CT for staging
  - Surgical resection with postoperative chemotherapy depending on stage is standard of care for nonmetastatic
  - Metastases to the liver, lung, or peritoneum may be resectable
- Anal squamous cell carcinoma (ASCC): 10 k cases per year
  - Risk triples after age 50, 77% nonmetastatic at diagnosis, median age is 63
  - Anoscopy for diagnosis, PET/CT for staging
  - Chemoradiation is standard for nonmetastatic, chemotherapy for metastatic
  - Surgical resection only for T1, low-risk tumors or salvage APR

Diagnosis

- *Symptomatic cases*
  - Blood per rectum is most common early symptom, followed by constipation
  - Anemia is a common laboratory finding
  - Locally advanced tumors may cause large bowel obstruction requiring urgent colostomy creation

---

A. Uppal (✉)
Emory University, Atlanta, GA, USA

- Late-stage symptoms include abdominal distension (from ascites or carcinomatosis), jaundice (from liver metastases obstructing the biliary system), weight loss, anorexia, and rarely dyspnea (from lung metastases)
- *Screening for colorectal cancer*
  - Colonoscopy starting at age 45 and repeated every 5–10 years is recommended for average risk (no family history of polyps or cancer, no predisposing syndrome)
  - Annual FIT with colonoscopy if positive is an acceptable alternative
- *Screening for anal squamous cell carcinoma*
  - High-resolution anoscopy recommended for HIV-positive patients
    - Reduces risk of death from anal cancer
  - Anal pap smear is not routinely recommended.
    - Does not reduce risk of anal cancer or death from it
- *Risk Factors* [1]
  - Familial adenomatous polyposis (FAP): Nearly 100% risk by age 40
    - 1% of all CRC, due to autosomal dominant APC mutation
    - Prophylactic total proctocolectomy is standard treatment by ages 18–20
    - Increased risk of gastric and duodenal cancer
  - Hereditary nonpolyposis colorectal cancer (HNPCC): 70–80% lifetime risk
    - 5% of all CRC, due to MLH1, MSH2, MSH6, PMS2, or POLE mutation
    - Diagnosed with tumor and blood testing for microsatellite instability/deficiency in mismatch repair
    - Median age at diagnosis is 45 years old
    - Total or segmental colectomy is a standard treatment for resectable cases
    - Immunotherapy is a standard treatment for unresectable cases
    - Increased risk of endometrial, ovarian, ureteral, gastric, biliary, pancreatic, small bowel, and CNS cancers
  - Inflammatory bowel disease (4–20× risk)
  - Age (8x increase for 55–65 years old compared to <55 years old)
  - Family history (especially <60 years old)
  - Obesity (men: HR 1.2–1.8 for BMI >30, women: HR 2.0 for waist >40in) [3, 4].
  - Smoking history (HR 1.2–1.3 depending on current status and years duration) [2]
  - Other genetic syndromes include MYH-associated polyposis (MAP), PTEN-associated (Cowden), Peutz-Jeghers and Juvenile Polyposis

Evaluation and Staging (Table 10.1)

Colon colonoscopy with biopsies, CT chest, abdomen, and pelvis, CEA, MSI testing

- MSI (microsatellite-instability) testing is PCR-based
- Deficient mismatch (dMMR) testing is IHC-based
- MRI with contrast is useful if CT is indeterminate for liver lesions
- M stage for all depend on organs involved ((a) one site, (b) more than one site, (c) peritoneum with or without other sites)

Table 10.1 Staging of colon and rectal adenocarcinomas. Used with permission of the American College of Surgeons, Chicago, Illinois. The original source for this information is the AJCC Cancer Staging System (2023)

T staging		AJCC staging
T0	No evidence of tumor	Stage I: T1/T2 and N0
Tis	Intraepithelial tumor without invasion of the lamina propria	Stage I: T3/T4 and N0
T1	Tumor invades the lamina propria, muscularis mucosa, or submucosa	Stage III: T1–T4 and N1–N3
T2	Tumor invades the muscularis propria	Stage IV: T1–T4, N1–N3, and M1a–M1c
T3	Tumor penetrates the subserosal connective tissue without invasion of the visceral peritoneum (serosa) or surrounding structures	
T4	Tumor invades the serosa or surrounding structures	
N staging		
N0	No regional lymph node involvement	
N1	Metastases in 1–2 regional lymph nodes or tumor deposits present with 0 nodal metastases (N1c)	
N2	Metastases in 3–6 regional lymph nodes	
N3	Metastases in 7+ regional lymph nodes	
M staging		
M0	No distant metastases	
M1a	Distant metastases in one organ	
M1b	Distant metastases in two or more organs not including peritoneum	
M1c	Distant metastases to peritoneum with or without other organs	

Rectum Above and MRI pelvis for T stage, N stage, EMVI, and pelvic sidewall evaluation

- Endoscopic ultrasound is acceptable if MRI is unavailable.

Anal Anoscopy with biopsies, HPV status, p16 IHC, MRI pelvis, and PET-CT

- HPV+/p16+ has better response to therapy.

Clinical staging: Colorectal
- T1–T4 based on depth of invasion (often cannot determine for colon)
- N0–N2 based on number of nodes (often cannot determine for colon)

Clinical staging: Anal (Table 10.2)
- T1–T3 depending on size of tumor
- N0 or N1 based on any nodal metastases

Due to high median age at diagnosis and efficacy of treatment, overall survival for nonmetastatic patients depends on age (Table 10.2)

- OS in <65 year olds is much higher than >65 year olds

Table 10.2 Staging of anal squamous cell carcinomas. Used with permission of the American College of Surgeons, Chicago, Illinois. The original source for this information is the AJCC Cancer Staging System (2023)

T staging		AJCC staging
T0	No evidence of tumor	Stage I: T1 N0
T1	Intraepithelial tumor without invasion of the lamina propria	Stage II: T1 N1 or T2, N0–N1
T1	Tumor <2 cm	Stage III: T3–T4, N0–N1
T2	Tumor 2-5 cm	Stage IV: T1–T4, N0–N1, M1
T3	Tumor >5 cm	
N staging		
N0	No regional lymph nodes involvement	
N1	Metastases to lymph nodes	
M staging		
M0	No distant metastases	
M1	Distant metastases in one organ	

Choice of Therapy

Colon Stages I–III undergo resection followed by chemotherapy if indicated

- Stage I (T1 or T2, N0): no therapy
- Stage II low risk (T3 or T4, N0, LVI-, PNI-, well or moderately differentiated): no therapy
- Stage II high risk (T3 or T4, N0 with any of above three factors or less than 12 lymph nodes evaluated): 3 months FOLFOX (5-FU, Leucovorin, Oxaliplatin) or XELOX (Xeloda: capecitabine, Oxaliplatin)
- Stage III: 3–6 months FOLFOX or XELOX

Rectal Depends on T and N status, distance from anal verge, and other risk factors

- Stage I (T1 or T2, N0): resection
- Stage II (T3 or T4, N0): 5-FU-based chemoradiation to 54Gy if <10 cm from anal verge or threatened margin and then resection
- Stage III (T1–4, N+): 5-FU-based chemoradiation to 54Gy followed by four months FOLFOX, followed by resection
- Risk factors for distant metastases: T4, N+, extramural vascular invasion (EMVI), tumor deposits, poorly differentiated grade, and signet ring cell histology
- Pelvic sidewall nodes (obturator, internal iliac) are generally resected if >5 mm after neoadjuvant therapy

Anal Depends on T and N stage

- Stage I (T1, N0): wide local excision if anatomically feasible, low-grade, no PNI or LVI
- All other nonmetastatic cases: Chemoradiation with 54Gy external beam, 5-FU, and either mitomycin or cisplatin

Stage IV (all types) Resectability depends on many biologic and technical factors

- Isolated CRC metastases to the liver, lung, or peritoneum should be evaluated for resection and systemic therapy in a multidisciplinary setting.
- Metastatic anal SCC is rarely resectable.

Microsatellite-instability high (MSI-H) Consider checkpoint blockade if unresectable

- Metastatic: Median OS of four years [5]

Surgical Therapy

Colon Partial colectomy for patients without genetic syndrome or inflammatory bowel disease

- Total colectomy or proctocolectomy generally recommended for these exceptions
- Goal is to remove entire draining lymph node basin and at least 12 lymph nodes
- Leak rate for right-sided (ileocolic) anastomosis: 1–2%
- Leak rate for colorectal anastomosis: 5–10%

Rectal low anterior resection (LAR) or abdominoperineal resection (APR)

- Goal is to remove draining lymph nodes and mesorectum without defects in mesorectal fascia (total mesorectal excision)
- At least 5 cm of mesorectum distal to tumor is needed
- For low rectal tumors, 1 cm with TME is adequate margin.
- Diverting ileostomy recommended for LAR after neoadjuvant radiotherapy, tumors <5 cm from anal verge or other risk factors for poor anastomotic healing
  - Leak rate varies from 3% to 15% depending on risk factors
- Multivisceral, extra-TME, and pelvic lymph node resections should be performed at specialized centers

Anal Wide local excision in low-risk T1, otherwise salvage APR after chemoradiation if residual tumor after 12 weeks

Vascular anatomy
- Right colectomy: ileocolic vessels and right colic at origins from SMV and SMA, right branch of middle colic
- Extended right: ileocolic, right colic, and middle colic at origins from SMV and SMA
- Left/splenic: left branch of middle colic, left ascending, and IMV at origin

- Sigmoid: IMA and IMV at origins
- Rectal and anal: IMA, IMV at origins, and middle rectals during total mesorectal excision
- Transverse colectomy is rarely performed and suboptimal for lymph node retrieval.

Extent of lymphadenectomy
- Right colon: D2 includes nodes along named vessels, D3 includes nodes along SMV, and complete mesocolic excision includes all tissue overlying right side of SMV
- Left colon, rectum, and anus: all nodes from IMA origin should be included.
- Common sites of locoregional recurrence in rectal cancer are missed pelvic lymph nodes (obturator or iliac), especially for <10 cm from anal verge.

Nonoperative management for rectal cancer should be performed at specialized centers

- Considered when tumor and nodes have complete clinical response:
  - Palpation: no palpable tumor
  - Endoscopy: no residual nodularity or mucosal abnormality other than white scar or telangiectasia
  - MRI: scar without evidence of tumor on diffuse-weighted sequences, no abnormal lymphadenopathy
- Surveillance every 3–4 months for at least five years
  - 15–30% regrowth rate requiring resection
  - 5% distant metastasis risk

Systemic Therapy for Nonmetastatic Cancer

Decision for systemic therapy driven by recurrence and mortality risk (Table 10.3)
- Stage II high risk (T4, LVI, PNI, poor differentiation, high tumor budding or <12 nodes resected):
- Stage III (any positive nodes)

5-Fluorouracil / Leucovorin [6, 7] backbone of chemotherapy (Table 10.4)

- 40% relative risk reduction in death compared to observation (39% vs 55% five-year OS)
  - Neutropenia, nausea, and fatigue are common.
- Capecitabine is the orally available prodrug:
  - Neutropenia and hand/foot syndrome (peeling of skin)
  - Risk of severe enterocolitis with poor metabolism (<5% of patients)

Table 10.3 Survival by pathologic stage and age

Stage	Colon five-year OS (%)	Rectum five-year OS (%)	Anus five-year OS
Age < 65			
Stage I/stage II	93.4–96.9	93.3–95.3	84.4–89.9
Stage III	77.9–83.3	77.0–80.6	63.6–74.9
Stage IV	17.0–24.5	18.2–24.1	17.2–35.6
Age 65+			
Stage I/II	88.3–89.7	82.2–84.5	78.1–83.1
Stage III	67.9–69.4	64.8–67.3	59.2–65.4
Stage IV	9.7–10.7	12.3–14.3	26.8–35.0

Source: National Institutes of Health Surveillance, Epidemiology and End Results (SEER) Explorer https://seer.cancer.gov/statistics-network/explorer/ updated: 2024 Jun 27

Table 10.4 Adjuvant therapy trials

Trial	Cohorts	Results
NSABP C06 [25]	Stage III CRC	Five-year OS
	5FU/LV	55%
	Observation	39%
MOSAIC [26]	Stage III CRC	Five-year DFS
	5FU/LV	64%
	FOLFOX	69%

Oxaliplatin [8, 14]

- 18% relative risk reduction for recurrence: 69% five-year DFS versus 64% for 5-FU alone
  - OS was not affected (likely due to age at diagnosis)
- A six-month therapy is a preferred duration.
  - Three months acceptable for T1/T2 and N1 tumors [9]
- Paresthesia of feet and hands can be permanent, especially after three months.

Management of Metastatic Cancer

Mutation testing should be performed in all cases:
- Minimum of MSI/MMR, KRAS, NRAS, and BRAF
- BRAF V600E mutations respond to encorafenib, bimetinimb, and cetuximab [10]
- KRAS mutations do not respond to anti-EGFR therapy (cetuximab, panitumumab)

Systemic Therapy for Metastatic Disease

- FOLFOX (5-FU, Leucovorin, Oxaliplatin) and FOLFIRI (5-FU, Leucovorin, Irinotecan) have similar efficacy [11]
  - FOLFOX: Constipation and neurotoxicity
  - FOLFIRI: Diarrhea and neutropenia

- FOLFIRINOX can be considered for patients <70 with excellent performance status
- 2–3 months PFS benefit but more GI toxicity
- Targeted therapies (anti-VEGF, bevacizumab, or anti-EGFR, cetuximab and panitumumab) have modest 1–2-month PFS benefit but are well tolerated.
  - Bevacizumab should be held six weeks prior to planned surgery due to risk of anastomotic leak.

Left-sided CRC generally better response and prognosis

- KRAS or NRAS-mutated tumors: FOLFOX or FOLFIRI + bevacizumab
- KRAS and NRAS wild-type tumors: FOLFOX or FOLFIRI + panitumumab or cetuximab

Right-sided CRC higher rates of BRAF mutation and worse prognosis

- BRAF-mutated tumors: FOLFOX+Bevacizumab or encorafenib, bimetinimb, and cetuximab
- Right-sided tumors do not respond to anti-EGFR therapy.

MSI-H/pMMR tumors checkpoint blockade (anti-PD1 or anti-CTLA4) provide disease control

- Median PFS 16 versus 8 months, median OS of 61% versus 50% with 83% having over 2 years of response to immunotherapy [12]

Surgical Resection of Liver and Lung Metastases

- Risk stratification based on patient condition, risk of operation, future organ remnant, and biology
- Liver: CEA >200 at diagnosis, 2+ tumors, largest >5 cm, N+ primary, and DFI < 12 months are all risk factors for recurrence [15]
  - A five-year OS 60% if 0 risk factors, 40% with 1–2, 20% with 3–4, 14% with all 5
  - Liver remnant <30% is at risk of liver failure, consider portal vein embolization of most affected lobe to hypertrophy remaining tissue
- Lung: Similar criteria are associated with survival, with similar five-year OS [16]
  - Preoperative PFTs are important to risk stratify resection
  - Stereotactic radiotherapy (SBRT) can be considered instead

Surgical Resection of Peritoneal Metastases

- Peritoneal Cancer Index (PCI) risk-stratified risk of recurrence [17]
  - Abdomen divided into 13 sections (9-square grid +4 sections of small bowel)

- Tumor <5 mm scores 1, 5 mm–5 cm scores 2, >5 cm or confluent scores 3
- PCI score of 0–10 is lower risk (five-year OS of 50%)
- PCI score of 11 or higher has lower OS (20–25%)
- Completeness of cytoreduction is the most important prognostic factor [18]
• Median disease-free survival is <18 months regardless of PCI [19]
  - 20–25% of low-PCI group will be disease-free at five years
• Role of Heated Intraperitoneal Chemotherapy (HIPEC) is unclear
  - Randomized trial of oxaliplatin HIPEC showed no difference in OS or DFS
  - Retrospective comparisons of oxaliplatin and mitomycin-C HIPEC show no clear difference [20, 21]

Radiotherapy

Rectal cancer neoadjuvant radiation is the standard of care for T3-T4 or N+ tumors (Table 10.5)

• Short course: 25Gy over five doses
  - RAPIDO study: short-course followed by FOLFOX reduced the risk of distant metastases, but potential risk of local recurrence compared to long course
• Long course: 54Gy over 28 doses with capecitabine
  - OPRA study: long course followed by FOLFOX reduced the risk of distant metastases and increased organ preservation

Anal cancer definitive chemoradiation with either 5-FU and MMC or 5-FU and Cisplatin

• Reevaluate at three-month posttherapy for response
  - Complete response: q6–12 month anoscopy, q6-month imaging and exam
• Persistent disease: reevaluate for APR after 1–3 months
  - Progression: salvage APR
  - Stable: APR or continue monitoring q3 months for progression

Table 10.5 Neoadjuvant Rectal Cancer Trials

Trial	Cohorts	Results
OPRA[27]	Stages II–III, lower risk	Three-year DFS
	CXRT then FOLFOX	76%
	FOLFOX then CXRT	76%
RAPIDO [28]	Stage II–III, high risk	Three-year metastasis-free survival
	CXRT +/− adj FOLFOX	73%
	RT and neoadj FOLFOX	80%
PRODIGE 23 [29]	Stage II–III, high risk	Seven-year OS
	CXRT, adjuvant FOLFIRINOX	76%
	FOLFIRINOX then CXRT and adjuvant FOLFOX or capecitabine	82%

Unusual Scenarios

Large Intestinal Neuroendocrine Tumors:
- Low grade and < 1 cm: polypectomy or transanal excision is sufficient
  - No specific surveillance required beyond colonoscopy in one year
- High grade or > 1 cm: higher risk of lymphadenopathy or metastatic disease, surgical treatment similar to adenocarcinoma
  - Surveillance similar to adenocarcinoma

Adenocarcinoma Within a Polyp:
- Polypectomy is sufficient if >2 mm margin, no LVI, and no poor differentiation
- Colonoscopy in 3–6 months and then at one-year postpolypectomy

Bibliography

1. Haggar FA, Boushey RP. Colorectal cancer epidemiology: incidence, mortality, survival, and risk factors. Clin Colon Rectal Surg. 2009;22(4):191–7. https://doi.org/10.1055/s-0029-1242458. PMID: 21037809; PMCID: PMC2796096.
2. Gram IT, Park SY, Wilkens LR, Haiman CA, Le Marchand L. Smoking-related risks of colorectal cancer by anatomical subsite and sex. Am J Epidemiol. 2020;189(6):543–53. https://doi.org/10.1093/aje/kwaa005. PMID: 31971226; PMCID: PMC7368133.
3. Campbell PT, Cotterchio M, Dicks E, Parfrey P, Gallinger S, McLaughlin JR. Excess body weight and colorectal cancer risk in Canada: associations in subgroups of clinically defined familial risk of cancer. Cancer Epidemiol Biomarkers Prev. 2007;16(9):1735–44. https://doi.org/10.1158/1055-9965.EPI-06-1059. PMID: 17855691.
4. Moore LL, Bradlee ML, Singer MR, Splansky GL, Proctor MH, Ellison RC, Kreger BE. BMI and waist circumference as predictors of lifetime colon cancer risk in Framingham Study adults. Int J Obes Relat Metab Disord. 2004;28(4):559–67. https://doi.org/10.1038/sj.ijo.0802606. PMID: 14770200.
5. Le DT, Diaz LA Jr, Kim TW, Van Cutsem E, Geva R, Jäger D, Hara H, Burge M, O'Neil BH, Kavan P, Yoshino T, Guimbaud R, Taniguchi H, Élez E, Al-Batran SE, Boland PM, Cui Y, Leconte P, Marinello P, André T. Pembrolizumab for previously treated, microsatellite instability-high/mismatch repair-deficient advanced colorectal cancer: final analysis of KEYNOTE-164. Eur J Cancer. 2023;186:185–95. https://doi.org/10.1016/j.ejca.2023.02.016. Epub 2023 Feb 24. PMID: 37141828.
6. Moertel CG, Fleming TR, Macdonald JS, Haller DG, Laurie JA, Goodman PJ, Ungerleider JS, Emerson WA, Tormey DC, Glick JH, et al. Levamisole and fluorouracil for adjuvant therapy of resected colon carcinoma. N Engl J Med. 1990;322(6):352–8. https://doi.org/10.1056/NEJM199002083220602. PMID: 2300087.
7. Moertel CG, Fleming TR, Macdonald JS, Haller DG, Laurie JA, Tangen CM, Ungerleider JS, Emerson WA, Tormey DC, Glick JH, et al. Intergroup study of fluorouracil plus levamisole as adjuvant therapy for stage II/Dukes' B2 colon cancer. J Clin Oncol. 1995;13(12):2936–43. https://doi.org/10.1200/JCO.1995.13.12.2936. PMID: 8523058.
8. Yothers G, O'Connell MJ, Allegra CJ, Kuebler JP, Colangelo LH, Petrelli NJ, Wolmark N. Oxaliplatin as adjuvant therapy for colon cancer: updated results of NSABP C-07 trial, including survival and subset analyses. J Clin Oncol. 2011;29(28):3768–74. https://doi.org/10.1200/JCO.2011.36.4539. Epub 2011 Aug 22. PMID: 21859995; PMCID: PMC3188282.
9. Grothey A, Sobrero AF, Shields AF, Yoshino T, Paul J, Taieb J, Souglakos J, Shi Q, Kerr R, Labianca R, Meyerhardt JA, Vernerey D, Yamanaka T, Boukovinas I, Meyers JP, Renfro LA,

Niedzwiecki D, Watanabe T, Torri V, Saunders M, Sargent DJ, Andre T, Iveson T. Duration of adjuvant chemotherapy for stage III colon cancer. N Engl J Med. 2018;378(13):1177–88. https://doi.org/10.1056/NEJMoa1713709. PMID: 29590544; PMCID: PMC6426127.
10. Kopetz S, Grothey A, Yaeger R, Van Cutsem E, Desai J, Yoshino T, Wasan H, Ciardiello F, Loupakis F, Hong YS, Steeghs N, Guren TK, Arkenau HT, Garcia-Alfonso P, Pfeiffer P, Orlov S, Lonardi S, Elez E, Kim TW, Schellens JHM, Guo C, Krishnan A, Dekervel J, Morris V, Calvo Ferrandiz A, Tarpgaard LS, Braun M, Gollerkeri A, Keir C, Maharry K, Pickard M, Christy-Bittel J, Anderson L, Sandor V, Tabernero J. Encorafenib, Binimetinib, and Cetuximab in *BRAF* V600E-mutated colorectal cancer. N Engl J Med. 2019;381(17):1632–43. https://doi.org/10.1056/NEJMoa1908075. Epub 2019 Sep 30. PMID: 31566309.
11. Tournigand C, André T, Achille E, Lledo G, Flesh M, Mery-Mignard D, Quinaux E, Couteau C, Buyse M, Ganem G, Landi B, Colin P, Louvet C, de Gramont A. FOLFIRI followed by FOLFOX6 or the reverse sequence in advanced colorectal cancer: a randomized GERCOR study. J Clin Oncol. 2004;22(2):229–37. https://doi.org/10.1200/JCO.2004.05.113. Epub 2003 Dec 2. Corrected and republished in: J Clin Oncol 2023 Jul 1;41(19):3469–3477. PMID: 14657227.
12. Diaz LA Jr, Shiu KK, Kim TW, Jensen BV, Jensen LH, Punt C, Smith D, Garcia-Carbonero R, Benavides M, Gibbs P, de la Fourchardiere C, Rivera F, Elez E, Le DT, Yoshino T, Zhong WY, Fogelman D, Marinello P, Andre T, KEYNOTE-177 Investigators. Pembrolizumab versus chemotherapy for microsatellite instability-high or mismatch repair-deficient metastatic colorectal cancer (KEYNOTE-177): final analysis of a randomised, open-label, phase 3 study. Lancet Oncol. 2022;23(5):659–70. https://doi.org/10.1016/S1470-2045(22)00197-8. Epub 2022 Apr 12. PMID: 35427471; PMCID: PMC9533375.
13. Mai S, Welzel G, Ottstadt M, Lohr F, Severa S, Prigge ES, Wentzensen N, Trunk MJ, Wenz F, von Knebel-Doeberitz M, Reuschenbach M. Prognostic relevance of HPV infection and p16 overexpression in squamous cell anal cancer. Int J Radiat Oncol Biol Phys. 2015;93(4):819–27. https://doi.org/10.1016/j.ijrobp.2015.08.004. Epub 2015 Aug 7. PMID: 26530750.
14. André T, Shiu KK, Kim TW, Jensen BV, Jensen LH, Punt C, Smith D, Garcia-Carbonero R, Benavides M, Gibbs P, de la Fouchardiere C, Rivera F, Elez E, Bendell J, Le DT, Yoshino T, Van Cutsem E, Yang P, Farooqui MZH, Marinello P, Diaz LA Jr, KEYNOTE-177 Investigators. Pembrolizumab in microsatellite-instability-high advanced colorectal cancer. N Engl J Med. 2020;383(23):2207–18. https://doi.org/10.1056/NEJMoa2017699. PMID: 33264544.
15. Fong Y, Fortner J, Sun RL, Brennan MF, Blumgart LH. Clinical score for predicting recurrence after hepatic resection for metastatic colorectal cancer: analysis of 1001 consecutive cases. Ann Surg. 1999;230(3):309–18; discussion 318–21. https://doi.org/10.1097/00000658-199909000-00004. PMID: 10493478; PMCID: PMC1420876.
16. Ziranu P, Ferrari PA, Guerrera F, Bertoglio P, Tamburrini A, Pretta A, Lyberis P, Grimaldi G, Lai E, Santoru M, Bardanzellu F, Riva L, Balconi F, Della Beffa E, Dubois M, Pinna-Susnik M, Donisi C, Capozzi E, Pusceddu V, Murenu A, Puzzoni M, Mathieu F, Sarais S, Alzetani A, Luzzi L, Solli P, Paladini P, Ruffini E, Cherchi R, Scartozzi M. Clinical score for colorectal cancer patients with lung-limited metastases undergoing surgical resection: Meta-Lung Score. Lung Cancer. 2023;184:107342. https://doi.org/10.1016/j.lungcan.2023.107342. Epub 2023 Aug 9. PMID: 37573705.
17. Quénet F, Elias D, Roca L, Goéré D, Ghouti L, Pocard M, Facy O, Arvieux C, Lorimier G, Pezet D, Marchal F, Loi V, Meeus P, Juzyna B, de Forges H, Paineau J, Glehen O; UNICANCER-GI Group and BIG Renape Group. Cytoreductive surgery plus hyperthermic intraperitoneal chemotherapy versus cytoreductive surgery alone for colorectal peritoneal metastases (PRODIGE 7): a multicentre, randomised, open-label, phase 3 trial. Lancet Oncol. 2021;22(2):256–266. https://doi.org/10.1016/S1470-2045(20)30599-4. Epub 2021 Jan 18. PMID: 33476595.
18. Elias D, Gilly F, Boutitie F, Quenet F, Bereder JM, Mansvelt B, Lorimier G, Dubè P, Glehen O. Peritoneal colorectal carcinomatosis treated with surgery and perioperative intraperitoneal chemotherapy: retrospective analysis of 523 patients from a multicentric French study. J Clin Oncol. 2010;28(1):63–8. https://doi.org/10.1200/JCO.2009.23.9285. Epub 2009 Nov 16. Erratum in: J Clin Oncol. 2010 Apr 1;28(10):1808. PMID: 19917863.

19. Sluiter NR, Rovers KP, Salhi Y, Vlek SL, Coupé VMH, Verheul HMW, Kazemier G, de Hingh IHJT, Tuynman JB. Metachronous peritoneal metastases after adjuvant chemotherapy are associated with poor outcome After Cytoreduction and HIPEC. Ann Surg Oncol. 2018;25(8):2347–56. https://doi.org/10.1245/s10434-018-6539-x. Epub 2018 May 31. PMID: 29855834; PMCID: PMC6028868.
20. Bakkers C, van Erning FN, Rovers KP, Nienhuijs SW, Burger JW, Lemmens VE, Aalbers AG, Kok NF, Boerma D, Brandt AR, Hemmer PH, van Grevenstein WM, de Reuver PR, Tanis PJ, Tuynman JB, de Hingh IH. Long-term survival after hyperthermic intraperitoneal chemotherapy using mitomycin C or oxaliplatin in colorectal cancer patients with synchronous peritoneal metastases: a nationwide comparative study. Eur J Surg Oncol. 2020;46(10 Pt A):1902–7. https://doi.org/10.1016/j.ejso.2020.04.018. Epub 2020 Apr 18. PMID: 32340819.
21. Prada-Villaverde A, Esquivel J, Lowy AM, Markman M, Chua T, Pelz J, Baratti D, Baumgartner JM, Berri R, Bretcha-Boix P, Deraco M, Flores-Ayala G, Glehen O, Gomez-Portilla A, González-Moreno S, Goodman M, Halkia E, Kusamura S, Moller M, Passot G, Pocard M, Salti G, Sardi A, Senthil M, Spiliotis J, Torres-Melero J, Turaga K, Trout R. The American Society of Peritoneal Surface Malignancies evaluation of HIPEC with Mitomycin C versus Oxaliplatin in 539 patients with colon cancer undergoing a complete cytoreductive surgery. J Surg Oncol. 2014;110(7):779–85. https://doi.org/10.1002/jso.23728. Epub 2014 Aug 2. PMID: 25088304.
22. Amin MB, et al. American joint committee on cancer (AJCC) cancer staging manual. 8th ed. American Joint Committee on Cancer, Springer; 2017.
23. Goodman KA, et al. AJCC cancer staging system: anus. 9th ed. American Joint Committee on Cancer, Springer; 2022.
24. SEER*Explorer: An interactive website for SEER cancer statistics [Internet]. Surveillance Research Program, National Cancer Institute; 2024 Apr 17. [updated: 2024 Jun 27; cited 2024 Sep 16]. Available from: https://seer.cancer.gov/statistics-network/explorer/.
25. Lembersky BC, Wieand HS, Petrelli NJ, O'Connell MJ, Colangelo LH, Smith RE, Seay TE, Giguere JK, Marshall ME, Jacobs AD, Colman LK, Soran A, Yothers G, Wolmark N. Oral uracil and tegafur plus leucovorin compared with intravenous fluorouracil and leucovorin in stage II and III carcinoma of the colon: results from National Surgical Adjuvant Breast and Bowel Project Protocol C-06. J Clin Oncol. 2006;24(13):2059–64. https://doi.org/10.1200/JCO.2005.04.7498. PMID: 16648506.
26. André T, Boni C, Navarro M, Tabernero J, Hickish T, Topham C, Bonetti A, Clingan P, Bridgewater J, Rivera F, de Gramont A. Improved overall survival with oxaliplatin, fluorouracil, and leucovorin as adjuvant treatment in stage II or III colon cancer in the MOSAIC trial. J Clin Oncol. 2009;27(19):3109–16. https://doi.org/10.1200/JCO.2008.20.6771. Epub 2009 May 18. PMID: 19451431.
27. Verheij FS, Omer DM, Williams H, Lin ST, Qin LX, Buckley JT, Thompson HM, Yuval JB, Kim JK, Dunne RF, Marcet J, Cataldo P, Polite B, Herzig DO, Liska D, Oommen S, Friel CM, Ternent C, Coveler AL, Hunt S, Gregory A, Varma MG, Bello BL, Carmichael JC, Krauss J, Gleisner A, Guillem JG, Temple L, Goodman KA, Segal NH, Cercek A, Yaeger R, Nash GM, Widmar M, Wei IH, Pappou EP, Weiser MR, Paty PB, Smith JJ, Wu AJ, Gollub MJ, Saltz LB, Garcia-Aguilar J. Long-term results of organ preservation in patients with rectal adenocarcinoma treated with total neoadjuvant therapy: the randomized phase II OPRA trial. J Clin Oncol. 2024;42(5):500–6. https://doi.org/10.1200/JCO.23.01208. Epub 2023 Oct 26. PMID: 37883738.
28. Bahadoer RR, Dijkstra EA, van Etten B, Marijnen CAM, Putter H, Kranenbarg EM, Roodvoets AGH, Nagtegaal ID, Beets-Tan RGH, Blomqvist LK, Fokstuen T, Ten Tije AJ, Capdevila J, Hendriks MP, Edhemovic I, Cervantes A, Nilsson PJ, Glimelius B, van de Velde CJH, Hospers GAP. RAPIDO collaborative investigators. Short-course radiotherapy followed by chemotherapy before total mesorectal excision (TME) versus preoperative chemoradiotherapy, TME, and optional adjuvant chemotherapy in locally advanced rectal cancer (RAPIDO): a randomised, open-label, phase 3 trial. Lancet Oncol. 2021;22(1):29–42. https://doi.org/10.1016/

S1470-2045(20)30555-6. Epub 2020 Dec 7. Erratum in: Lancet Oncol. 2021 Feb;22(2):e42. PMID: 33301740.

29. Conroy T, Bosset JF, Etienne PL, Rio E, François É, Mesgouez-Nebout N, Vendrely V, Artignan X, Bouché O, Gargot D, Boige V, Bonichon-Lamichhane N, Louvet C, Morand C, de la Fouchardière C, Lamfichekh N, Juzyna B, Jouffroy-Zeller C, Rullier E, Marchal F, Gourgou S, Castan F, Borg C, Unicancer Gastrointestinal Group and Partenariat de Recherche en Oncologie Digestive (PRODIGE) Group. Neoadjuvant chemotherapy with FOLFIRINOX and preoperative chemoradiotherapy for patients with locally advanced rectal cancer (UNICANCER-PRODIGE 23): a multicentre, randomised, open-label, phase 3 trial. Lancet Oncol. 2021;22(5):702–15. https://doi.org/10.1016/S1470-2045(21)00079-6. Epub 2021 Apr 13. PMID: 33862000.

Melanoma

Jessica S. Crystal and Susan B. Kesmodel

Introduction

- Epidemiology
  - Malignant melanoma represents only about 1% of all skin cancer cases but accounts for most of the deaths from skin cancer [1].
  - In 2023, approximately 97,610 people will be diagnosed with malignant melanoma, 89,070 people will be diagnosed of melanoma in situ, and 7990 people will die of melanoma in the United States [1].
    - This is likely an underestimate of the true annual incidence, as many superficial and in situ melanomas are not reported.
  - Increasing incidence: rate of 33% for men and 23% for women from 2002 to 2006 [2].
  - Median age of diagnosis 59 years.
  - One of the most deadly skin cancers.

Clinical Presentation and Prognostication

- Signs/Symptoms:
  - Assessment of pigmented lesions for suspicious features
    - Asymmetry
    - Border (irregular, uneven)
    - Color (more than one color)

J. S. Crystal (✉) · S. B. Kesmodel
Division of Surgical Oncology, Dewitt Daughtry Department of Surgery, University of Miami Miller School of Medicine, Miami, FL, USA
e-mail: Jessica.Crystal@med.miami.edu

- Diameter (> 6 mm)
    - Evolution (changes in size, shape, or color)
  - Bleeding
  - Pruritus
  - Constitutional symptoms (e.g., headache, dizziness, weight loss, GI bleeding, etc.)
- Physical Exam Findings
  - Suspicious pigmented lesions
  - Enlarged regional nodes
- Risk Factors
  - Personal/Hereditary Factors [3–11]
    - Male Sex
    - Age > 50 years
    - Skin type
      - Fitzpatrick skin type I
        - Pale skin, blue/green eyes, and red/blond hair
        - Always burns
      - Fitzpatrick skin type II
        - Fair skin and blue eyes
        - Burns easily
    - History of blistering sunburns
    - Personal history of prior melanoma, actinic keratosis, nonmelanoma skin cancers (basal cell and squamous cell carcinoma)
    - Multiple clinically atypical moles (particularly large nevi)
    - Dysplastic nevi
    - Immunosuppression
      - Solid organ transplant
      - Hematopoietic cell transplantation
      - HIV/AIDS
    - Family history of melanoma (especially if multiple); pancreatic, renal, and/or breast cancer; astrocytoma; uveal melanoma; and/or mesothelioma
    - Inherited genetic mutations
      - CDKN2a, CDK4, MC1R, BAP1 [especially for uveal melanoma], TERT, MITF, PTEN, and BRCA
    - Xeroderma pigmentosum
  - Environmental Factors [12–14]
    - Excess sun exposure
    - UV-based artificial tanning
- Pathologic Features [14–18]
  - Histologic subtype (if desmoplastic, specify pure vs. mixed)
  - Breslow thickness (reported to nearest 0.1 mm)
  - Ulceration
  - Mitotic rate (number of mitoses per mm^2)
  - Microsatellites

- Macroscopic satellites
- Lymphovascular/angiolymphatic invasion
- Regression
- Neurotropism
- Margin status (peripheral and deep)
- Prognostic Factors [3, 19]
  - Patient-specific factors
    - Older age
    - Gender
  - Tumor-Specific Factors
    - Breslow tumor thickness
    - Ulceration
    - Mitotic rate
    - Lymphovascular invasion (LVI)
    - Microsatellites
    - Nodal status
  - Molecular Testing—Gene Expression Profile (GEP)
    - Some of these tests may be used to assist in distinguishing lesions of uncertain biologic potential or uncertain histopathology [20–22].
    - Commercially available GEP testing is being advertised as a means to prognosticate melanoma biopsies. There is no randomized controlled trial evidence supporting that GEP testing is superior to the aforementioned known prognostic factors (like thickness, ulceration, and nodal status). As such, currently, there are no established guidelines on how to use GEP testing to direct clinical management [23–25].

Evaluation and Clinical Staging

- Diagnostic Tests:
  - Principles of Biopsy of Suspicious Skin Lesions: [26]
    - Suspicious skin lesions should be biopsied. Appearance of lesion should dictate approach.
    - When possible, perform a full-thickness biopsy by elliptical, incisional, punch, or shave biopsy, depending on the size and location of the lesion. With excisional biopsy, it is important to use narrow margins (1–3 mm) to allow for future lymphatic mapping if needed.
    - Should consider the orientation of the biopsy to optimize the subsequent definitive wide local excision.
    - If unable to do full excision due to the size or location of the lesion, perform an incisional or punch biopsy of the thickest or most abnormal portion of the lesion on clinical exam.
      - Multiple (scouting) biopsies of larger lesions to guide management may be helpful.

- If biopsy is felt to be discordant with clinical appearance or potentially understages the lesion, consider obtaining additional biopsies or full excisional biopsy for diagnosis.
- If concern for true scar recurrence, recommend biopsy of abnormal area.
– Principles of Biopsy of Clinically Negative Lymph Nodes
  - Sentinel Lymph Node Biopsy (SLNB)
    – Minimally invasive surgical technique to determine spread of melanoma to regional lymph node basins.
      - Preoperative dynamic lymphoscintigraphy (often with technetium 99), intraoperative identification using dye (most commonly isosulfan blue), and a gamma probe to detect radiolabeled lymph nodes.
    – For patients with clinical stage I/stage II disease, SLN status serves as the most significant prognostic factor [26].
    – When possible, SLNB should be performed at the time wide local excision (WLE) (to avoid disruption to the draining lymphatics), although it can be successfully performed after WLE [27].
    – Recommended for patients with clinical stage IB-II:
      - < 0.8 mm with ulceration
      - ≥ 0.8 mm with or without ulceration
      - Consideration of performing SLNB for patients with thinner, nonulcerated melanoma where there is a positive deep margin on biopsy.
      - Consideration of performing SLNB for patients whose risk of a positive SLN is >5% (Breslow depth ≥ 0.5 mm with other risk factors including age ≤ 42 years, head/neck location, presence of lymphovascular invasion, and/or mitotic index ≥$2/mm^2$, immunosuppression).
    – SLNB can provide regional nodal disease control (see Treatment section for details) [28].
    – It is important for the surgeon to assess the risk/benefit ratio of this procedure in each patient. Must take into account each patient's risk of SLN positivity, comorbidities, and whether the information will change management.
      - Can also use online tools to calculate the risk of SLN-positive disease.
    – Currently GEP testing should not replace SLNB nor should surveillance ultrasounds [29].
– Principles of Biopsy of Clinically Suspicious Lymph Nodes [30]
  - If an abnormal lymph node is found on physical exam or incidentally on imaging, biopsy should be obtained.
    – When possible core biopsy is preferred over fine-needle aspiration (FNA).
    – If percutaneous biopsy is not possible, can consider excisional biopsy.
– Principles of Biopsy of In-Transit Lesions:
  - Similar principles to biopsy of suspicious skin lesions (see above)
– Principles of Biopsy of Suspicious Metastases
  - Obtain biopsy to confirm distant metastasis
    – When possible, try to limit the morbidity of the procedure while obtaining staging information.

- Options include core (preferred), FNA, incisional, or excisional biopsy.
        - If needed consider determining presence of *BRAF* or *KIT* mutations (if patient is being considered for targeted therapy) or broader genomic profiling to allow for clinical trials (if indicated).
- Labs:
    - Routine lab tests are not recommended for node-negative melanoma
    - Otherwise are performed at the discretion of the treating clinician to assess patient-reported signs or symptoms.
    - Lactate dehydrogenase (LDH) when metastatic disease is found.
- Imaging:
    - Routine imaging (cross-sectional imaging with CT with IV contrast of the chest, abdomen, pelvis (and neck if needed), and/or PET/CT) is not recommended for node-negative melanoma (stages 0, IA, IB, and II), unless needed for surgical planning.
        - Some practitioners may consider systemic staging for patients who are going to be getting adjuvant immunotherapy ($\geq$T3B tumors).
    - Appropriate imaging should be performed at the discretion of the treating clinician to evaluate any signs or symptoms concerning for metastatic disease regardless of stage.
    - While ultrasound (US) of the nodal basin may assist with staging, it is not a substitute for the SLNB.
        - Nodal basin US should assist in assessing suspicious lymph nodes identified on physical exam.
        - Characteristics of abnormal lymph nodes:
            - Hypoechoic islands in the cortex
            - Asymmetrical focal cortical thickening
            - Peripheral vascularity (especially when perfusion is associated with the area of cortical thickening)
        - Abnormal lymph nodes or lesions should be further evaluated with core needle biopsy for histologic confirmation.
    - For patients with Stage IIIA (sentinel lymph node positive):
        - Cross-sectional whole body imaging can be considered.
    - For patients with stage IIIB/C/D:
        - Cross-sectional whole body imaging with or without brain imaging with MRI brain.
    - For patients with scar recurrence (persistent disease):
        - Imaging appropriate to tumor characteristics and melanoma staging.
    - For patients with local satellite/intransit recurrence:
        - Imaging to evaluate the extent of disease and any specific signs or symptoms.
        - Cross-sectional whole body imaging should be considered in these patients since this is a stage IIIC disease.
    - For patients with stage IV or recurrence with distant metastatic disease:
        - Cross-sectional whole body imaging and brain imaging.
- TNM staging (see Table 11.1) and survival (Table 11.2).

Table 11.1 AJCC 8th Edition Staging of Melanoma

T category	Thickness	Ulceration
TX: Primary tumor thickness cannot be assessed (e.g., diagnosis by curettage)	N/A	N/A
T0: No evidence of primary tumor (e.g., unknown primary or completely regressed melanoma)	N/A	N/A
Tis (melanoma in situ)	N/A	N/A
T1	≤1 mm	Unknown or unspecified
T1a	<0.8 mm	Without ulceration
T1b	<0.8 mm	With ulceration
	0.8–1.0 mm	With or without ulceration
T2	>1.0–2.0 mm	Unknown or unspecified
T2a	>1.0–2.0 mm	Without ulceration
T2b	>1.0–2.0 mm	With ulceration
T3	>2.0–4.0 mm	Unknown or unspecified
T3a	>2.0–4.0 mm	Without ulceration
T3b	>2.0–4.0 mm	With ulceration
T4	>4.0 mm	Unknown or unspecified
T4a	>4.0 mm	Without ulceration
T4b	>4.0 mm	With ulceration

N category	Number of tumor involved lymph nodes	Presence of intransit, satellite, and/or microsatellite metastases
NX	Regional nodes not assessed (e.g., SLN biopsy not performed, regional nodes previously removed for another reason) Exception: When there are no clinically detected regional metastases in a pT1 cM0 melanoma, assign cN0 instead of pNX.	No
N0	No regional metastases detected	No
N1	One tumor-involved node or intransit, satellite, and/or microsatellite metastases with no tumor-involved nodes	
N1a	One clinically occult (i.e., detected by SLN biopsy)	No
N1b	One clinically detected	No
N1c	No regional lymph node disease	Yes
N2	Two or three tumor-involved nodes or intransit, satellite, and/or microsatellite metastases with one tumor-involved node	
N2a	Two or three clinically occult (i.e., detected by SLN biopsy)	No
N2b	Two or three, at least one of which was clinically detected	No
N2c	One clinically occult or clinically detected	Yes
N3	Four or more tumor-involved nodes or intransit, satellite, and/or microsatellite metastases with two or more tumor-involved nodes, or any number of matted nodes without or with intransit, satellite, and/or microsatellite metastases	
N3a	Four or more clinically occult (i.e., detected by SLN biopsy)	No
N3b	Four or more, at least one of which was clinically detected, or presence of any number of matted nodes	No
N3c	Two or more clinically occult or clinically detected and/or presence of any number of matted nodes	Yes

(continued)

Table 11.1 (continued)

M category	Anatomic site	LDH level
M0	No evidence of distant metastasis	Not applicable
M1	Evidence of distant metastasis	
M1a	Distant metastasis to skin, soft tissue including muscle, and/or nonregional lymph node	Not recorded or unspecified
M1a (0)		Not elevated
M1a (1)		Elevated
M1b	Distant metastasis to lung with or without M1a sites of disease	Not recorded or unspecified
M1b (0)		Not elevated
M1b (1)		Elevated
M1c	Distant metastasis to non-CNS visceral sites with or without M1a or M1b sites of disease	Not recorded or unspecified
M1c (0)		Not elevated
M1c (1)		Elevated
M1d	Distant metastasis to CNS with or without M1a, M1b, or M1c sites of disease	Not recorded or unspecified
M1d (0)		Not elevated
M1d (1)		Elevated

AJCC Prognostic Stage Groups Clinical Staging (cTNM)			
	T	N	M
Stage 0	Tis	N0	M0
Stage IA	T1a	N0	M0
Stage IB	T1b	N0	M0
	T2a	N0	M0
Stage IIA	T2b	N0	M0
	T3a	N0	M0
Stage IIB	T3b	N0	M0
	T4a	N0	M0
Stage IIC	T4b	N0	M0
Stage III	Any T, Tis	$\geq$N1	M0
Stage IV	Any T	Any N	M1

Pathologic staging (pTNM)			
	T	N	M
Stage 0	Tis	N0	M0
Stage IA	T1a	N0	M0
	T1b	N0	M0
Stage IB	T2a	N0	M0
Stage IIA	T2b	N0	M0
	T3a	N0	M0
Stage IIB	T3b	N0	M0
	T4a	N0	M0
Stage IIC	T4b	N0	M0
Stage IIIA	T1a/b, T2	N1a, N2a	M0
Stage IIIB	T0	N1b, N1c	M0
	T1a/b, T2aN1b/c, N2b		M0

(continued)

Table 11.1 (continued)

Pathologic staging (pTNM)			
	T	N	M
	T2b, T3a	N1a/b/c, N2a/b	M0
Stage IIIC	T0	N2b/c, N3b/c	M0
	T1a/b, T2a/b, T3a	N2c, N3a/b/c	M0
	T3b, T4a	Any N ≥ N1	M0
	T4b	N1a/b/c, N2a/b/c	M0
Stage IIID	T4b	N3a/b/c	M0
Stage IV	Any T, Tis	Any N	M1

Table 11.2 Melanoma-specific survival according to stage [31]

Stage	Five-year MSS	Ten-year MSS
IA	99%	98%
IB	97%	94%
IIA	94%	88%
IIB	87%	82%
IIC	82%	75%
IIIA	93%	88%
IIIB	83%	77%
IIIC	69%	60%
IIID	32%	24%

Please note that stage IIIA has a worse prognosis than IIB–IIC. For metastatic disease, survival rates are 20–30% at five years since the advent of immunotherapy and targeted therapies

Treatment

- Local Disease
  - Surgery
    - WLE (to level of the fascia, or at least 3 cm in areas such as the buttock or breast, in stages I–III) Margins discussed in Tables 11.3 and 11.4. For subtypes like a pure desmoplastic melanoma, risk of positive SLNB is <5%.
    - *MelMarT-II (NCT 03860883) is an ongoing RCT looking at AJCC 8th edition pT2b-T4b patients randomized to 1 versus 2 cm margins due to risk of distant disease as opposed to locoregional control.*
    - Addition of SLNB:
      - <0.8 mm thick with ulceration or ≥ 0.8 mm ± ulceration
        - If there is uncertainty about the true depth of the melanoma (eg, due to positive deep margins or inadequate sampling of a larger lesion), may consider SLNB.
      - For patients with >10% risk of SLN metastases
      - When risk is 5–10%, SLN should be discussed with the patient. Features which increase risk of SLN positivity include age ≤ 42 years, head/neck location, LVI, and/or mitotic index ≥2/mm [39].
        - Can use available normograms to calculate risk [40].

Table 11.3 Margins for wide local excision of melanoma

Breslow thickness	Recommended excision margin
Melanoma in situ	0.5 to 1 cm
≤1 mm (T1)	1 cm
>1 to 2 mm (T2)	1 to 2 cm
>2 mm (T3 to T4)	2 cm

Table 11.4 RCT for surgical margins in cutaneous melanoma

Trial	Patients	Margins	Results
Kunishige et al. [32]	N = 1120 Melanoma in situ	3 mm margin followed by 3 mm→ if positive margin resect another 3 mm	86% with negative margins at 6 mm 97% at 9 mm Local recurrence 0.8% at 5 years
WHO (1988) [33]	N = 703 ≤2 mm Excluded face and digits	1 v 3 cm	Local recurrence rate 2.6% vs 0.1% OS 89.6% vs 90.3% In the group < 1 mm, there were no recurrences at 55 months→ recommend 1 cm margins < 1 mm thickness
Intergroup [34]	N = 740 1–4 mm	2 v 4 cm All head and neck received 2 cm margins for technical feasibility	OS 70% vs 77% (NS) Local recurrence 2.1% vs 2.6% (NS)
Swedish melanoma trial I [35]	N = 989 0.8–2.0 mm	2 vs 5 cm	Local recurrence rates < 1% which was too low to draw conclusions
European melanoma trial [36]	N = 337 ≤2 mm Excluded digits and acral melanomas	2 vs 5 cm	DFS 85% vs 83% (NS) OS 87% vs 86% (NS) Local recurrence 0.6% vs 2.4% (NS)
UK melanoma trial [37]	N = 900 ≥ 2 mm Excluded palms of hands and soles of feet	1 v 3 cm	1 cm group with more LRR (38% vs 32%, p = 0.05) and 24% increased risk of death This was the first trial to show that wider may be better in thicker melanomas Note that these patients did not have a SLNB
Swedish melanoma trial II [38]	N = 936 ≥ 2 mm	2 vs 4 cm	OS 65% in both groups (NS) LRR 4.3% vs 1.9% (NS) 2 cm margin is safe for thick melanomas

NS not significant

- At the present time, the use of GEP to determine need for SLNB requires further investigation and should not directly drive decision-making.
- SLNB is performed for staging, prognosis even in those with intransit disease, and locoregional control/survival benefit in intermediate to thick melanomas.

Table 11.5 Immunotherapy trials in thick primaries

Trial	Patients	Results
KEYNOTE 716 [41]	Resected stage IIB or IIC melanoma received either pembrolizumab or placebo every 3 weeks for 17 cycles or until disease recurrence or unacceptable toxicity	15% of patients in the pembrolizumab group and 24% in the placebo group had a first recurrence or died (HR 0·61 [95% CI 0·45–0·82]) RFS was not yet reached. OS not evaluated
CheckMate 76K [42]	Resected stage IIB or IIC melanoma received either nivolumab or placebo every 4 weeks for 12 months	7.8-month follow-up, nivolumab patients had a significantly improved RFS versus placebo (hazard ratio (HR) = 0.42; 95% confidence interval (CI): 0.30–0.59; $P < 0.0001$) 12-month RFS of 89.0% versus 79.4% and benefit observed across subgroups. Nivolumab patients also had improved distant metastases-free survival

- Adjuvant systemic therapy
    - If final pathology shows pT1a–3a N0 (path stages I–IIA): clinical trial for stage II disease or observation.
    - For patients with pT3b-T4b N0 (stages IIB and IIC disease) status post resection, consider adjuvant immunotherapy.
    - Randomized controlled trials for immunotherapy in thick primaries are listed in Table 11.5.
- Radiation: No benefit in comparison to WLE; however may consider definitive radiation to treat melanoma in situ, lentigo maligna-type (i.e., high-cumulative sun damage) in patients who cannot tolerate surgical resection (due to comorbidities or extent of resection needed relative to critical anatomic structures [43, 44]
- Locally Advanced Disease
    - SLNB Positive
        - Multicenter Selective Lymphadenectomy Trial-I (MSLT-I) was a large randomized controlled trial that showed that lymphatic mapping with SLNB is useful in determining prognosis of melanoma and its influence on survival. Patient with SLNB positive disease had improved melanoma outcomes when SLNB was used to stage nodal disease, instead of observation and lymph node dissection when lymph node metastases became clinically present [45, 46].
            - Ten-year disease-free survival rates were significantly improved in the biopsy group as compared with the observation group, in patients with intermediate-thickness melanoma (1.20–3.50 mm) (71.3 ± 1.8% vs. 64.7 ± 2.3%; hazard ratio for recurrence or metastasis, 0.76; $P = 0.01$) and those with thick melanomas, defined as >3.50 mm (50.7 ± 4.0% vs. 40.5 ± 4.7%; hazard ratio, 0.70; $P = 0.03$).
            - When management was directed by SLNB in patients with intermediate-thickness melanomas and nodal metastases, there was an improved

ten-year distant disease-free survival (HR 0.62; $P = 0.02$) and ten-year melanoma-specific survival (HR 0.56; $P = 0.006$).
- Surgery with completion lymph node dissection (CLND) versus active surveillance without additional nodal surgery with radiographic nodal surveillance.
- Active surveillance is the preferred approach based on the results of MSLT-II and German Dermatologic Cooperative Oncology Group — Selective Lymphadenectomy Trial (DeCOG-SLT) and their follow-up studies [28, 47, 48] (Table 11.6). These two large randomized controlled trials showed no difference in OS when comparing these two approaches in patients with positive SLNB.
- For patients where active surveillance is not possible, perform CLND.
- Adjuvant systemic therapy (Table 11.7): Use depends on risk of recurrence.
  - Targeted Therapy

Table 11.6 RCT of completion lymph node dissections

Trial	Patients	Results
MSLTII	Phase 3 Sentinel lymph node biopsy positive	At a median follow-up of 43 months, 3-year melanoma-specific survival was similar in the CLND group and the observation group (86 ± 1.3% and 86 ± 1.2%, respectively, $P = 0.42$)
DeCOG-SLT	Phase 3 Sentinel lymph node positive *Head and neck melanoma excluded	Trial was underpowered At a median follow-up of 72 months, analysis of the observation and CLND arms showed no significant treatment-related difference in five-year DMFS between the (67.6% vs. 64.9%, respectively, HR 1.08; $P = 0.87$), five-year RFS and OS also showed no difference (HR, 1.01 and 0.99, respectively).

Table 11.7 RCT of adjuvant use of checkpoint inhibitors

Trial	Patients	Results
Checkmate 238 [49]	Phase 3 Stage IIIB-C/IV without brain metastases (NO stage IIIA patients included) Ipilimumab or nivolumab up to 12 months	A four-year RFS (51.7% (95% CI 46.8–56.3) in the nivolumab group and 41.2% (36.4–45.9) in the ipilimumab group (hazard ratio [HR] 0.71 [95% CI 0.60–0.86]; $p = 0.0003$)) A four-year DMFS (59.2% (95% CI 53.7–64.2) with nivolumab and 53.3% (47.7–58.5) with ipilimumab, with an absolute risk difference of 5.9% (95% CI 2.8–10.7)
KEYNOTE-054 [50]	Phase 3 Stage IIIA–IIIC Pembrolizumab v placebo up to 12 months	Improved RFS in the pembrolizumab group 59.8% (95% CI 55.3–64.1) than the placebo group 41.4% (37.0–45.8) Improved 3.5-year DMFS 65.3% [95% CI 60.9–69.5] in the pembrolizumab group versus 49.4% [44.8–53.8] in the placebo group; HR 0.60 [95% CI 0.49–0.73]; $p < 0.0001$

- *Single Agent Vemurafenib for adjuvant treatment*
    - BRIM8: Trial evaluating patients with AJCC 7th Edition stage IIC-III disease and BRAF V600-activating mutation who received adjuvant treatment with the BRAF inhibitor vemurafenib monotherapy compared to placebo. The study showed improved DFS and possibly DMFS but no OS benefit [51].
- Dabrafenib/trametinib for patients with BRAF V600 activating mutation.
    - COMBI-AD: Trial in patients with resected stage III disease and BRAF V600 E/K mutation. Compared adjuvant treatment with dabrafenib/trametinib (BRAF/MEK inhibitor combination) compared to placebo. At a median follow-up of five years, combination of dabrafenib plus trametinib improved both five-year RFS (52 versus 36 percent; HR 0.51, 95% CI 0.42–0.61) and DMFS at five years (65 versus 54 percent, HR 0.55, 95% CI 0.44–0.7) compared to placebo. There was also improved OS at three years (86 versus 77%; HR 0.57, 95% CI 0.42–0.79) and this occurred regardless of baseline factors. [44, 52]
    - Studies showed that there was an increase in hyperproliferative cutaneous adverse events in the adjuvant vemurafenib arm compared to placebo in BRIM8. This was not shown in the COMBI-AD trial [51, 52].
    - Consequently, since the safety and efficacy of the combo BRAF/MEK inhibitor therapy is better than monotherapy, single agent vemurafenib is no longer approved for treatment of melanoma at this time.
- Many of the clinical trials evaluating immune checkpoint inhibitors or BRAF-targeted therapies included SLN+ patients who had greater nodal disease burden, at least 1 mm in diameter, who were felt to be higher risk. Also, for these studies, AJCC 7th Edition staging was commonly used. As such, the patients listed as stage IIIA disease were a higher risk group than the current AJCC 8th Edition stage IIIA patients as current staging incorporates Breslow thickness into stage III (AJCC 7th Edition stage IIIA five-year melanoma-specific survival is 78%, compared to 93% for AJCC 8th Edition) [53].
- Risks of toxicity of adjuvant therapy may outweigh benefits in very-low-risk stage IIIA disease (nonulcerated primary ≤2 mm thickness, SLN metastasis <1 mm).
- There are no head-to-head trials comparing nivolumab to pembrolizumab, but given the aforementioned trials showed similar outcomes from a survival standpoint and safety profile, there is no preference for one checkpoint inhibitor over the other. Likewise, there are no randomized controlled trials directly comparing checkpoint inhibitors to targeted therapy, and therefore both options are considered effective treatments.

- Clinically positive node[s]: Defined as clinically identified lymph nodes on radiographic imaging or physical exam and confirmed by biopsy.
  - Surgery:
    - Resectable nodal disease: WLE of primary tumor (if found) + therapeutic lymph node dissection (TLND).
    - If unresectable, proceed with systemic therapy.
  - Systemic Therapy
    - Adjuvant Therapy
      - Similar approach to systemic therapy in SLN-positive patients (see above).
      - Can also consider dual agent therapy
    - Advanced Disease
      - Checkpoint inhibition (Table 11.8)
      - Neoadjuvant therapy (Table 11.9)
      - Neoadjuvant therapy is now used in both resectable and unresectable advanced stage melanomas.
  - Radiation: Consider radiation therapy to nodal basin in patients with an elevated risk of regional recurrence. This may reduce the risk of regional recurrence but is not associated with improved RFS or OS. The decision to use radiation therapy should be balanced between the toxicity of radiation (lymphedema and oropharyngeal complications) compared to benefits, especially in the setting of the current effective systemic therapies [60–63].
    - Risk factors for regional nodal recurrence [58, 60, 61]:
      - Gross and/or histologic extracapsular extension of melanoma in clinically (macroscopic) involved node(s)
      - ≥ 1 parotid node
      - ≥ 2 cervical or axillary nodes

Table 11.8 Checkpoint inhibition in advanced stage melanoma

Trial	Patients	Results
Checkmate 067 [54]	*Phase 3 Untreated stages III–IV Nivolumab (mg/kg) + ipilimumab (3 mg/kg) × 4 doses and then nivolumab alone versus nivolumab alone versus ipilimumab alone*	Median PFS NR in the ipilimumab/nivolumab group, 37.6 months in the nivolumab group, and 19.9 months in the ipilimumab group OS at three years was 58% in the ipilimumab/nivolumab group, 52% in the nivolumab group, and 34% in the ipilimumab group
RELATIVITY-047 [55]	*Phases 2–3 Stages III–IV Relatlimab (Lag3 inhibitor) + nivolumab versus nivolumab single agent*	Median PFS was 10.1 months (95% confidence interval [CI], 6.4–15.7) in the combo arm and 4.6 months (95% CI, 3.4–5.6) with nivolumab alone (hazard ratio for progression or death, 0.75 [95% CI, 0.62–0.92]; $P = 0.006$) *This did come at the cost of increased adverse events in the relatlimab/nivolumab (18.9 versus 9.7%)

Table 11.9 Neoadjuvant therapy in advanced stage melanoma

Trial	Patients	Results
SWOG S1801 [56]	Phase 2 Stages IIIB–IVC resectable Three doses of neoadjuvant pembrolizumab + surgery + 15 adjuvant doses v surgery + 1 year adjuvant pembrolizumab	The neoadjuvant arm had a significantly longer event-free survival (72% vs. 49%)
OpACIN-neo [57, 58]	Phase 2 Stage III Resectable (no intransits) Group A: Two cycles ipilimumab 3 mg/kg + nivolumab 1 mg/kg Q3weeks Group B: Two cycles 2 cycles ipilimumab 1 mg/kg + nivolumab 3 mg/kg Q3weeks Group C: Two cycles of ipilimumab 3 mg/kg Q3W followed by 2 cycles of nivolumab 3 mg/kg Q2 weeks	Group B was well tolerated with high pathologic complete response rates Radiological response in 63% [95% CI 44–80] Group A, 57% [95% CI 37–75] Group B 35% Group C[95% CI 17–57] Pathological response in 80% [95% CI 61–92] Group A, 77% [95% CI 58–90] Group B, and 65% [95% CI 44–83] Group C Grades III and IV events was 40% group A, 20% Group B, and 50% Group C Pathologic response to neoadjuvant therapy also appeared to be a reliable surrogate for RFS and OS
PRADO [59]	Extension of OpACIN-neo Stage IIIB–IIID (no intransits) Major pathologic response (MPR, ≤10% viable tumor) in their index lymph node → TLND and adjuvant therapy were excluded Partial pathologic response (pPR;>10–≤50% viable tumor) →t TLND only No pathologic response (pNR;>50% viable tumor→ TLND and received adjuvant systemic therapy ± synchronous radiotherapy	The pRR was 72%. Relapse-free survival and distant metastasis-free survival rates were – 93% and 98% in patients with MPR –64% and 64% in patients with pPR –71% and 76% in patients with pNR This trial provides support for individualizing treatment based on response to neoadjuvant systemic therapy

- ≥3 inguinofemoral nodes
- ≥3 cm cervical or axillary node
- ≥4 cm inguinofemoral node
- Lymphatic Mets:
    - Microsatellites: one or more discontinuous nests of neoplastic cells >0.05 mm, clearly separated from normal dermis
    - Satellite metastases: cutaneous and /or subcutaneous intralymphatic metastases occurring within 2 cm of from the primary melanoma)
    - Intransit metastases: cutaneous and/or subcutaneous metastases at a distance >2 cm from the primary melanoma in the region between the primary and first echelons of regional lymph nodes

- Microscopic Satellites: Defined as microscopic lymphatic metastasis that are discontinuous from the primary tumor.
  - Microscopic satellites in biopsy specimen from primary lesion:
    - Surgery: WLE and discuss/offer SLNB
    - Systemic Therapy:
      - If SLNB negative, can consider adjuvant PD-1 immunotherapy including pembrolizumab or nivolumab, observation, or a clinical trial.
      - If SLNB positive, adjuvant systemic therapy as per node-positive discussion (see above)
    - Radiation principles as per above for positive nodal disease
  - Microscopic satellites positive in wide excision specimen and SLNB negative or not performed:
    - Surgery: Consider delayed SLNB.
      - If SLNB negative, can consider adjuvant PD-1 immunotherapy including pembrolizumab or nivolumab, observation, or a clinical trial.
      - If SLNB positive, adjuvant systemic therapy as per node-positive discussion (see above)
  - Microscopic satellites in wide excision specimen and SLNB positive: see discussion for SLNB-positive disease.
- Intransit Disease:
  - Limited resectable disease
    - Surgery: Complete excision to clear margins (preferred management of small number of resectable intransit metastases if able to achieve negative margins). No evidence to support exact margin. Can consider SLNB if it would change management [64].
    - Intralesional Injection: Talimogene laherparepvec (T-VEC) which is a modified oncolytic herpes simplex virus-1 (see explanation below)
    - Systemic therapy to follow surgery with nivolumab, pembrolizumab, or dabrafenib/trametinib for patients with *BRAF* V600-activating mutations.
  - Unresectable disease
    - Systemic therapy: with nivolumab, pembrolizumab, or dabrafenib/trametinib for patients with *BRAF* V600-activating mutations.
    - Local therapy:
      - Intralesional injection:
        - T-VEC (oncolytic virus): Inject the first dose of T-VEC at 10^6 pfu/mL (to seroconvert HSV-seronegative patients). Subsequent T-VEC doses of 10^8 pfu/mL were administered three weeks after the first dose and then once every two weeks. Total T-VEC volume was up to 4.0 mL per treatment session. Injected volume per lesion ranged from 0.1 mL for lesions <0.5 cm to 4.0 mL for lesions >5 cm in longest diameter.

- OPTiM study: Randomized open-label phase III trial. Patients with unresectable, injectable disease (stage IIIB-IVM1c) randomized to receive intratumoral T-VEC or subcutaneous GM-CSF. T-VEC durable response rate was better (16.3%; 95% CI, 12.1–20.5%) than GM-CSF (2.1%; 95% CI, 0–4.5%]; odds ratio, 8.9; $P < 0.001$). Overall response rate was also higher in the T-VEC arm (26.4%; 95% CI, 21.4% to 31.5% v 5.7%; 95% CI, 1.9% to 9.5%). Median OS was 23.3 months (95% CI, 19.5 to 29.6 months) with T-VEC and 18.9 months (95% CI, 16.0–23.7 months) with GM-CSF (hazard ratio, 0.79; 95% CI, 0.62 to 1.00; $P = 0.051$) Treatment with T-VEC worked best in untreated patients or those with stage IIIB, IIIC, or IVM1a disease [65, 66]. T-VEC injection resulted in shrinking and resolution of injected lesions, noninjected lesions, and visceral metastasis [67]. Most common adverse effects: fatigue, chills, and pyrexia.
- There is mixed data regarding benefit of combination of T-VEC with immunotherapy. It is our practice to not combine them.
  – MASTERKEY-265: Study combining pembrolizumab and T-VEC did not show improvement in PFS or OS [68].
  – Study combining T-VEC and ipilimumab vs ipilimumab alone showed objective response rate was significantly higher with T-VEC plus ipilimumab versus ipilimumab alone [69]. But given that ipilimumab is not the preferred first-line immune checkpoint inhibitor, and because the improvements in response did not result in improved PFS, this is not frequently used.
- IL-2 (Useful in certain circumstances): Complete response rate in IL-2-injected lesions may be as high as 70% and the treatment is less toxic than IV [70].
- Topical imiquimod for superficial dermal lesions (useful in certain circumstances).
– Regional Therapy:
  - Isolated limb perfusion/infusion (ILP/ILI):
  - ILP: isolation of the inflow and outflow of the extremity and administration of a concentrated chemotherapy via an extracorporeal bypass circuit, with an oxygenator to maintain physiologic pH and oxygenation.
    – Delivery of high-dose cytotoxic chemotherapy (usually melphalan) limited to the affected limb, while trying to reduce the side effects to the rest of the body).
    – Usually performed under hyperthermic conditions to improve effectiveness (felt to promote venodilation, but no proof of

overall survival benefit), but at the cost of potential increased adverse events [71].
- Can achieve good disease control. A large systematic review of ILP studies from 1990 to 2008 showed an overall response rate (ORR) of 90% (64–100%), and median complete response rate of 58% (25–89%). This is a complex procedure which requires experience and has potential for limb toxicity. Therefore, this surgery should only be performed at experienced centers and should be avoided in patients with multiple comorbidities or who are frail [72].
- ILI: technique that accesses the lower-extremity vessels percutaneously and does not require the use of the bypass circuit. It uses mild hyperthermia (39 °C), hypoxemia, and acidemia within the limb and uses a slower infusion of the same chemotherapeutic agent with a shorter exposure time of 30 minutes.
  - ILI was adopted in the 1990s to simplify the approach to perfusion of the limb and make it less invasive and in turn less toxic/morbid. This treatment can be repeated if there is recurrence or progression.
  - There is mixed data as to the response rate. The largest studies showed ORR of 64–75% [73, 74].
- Complications:
  - Local skin reactions
  - Systemic toxicity from chemo (small amounts) reaching the systemic circulation
  - Extremity compartment syndrome
  - Amputation
- Radiation therapy: to be used for symptomatic unresectable regional recurrences when no better options are available.
- Recurrence:
  - WLE Scar Recurrence
    - Surgery: Reexcise tumor site to appropriate margin. Consider SLNB dependent on pathology of scar recurrence.
    - Further treatment based upon clinical stage of surgery.
  - Local satellite/intransit recurrence: See above discussion of management of local satellite/intransit recurrence.
  - Nodal recurrence (without distant metastatic disease):
    - No prior lymph node dissection
      - If resectable either therapeutic lymph node dissection (TLND) or neoadjuvant therapy followed by TLND
      - Adjuvant systemic therapy: nivolumab, pembrolizumab, or dabrafenib/trametinib (for *BRAF* V600 activating mutation); consider ipilimumab if prior exposure to anti PD-1

- Can consider radiation therapy for select high-risk patients based upon location, size, number of involved nodes, and presence of extracapsular extension.
• Prior lymph node dissection:
  - If resectable: excise recurrence and if prior node dissection was incomplete, perform complete dissection, or consider neoadjuvant therapy.
    • Adjuvant systemic therapy: nivolumab, pembrolizumab, or dabrafenib/trametinib (for *BRAF* V600-activating mutation), consider ipilimumab if prior exposure to anti-PD-1
    • Can consider radiation therapy for select high-risk patients based upon location, size, number of involved nodes, and presence of extracapsular extension.
  - If unresectable: systemic therapy and/or palliative RT and/or intralesional TVEC.
• Metastatic Disease
  - Oligometastatic Disease
    • Multidisciplinary evaluation
    • Metastatic directed therapy:
      - Resection
        • Even before the advent of effective systemic therapy showing improved survival, studies showed survival benefit to complete curative resection of select stage IV patients with melanoma metastases [75, 76].
          - Howard et al. compared patients with metastatic disease who were given systemic therapy with or without metastasectomy. The median survival was 15.8 versus 6.9 months, and four-year survival was 20.8 versus 7.0% for patients receiving surgery with or without systemic medical therapy versus systemic medical therapy alone ($p < 0.0001$; hazard ratio 0.406). There was a benefit shown regardless if patients had M1a, M1b, or M1c disease.
        • Symptomatic metastatic disease may require surgical resection for palliation
      - Stereotactic ablative therapy
      - T-VEC/intralesional therapy
    • Systemic Therapy can be considered before and after resection (if resection is feasible) nivolumab, pembrolizumab, nivolumab/ipilimumab, or for *BRAF* V600-activating mutation: dabrafenib/trametinib, vemurafenib/cobimetinib, and encorafenib/binimetinib, consider ipilimumab if prior exposure to anti-PD-1.
  - Multivisceral disease (widely disseminated):
    • With or without brain metastases
      - Systemic therapy: if unresectable: nivolumab/ipilimumab, nivolumab/relatlimab, pembrolizumab, nivolumab, or for *BRAF* V600-activating mutations: Dabrafenib/trametinib, vemurafenib/cobimetinib, and encorafenib/binimetinib

- If there is progression, consider above, or can try other recommended regimens including ipilimumab alone, high-dose IL2, KIT inhibitor (for *KIT*-activating mutation), crizotinib or entrectinib (for *ROS1* fusions), larotrectinib or entrectinib (for *NTRK* fusions), binimetinib (for *NRAS* mutated tumors), combination therapy with pembrolizumab/lenvatinib, ipilimumab/intralesional T-VEC, combo BRAF/MEK + PD(L)-1 checkpoint inhibitors, or cytotoxic agents.
  - If limited extracranial lesions, consider intralesional T-VEC.
  - Consider palliative resection and/or RT for symptomatic intracranial disease
  - Palliative care

Summary Malignant melanoma represents a minority of skin cancers but a majority of the deaths from skin cancer. While the primary treatment for localized melanoma is surgical, immunotherapy and targeted therapy are important in the management of patients with more advanced disease. With these new effective systemic therapies, the management of locally advanced and metastatic disease will continue to evolve.

References

1. Cancer Facts & Figures 2023. Atlanta: American Cancer Society, Inc. 2022.
2. Jemal A, Saraiya M, Patel P, et al. Recent trends in cutaneous melanoma incidence and death rates in the United States, 1992-2006. J Am Acad Dermatol. 2011;65:S17–25 e11–13
3. Siegel RL, Miller KD, Fuchs BS, et al. Cancer Statistics, 2021. CA Cancer J Clin. 2021;71:7–33.
4. Naeyaert JM, Brochez L. Clinical practice. Dysplastic nevi. N Engl J Med. 2003;349:2233–40. Available at: http://www.ncbi.nlm.nih.gov/pubmed/14657431.
5. Rigel DS, Rivers JK, Kopf AW, et al. Dysplastic nevi. Markers for increased risk for melanoma. Cancer. 1989;63:386–9. Available at: http://www.ncbi.nlm.nih.gov/pubmed/2910446.
6. Evans RD, Kopf AW, Lew RA, et al. Risk factors for the development of malignant melanoma--I: Review of case-control studies. J Dermatol Surg Oncol. 1988;14:393–408. Available at: http://www.ncbi.nlm.nih.gov/pubmed/3280634.
7. Williams ML, Sagebiel RW. Melanoma risk factors and atypical moles. West J Med. 1994;160:343–50.
8. Omland SH, Gniadecki R, Haedersdal M, et al. Skin cancer risk in hematopoietic stem-cell transplant recipients compared with background population and renal transplant recipients: a population-based cohort study. JAMA Dermatol. 2015;152:1–7.
9. Olsen CM, Knight LL, Green AC. Risk of melanoma in people with HIV/AIDS in the pre- and post-HAART eras: a systematic review and meta-analysis of cohort studies. PLoS One. 2014;9:e95096.
10. Kraemer KH, Lee MM, Scotto J, Xeroderma pigmentosum. Cutaneous, ocular, and neurologic abnormalities in 830 published cases. Arch Dermatol. 1987;123:241–50.
11. Leachman SA, Lucero OM, Sampson JE, et al. Identification, genetic testing, and management of hereditary melanoma. Cancer Metastasis Rev. 2017;36:77–90.
12. Ivry GB, Ogle CA, Shim EK. Role of sun exposure in melanoma. Dermatologic Surg. 2006;32:481–92.
13. Colantonio S, Bracken MB, Beecker J. The association of indoor tanning and melanoma in adults: systematic review and meta-analysis. J Am Acad Dermatol. 2014;70:847–857 e841–818. Available at: http://www.ncbi.nlm.nih.gov/pubmed/24629998.

14. Gordon D, Gillgren P, Eloranta S, et al. Time trends in incidence of cutaneous melanoma by detailed anatomical location and patterns of ultraviolet radiation exposure: a retrospective population-based study. Melanoma Res. 2015;25:348–56.
15. Swetter SM, Tsao H, Bichakjian CK, et al. Guidelines of care for the management of primary cutaneous melanoma. J Am Acad Dermatol. 2019;80:208–50.
16. Scolyer R, Balamurgan T, Busam K, et al. Invasive melanoma, histopathology reporting guide, 2nd ed. Sydney: International Collaboration on Cancer Reporting; 2019. Available at: http://www.iccr-cancer.org/datasets/published-datasets/skin/invasive-melanoma.
17. Amin MB, Edge S, Greene F, et al., editors. AJCC Cancer Staging Manual (ed 8th). New York: Springer International Publishing; 2017.
18. Shon W, Frishberg DP, Gershenwald J, et al. Protocol for the examination of excision specimens from patients with melanoma of the skin, version 4.2.0.0. College of American Pathologists (CAP); 2020.
19. Khosrotehrani K, Dasgupta P, Byrom L, et al. Melanoma survival is superior in females across all tumour stages but is influenced by age. Arch Dermatol Res. 2015;307:731–40.
20. Emanuel PO, Andea AA, Vidal CI, et al. Evidence behind the use of molecular tests in melanocytic lesions and practice patterns of these tests by dermatopathologists. J Cutan Pathol. 2018;45:839–46.
21. Vidal CI, Armbrect EA, Andea AA, et al. Appropriate use criteria in dermatopathology: Initial recommendations from the American Society of Dermatopathology. J Cutan Pathol. 2018;45:563–80.
22. Clarke LE, Warf BM, Flake DD 2nd, et al. Clinical validation of a gene expression signature that differentiates benign nevi from malignant melanoma. J Cutan Pathol. 2015;42:244–52.
23. Zager JS, Gastman BR, Leachman S, et al. Performance of a prognostic 31-gene expression profile in an independent cohort of 523 cutaneous melanoma patients. BMC Cancer. 2018;18:130.
24. Kangas-Dick AW, Greenbaum A, Gall V, et al. Evaluation of a gene expression profiling assay in primary cutaneous melanoma. Ann Surg Oncol. 2021;28:4582–9.
25. Sabel MS. Genomic expression profiling in melanoma and the road to clinical practice. Ann Surg Oncol. 2022;29:764–6.
26. Krag DN, Meijer SJ, Weaver DL, et al. Minimal-access surgery for staging of malignant melanoma. Arch Surg. 1995;130(6):654.
27. Gannon CJ, Rousseau DL Jr, Ross MI, et al. Accuracy of lymphatic mapping and sentinel lymph node biopsy after previous wide local excision in patients with primary melanoma. Cancer. 2006;107(11):2647–52.
28. Multicenter Selective Lymphadenectomy Trials Study Group, Crystal JS, Thompson JF, Hyngstrom J, et al. Therapeutic value of sentinel lymph node biopsy in patients with melanoma: a randomized clinical trial. JAMA Surg. 2022;157:835–42.
29. Melanomarisk.org.au
30. National Comprehensive Cancer Network. Melanoma: Cutaneous (Version 3.2023). https://www.nccn.org/professionals/physician_gls/pdf/cutaneous_melanoma.pdf. Accessed 25 Nov 2023.
31. Gershenwald JE, Scolyer RA. Melanoma Staging: American Joint Committee on Cancer (AJCC) 8th edition and beyond. Ann Surg Oncol. 2018;25:2105–10.
32. Kunishige JH, Doan L, Brodland DG, Zitelli JA. Comparison of surgical margins for lentigo maligna versus melanoma in situ. J Am Acad Dermatol. 2019;81(1):204–12.
33. Veronesi U, Cascinelli N, Adamus J, et al. Thin stage I primary cutaneous malignant melanoma. Comparison of excision with margins of 1 or 3 cm. N Engl J Med. 1988;318(18):1159–62.
34. Balch CM, Urist MM, Karakousis CP, et al. Efficacy of 2-cm surgical margins for intermediate-thickness melanomas (1 to 4 mm). Results of a multi-institutional randomized surgical trial. Ann Surg. 1993;218(3):262–7; discussion 267–9.
35. Khayat D, Rixe O, Martin G, et al. French Group of Research on Malignant Melanoma. Surgical margins in cutaneous melanoma (2 cm versus 5 cm for lesions measuring less than 2.1-mm thick). Cancer. 2003;97(8):1941–6.

36. Cohn-Cedermark G, Rutqvist LE, Andersson R, et al. Long term results of a randomized study by the Swedish Melanoma Study Group on 2-cm versus 5-cm resection margins for patients with cutaneous melanoma with a tumor thickness of 0.8-2.0 mm. Cancer. 2000;89(7):1495–501.
37. Thomas JM, Newton-Bishop J, A'Hern R, et al. United Kingdom Melanoma Study Group; British Association of Plastic Surgeons; Scottish Cancer Therapy Network. Excision margins in high-risk malignant melanoma. N Engl J Med. 2004;350(8):757–66.
38. Utjés D, Malmstedt J, Teras J, et al. 2-cm versus 4-cm surgical excision margins for primary cutaneous melanoma thicker than 2 mm: long-term follow-up of a multicentre, randomised trial. Lancet. 2019;394(10197):471–7.
39. Shannon AB, Sharon CE, Straker RJ, et al. Sentinel lymph node biopsy in patients with T1a cutaneous malignant melanoma: A multicenter cohort study. J Am Acad Dermatol. 2023;88:52–9.
40. Lo SN, Ma J, Scolyer RA, et al. Improved risk prediction calculator for sentinel node positivity in patients with melanoma: the Melanoma Institute Australia nomogram. J Clin Oncol. 2020;38(24):2719–27.
41. Luke JJ, Rutkowski P, Queirolo P, et al. Pembrolizumab versus placebo as adjuvant therapy in completely resected stage IIB or IIC melanoma (KEYNOTE-716): a randomised, double-blind, phase 3 trial. Lancet. 2022;399(10336):1718–29.
42. Kirkwood JM, Del Vecchio M, Weber J, et al. Adjuvant nivolumab in resected stage IIB/C melanoma: primary results from the randomized, phase 3 CheckMate 76K trial. Nat Med. 2023;29(11):2835–43.
43. Hedblad MA, Mallbris L. Grenz ray treatment of lentigo maligna and early lentigo maligna melanoma. J Am Acad Dermatol. 2012;67:60.
44. Hellriegel W. Radiation therapy of primary and metastatic melanoma. Ann N Y Acad Sci. 1963;100:131.
45. Morton DL, Thompson JF, Cochran AJ, et al. Sentinel-node biopsy or nodal observation in melanoma. N Engl J Med. 2006;355:1307.
46. Morton DL, Thompson JF, Cochran AJ, et al. Final trial report of sentinel-node biopsy versus nodal observation in melanoma. N Engl J Med. 2014;370:599.
47. Faries MB, Thompson JF, Cochran AJ, et al. Completion dissection or observation for sentinel-node metastasis in melanoma. N Engl J Med. 2017;376(23):2211–22. PMID: 28591523
48. Leiter U, Stadler R, Mauch C, et al. German Dermatologic Cooperative Oncology Group. Final analysis of DeCOG-SLT trial: no survival benefit for complete lymph node dissection in patients with melanoma with positive sentinel node. J Clin Oncol. 2019;37(32):3000–8. PMID: 31557067
49. Ascierto PA, Del Vecchio M, Mandalá M, et al. Adjuvant nivolumab versus ipilimumab in resected stage IIIB-C and stage IV melanoma (CheckMate 238): 4-year results from a multicentre, double-blind, randomised, controlled, phase 3 trial. Lancet Oncol. 2020;21:1465.
50. Eggermont AMM, Blank CU, Mandalà M, et al. Adjuvant pembrolizumab versus placebo in resected stage III melanoma (EORTC 1325-MG/KEYNOTE-054): distant metastasis-free survival results from a double-blind, randomised, controlled, phase 3 trial. Lancet Oncol. 2021;22:643.
51. Maio M, Lewis K, Demidov L, et al. Adjuvant vemurafenib in resected, BRAF(V600) mutation-positive melanoma (BRIM8): a randomised, doubleblind, placebo-controlled, multicentre, phase 3 trial. Lancet Oncol. 2018;19:510–20.
52. Dummer R, Hauschild A, Santinami M, et al. Five-year analysis of adjuvant Dabrafenib plus Trametinib in stage III melanoma. N Engl J Med. 2020;383:1139.
53. Gershenwald JE, Scolyer RA, Hess KR, et al. Melanoma staging: Evidence-based changes in the American Joint Committee on Cancer eighth edition cancer staging manual. CA Cancer J Clin. 2017;67:472–92.
54. Wolchok JD, Chiarion-Sileni V, Gonzalez R, et al. Long-term outcomes with nivolumab plus ipilimumab or nivolumab alone versus ipilimumab in patients with advanced melanoma. J Clin Oncol. 2022;40(2):127–37.

55. Tawbi HA, Schadendorf D, Lipson EJ, et al. Relatlimab and nivolumab versus nivolumab in untreated advanced melanoma. N Engl J Med. 2022;386:24–34.
56. Patel SP, Othus M, Chen Y, et al. Neoadjuvant–adjuvant or adjuvant-only pembrolizumab in advanced melanoma. N Engl J Med. 2023;388:813.
57. Rozeman EA, Menzies AM, van Akkooi ACJ, et al. Identification of the optimal combination dosing schedule of neoadjuvant ipilimumab plus nivolumab in macroscopic stage III melanoma (OpACIN-neo): a multicentre, phase 2, randomised, controlled trial. Lancet Oncol. 2019;20:948.
58. Versluis JM, Menzies AM, Sikorska K, et al. Survival update of neoadjuvant ipilimumab plus nivolumab in macroscopic stage III melanoma in the OpACIN and OpACIN-neo trials. Ann Oncol. 2023;34:420.
59. Reijers ILM, Menzies AM, van Akkooi ACJ, et al. Personalized response-directed surgery and adjuvant therapy after neoadjuvant ipilimumab and nivolumab in high-risk stage III melanoma: the PRADO trial. Nat Med. 2022;28:1178.
60. Henderson MA, Burmeister BH, Ainslie J, et al. Adjuvant lymph-node field radiotherapy versus observation only in patients with melanoma at high risk of further lymph-node field relapse after lymphadenectomy (ANZMTG 01.02/ TROG 02.01): 6-year follow-up of a phase 3, randomised controlled trial. Lancet Oncol. 2015;16:1049–60.
61. Creagan ET, Cupps RE, Ivins JC, et al. Adjuvant radiation therapy for regional nodal metastases from malignant melanoma: a randomized, prospective study. Cancer. 1978;42:2206–10.
62. Beadle BM, Guadagnolo BA, Ballo MT, et al. Radiation therapy field extent for adjuvant treatment of axillary metastases from malignant melanoma. Int J Radiat Oncol Biol Phys. 2009;73:1376–82.
63. Lee RJ, Gibbs JF, Proulx GM, et al. Nodal basin recurrence following lymph node dissection for melanoma: implications for adjuvant radiotherapy. Int J Radiat Oncol Biol Phys. 2000;46:467–74.
64. Beasley GM, Speicher P, Sharma K, Seigler H, Salama A, Mosca P, Tyler DS. Efficacy of repeat sentinel lymph node biopsy in patients who develop recurrent melanoma. J Am Coll Surg. 2014;218(4):686–92.
65. Andtbacka RH, Kaufman HL, Collichio F, Amatruda T, Senzer N, Chesney J, Delman KA, Spitler LE, Puzanov I, Agarwala SS, Milhem M, Cranmer L, Curti B, Lewis K, Ross M, Guthrie T, Linette GP, Daniels GA, Harrington K, Middleton MR, Miller WH Jr, Zager JS, Ye Y, Yao B, Li A, Doleman S, VanderWalde A, Gansert J, Coffin RS. Talimogene Laherparepvec improves durable response rate in patients with advanced melanoma. J Clin Oncol. 2015;33(25):2780.
66. Andtbacka RHI, Collichio F, Harrington KJ, Middleton MR, Downey G, Öhrling K, Kaufman HL. Final analyses of OPTiM: a randomized phase III trial of talimogene laherparepvec versus granulocyte-macrophage colony-stimulating factor in unresectable stage III-IV melanoma. J Immunother Cancer. 2019;7(1):145.
67. Andtbacka RH, Ross M, Puzanov I, Milhem M, Collichio F, Delman KA, Amatruda T, Zager JS, Cranmer L, Hsueh E, Chen L, Shilkrut M, Kaufman HL. Patterns of Clinical Response with Talimogene Laherparepvec (T-VEC) in Patients with Melanoma Treated in the OPTiM Phase III Clinical Trial. Ann Surg Oncol. 2016;23(13):4169.
68. Chesney J, Ribas A, Long GV, Kirkwood JM, Dummer R, et al. Randomized, double-blind, placebo-controlled, global phase III trial of talimogene laherparepvec combined with pembrolizumab for advanced melanoma. J Clin Oncol. 2023;41(3):528–40.
69. Chesney J, Puzanov I, Collichio F, et al. Randomized, open-label phase II study evaluating the efficacy and safety of talimogene laherparepvec in combination with ipilimumab versus ipilimumab alone in patients with advanced, unresectable melanoma. J Clin Oncol. 2018;36:1658–67.
70. Byers BA, Temple-Oberle CF, Hurdle V, McKinnon JG. Treatment of in-transit melanoma with intra-lesional interleukin-2: a systematic review. J Surg Oncol. 2014;110:770–5.
71. Barbour AP, Thomas J, Suffolk J, et al. Isolated limb infusion for malignant melanoma: predictors of response and outcome. Ann Surg Oncol. 2009;16:3463–72.

72. Moreno-Ramirez D, de la Cruz-Merino L, Ferrandiz L, et al. Isolated limb perfusion for malignant melanoma: systematic review on effectiveness and safety. Oncologist. 2010;15:416–27.
73. Kroon HM, Coventry BJ, Giles MH, et al. Australian Multicenter Study of isolated limb infusion for melanoma. Ann Surg Oncol. 2016;23:1096.
74. Beasley GM, Caudle A, Petersen RP, et al. A multi-institutional experience of isolated limb infusion: defining response and toxicity in the US. J Am Coll Surg. 2009;208:706.
75. Sosman JA, Moon J, Tuthill RJ, et al. A phase 2 trial of complete resection for stage IV melanoma: results of Southwest Oncology Group Clinical Trial S9430. Cancer. 2011;117:4740.
76. Howard JH, Thompson JF, Mozzillo N, et al. Metastasectomy for distant metastatic melanoma: analysis of data from the first Multicenter Selective Lymphadenectomy Trial (MSLT-I). Ann Surg Oncol. 2012;19:2547.

Nonmelanoma Skin Cancers

12

Jason M. Lizalek and Juan A. Santamaria-Barria

Squamous Cell Skin Cancer

- **Introduction**
  - Cutaneous squamous cell cancer is the second most common nonmelanoma skin cancer, after basal cell cancer
  - Diagnosis is made by physical exam and confirmed via biopsy
  - Locally advanced disease can be assessed with US, CT, MRI, or PET/CT
  - Surgical resection is the current standard of care with a variety of systemic treatments and radiotherapy modalities available for patients with locally advanced, unresectable, and metastatic disease.
- **Diagnosis**
  - Symptoms may include bleeding, pruritus, and growing lesion
  - Physical exam findings concerning for regional metastatic disease:
    - Cervical, occipital, axillary, or inguinal lymphadenopathy
  - Risk factors [65]
    - Ultraviolet light-cumulative exposure
    - Age
    - Fair skin
    - Recreational tanning/tanning beds
    - Immunosuppression
    - HPV/HIV/AIDS
    - Ionizing radiation exposure

J. M. Lizalek · J. A. Santamaria-Barria (✉)
Division of Surgical Oncology, Department of Surgery, University of Nebraska Medical Center, Fred & Pamela Buffett Cancer Center, Omaha, NE, USA
e-mail: juan.santamaria@unmc.edu

© The Author(s), under exclusive license to Springer Nature Switzerland AG 2025
C. Schmidt, M. G. Kledzik (eds.), *Complex General Surgical Oncology*,
https://doi.org/10.1007/978-3-031-88954-7_12

- Chemical exposure
  - Arsenic
  - Polycyclic aromatic hydrocarbons (coal tar)
  - Nitrosamines
  - Alkylating agents
- Chronic inflammation (healing scars, burns, ulcers)
- Personal history of skin cancer
- Family history of skin cancer
- Benign sun-related skin disorders
  - Solar lentigines
- Premalignant lesions
  - Actinic keratoses
  - Squamous cell carcinoma in situ (Bowen's disease)
  - Keratoacanthoma
  - Cutaneous horn
- Psoralen/PUVA for psoriasis
- Genetic syndromes [36]
  - Xeroderma pigmentosum
  - Oculocutaneous albinism
  - Muir-Torre syndrome
  - Fanconi anemia
- Screening recommendations and total body skin exam
  - Immunosuppressed [97]
    - No skin cancer/field disease every 12 months
    - Field disease/one NMSC every 3–6 months
    - High-risk cSCC/multiple NMSC every 3 months
    - Metastatic SCC or melanoma every 1–3 months
    - Xeroderma pigmentosum [46]
      - 3–6 months
    - Oculocutaneous albinism
      - 6–12 months
    - Muir-Torre syndrome
      - Annual
    - Fanconi anemia
      - Annual
- Chemoprevention
  - Transplant, Xeroderma pigmentosa, psoriasis, and PUVA exposure
    - Oral retinoid prophylaxis may be effective in reducing development of new SCC (NCCN 2023 Squamous cell carcinoma)
    - Acitretin may be used in solid organ transplant recipients (SOTR) with history of SCC [91]
    - Consider side effect profile and teratogenesis in patients of childbearing age

- Nicotinamide (vitamin B3) did not lead to reduction in SCC incidence in SOTR at 12 months [3] (ONTRANS trial)
  - Immunocompetent, high-risk of recurrence or metastases
    - Nicotinamide B3, 500 mg BID, and 30% reduction in 12-month rate of new SCC [16] (ONTRAC trial)
- **Evaluation and Clinical Stage**
  - History and Physical Exam
    - History focusing on risk factors
    - Total body skin examination
      - Clinical exam findings consistent with cSCC
      - Induration
      - Adherent crust with ill-defined margins
        - Dermoscopy can aid in diagnosis with two vascular patterns: small, dotted vessels and glomerular vessels
    - Regional lymph node examination
  - Biopsy and pathology [91]
    - Punch, shave, and excisional biopsy all are acceptable.
    - Size and depth should be adequate to assess high-risk pathologic findings.
  - Regional lymph node examination
    - US for initial assessment of palpable regional lymph nodes
    - CT scan with contrast
      - Nodal basin can assess size, number, and location of lymph nodes.
      - Assessing invasion of bone (preferred), named nerve, or deep soft tissue.
    - MRI with contrast used to assess for peripheral nerve involvement or if there is suspicion of extensive disease
    - Sample clinically suspicious lymph nodes with FNA, core needle, or excisional biopsy
  - Systemic imaging to evaluate metastatic disease in locally advanced or positive regional disease:
    - CT chest, abdomen, and pelvis with contrast
    - FDG PET/CT skull to foot
    - Consider MRI brain if concern for subcortical involvement from bone invasion
    - Biopsy clinically suspicious lesions for locoregional or metastatic disease
      - FNA, core needle biopsy, or excisional biopsy
  - Risk factors for recurrence and metastases – Table 12.1 (NCCN cutaneous squamous cell cancer risk) [75]
  - TNM staging of head and neck (AJCC 8th edition) – Table 12.2 (American College of Surgeons)
  - AJCC Prognostic Stages – Table 12.3 (American College of Surgeons)
  - Brigham and Women's Hospital (BWH) system for prognostication of localized cSCC – Table 12.4 [37]

Table 12.1 Cutaneous squamous cell cancer stratification of risk factors for recurrence and metastases

Risk group	Low risk	High risk	Very high risk
H&P			
Location/size	Trunk, extremities ≤2 cm	Trunk, extremities >2 cm– ≤ 4 cm. Head, neck, hands, feet, pretibial, and anogenital (any size)	> 4 cm (any location)
Clinical extent	Well-defined	Poorly defined	
Primary vs. recurrent	Primary	Recurrent	
Immunosuppression	–	+	
Site of prior RT or chronic inflammatory process	–	+	
Rapidly growing tumor	–	+	
Neurologic symptoms	–	+	
Pathology			
Degree of differentiation	Well or moderately differentiated		Poor differentiation
Histologic features: Acantholytic (adenoid), Adenosquamous (showing mucin production), or metaplastic (carcinosarcomatous) subtypes	–	+	Desmoplastic SCC
Depth: thickness or level of invasion	< 2 mm thick and no invasion beyond subcutaneous fat	2–6 mm depth	> 6 mm or invasion beyond subcutaneous fat
Perineural involvement	–	+	Tumor cells within the nerve sheath of a nerve lying deeper than the dermis or measuring ≥0.2 mm
Lymphatic or vascular involvement	–	–	+

Table 12.2 TNM Staging classification of cutaneous carcinoma of the head and neck (AJCC 8th edition)

Tis	Carcinoma in situ
T1	≤2 cm
T2	>2 cm ≤ 4 cm
T3	>4 cm, or minor bone erosion, or perineural invasion or deep invasion (>6 mm)
T4	Gross cortical bone/marrow, skull base invasion, and/or skull base foramen invasion
T4a	Gross cortical bone/marrow invasion
T4b	Skull base invasion and/or skull base foramen involvement
N0	No regional lymph node metastasis
N1	Metastasis 1 ipsilateral LN, ≤3 cm and ENE-
N2	Metastasis 1 ipsilateral LN, ≤3 cm and ENE+ Or metastasis >3 cm ≤ 6 cm and ENE– Or metastasis in multiple ipsilateral LN, ≤6 cm and ENE- Or bilateral or contralateral LN, ≤6 cm and ENE-

(continued)

Table 12.2 (continued)

Tis	Carcinoma in situ
N2a	Metastasis 1 ipsilateral LN, ≤3 cm and ENE+
	Or metastasis >3 cm ≤ 6 cm and ENE−
N2b	Metastasis in multiple ipsilateral LN, ≤ 6 cm and ENE−
N2c	Metastasis in bilateral or contralateral LN, ≤ 6 cm and ENE−
N3	Metastasis in a LN > 6 cm and ENE−
	Or 1 ipsilateral LN > 3 cm and ENE+
	Or multiple ipsilateral, contralateral, or bilateral LN, any with ENE+
	Or single contralateral LN any size and ENE+
N3a	Metastasis in a LN > 6 cm and ENE−
N3b	Metastasis in 1 ipsilateral LN > 3 cm and ENE+
	Or multiple ipsilateral, contralateral, or bilateral LN, any with ENE+
	Or single contralateral LN any size and ENE+
M0	No distant metastasis
M1	Distant metastasis
G1	Well differentiated
G2	Moderately differentiated
G3	Poorly differentiated
G4	Undifferentiated

Table 12.3 Prognostic stage groups for cutaneous carcinoma of the head and neck (AJCC 8th edition)

	T	N	M
Stage 0	Tis	N0	M0
Stage I	T1	N0	M0
Stage II	T2	N0	M0
Stage III	T3	N0	M0
Stage IV	T1	N1	M0
	T2	N1	M0
	T3	N1	M0
	T1	N2	M0
	T2	N2	M0
	T3	N2	M0
	Any T	N3	M0
	T4	Any N	M0
	Any T	Any N	M1

Table 12.4 Brigham and Women's Hospital (BWH) system for prognostication of localized cutaneous squamous cell carcinoma

T stage	Number of high-risk factors[a]	10-year local recurrence, (%)	10-year nodal metastasis, (%)	10-year disease-specific death, (%)	10-year overall death, (%)
T1	0	0.6	0.1	0	32
T2a	1	5	3	1	32
T2b	2–3	21	21	10	51
T3	≥4	67	67	100	100

[a]Tumor diameter ≥2 cm, poorly differentiated histology, perineural invasion ≥0.1 mm, tumor invasion beyond fat, and excluding bone invasion

- **Choice of Therapy**
  - Local disease
    - Low risk = curettage and electrodessication, shave excision, standard excision, Mohs or PDEMA (peripheral and deep en face margin assessment), or definitive RT if not candidate for above
    - High-risk/very-high-risk = Mohs or PDEMA, standard excision, definitive RT, or systemic therapy
  - Positive regional lymph nodes
    - Head and neck = excision of primary tumor, unilateral or bilateral neck dissection, +/− parotidectomy, +/− RT, and +/− systemic therapy
    - Trunk and extremities = excision of primary tumor and regional lymph node dissection, +/− RT
  - Locally advanced unresectable, metastatic disease, or nonsurgical candidate
    - RT +/− systemic therapy
- **Nonoperative Therapy**
  - Curettage and electrodessication
    - Does not allow histologic margin assessment
    - First-line therapy for local, low-risk without dermal invasion
      - Recurrence rate 1.7% [45]
    - Contraindications as definitive therapy:
      - Areas of terminal hair growth – scalp, pubic or axillary regions, and beard area – due to potential follicular extension of tumor
      - If subcutaneous tissue reached requires surgical excision
      - Biopsy of lesion reveals high-risk pathologic features
  - Cryotherapy
    - Can be used for local, low-risk cSCC when other methods contraindicated or impractical
    - Recurrence rate 0.8% [45]
    - Unable to assess histologic margin control
  - Topical therapy – 5-fluorouracil or imiquimod – can consider for cSCC in situ
  - Photodynamic therapy – can consider for cSCC in situ
  - Definitive radiation therapy
    - 70–93 Gy for conventional fractionation
    - 56–88 Gy for hypofractionation
    - ~7-year local control rate and local recurrence rate, 87.2% and 7.2% [41]
- **Surgical Therapy**
  - Mohs
    - Allows for histologic examination of 100% of surgical margins with sequential thin excisions [80].
    - Preferred method for low-, high-, and very high-risk lesions (Connolly et al. 2012)
    - 2.3% local recurrence for primary and up to 16% for recurrence treated with Mohs [81]
  - Peripheral and Deep En face Margin Assessment (PDEMA)

- Techniques allow complete histopathologic marginal (deep and peripheral) assessment of tumor
  - Mohs
  - Tubingen muffin technique [56]
  - Tubingen torte technique [62]
- Low-risk
  - 4-mm margin for tumor <2 cm
  - 6-mm margin for tumor >2 cm
  - Wide local excision
    - Cure rates 90–98% [44]
  - Mohs or other PDEMA methods (preferred technique)
- High-risk/very-high risk
  - Wide local excision to 6–10 mm margins
    - Local recurrence 0–14%, regional metastases 0–13%
    - A five-year recurrence rate for primary vs. recurrence, 5.7% vs. 17.3%
  - Mohs or other PDEMA method (preferred technique)
    - Local recurrence rate = 1.2–4.1% [94]
- Sentinel lymph node biopsy [2]
  - Consider in very-high-risk or recurrent disease when clinically node negative and occult risk > 15% [96].
  - Rate of subclinical nodal positivity 7–21% [28, 42, 68]
  - False-negative rate 4.6% [58]
- Lymphadenectomy
  - Head and neck
    - Unilateral nodal disease – Excision of primary tumor and ipsilateral neck dissection
    - Bilateral nodal disease – Excision of primary tumor and bilateral neck dissection
    - Parotid nodal disease – Excision of primary tumor, superficial parotidectomy, and ipsilateral neck dissection
      - Consider role of total parotidectomy
    - A five-year overall survival, 45–50% and disease-specific rates, 60–72% [96]
  - Trunk and extremities
    - Excision of primary tumor and regional lymph node dissection
    - A five-year overall survival, 32–56% [96]
- Reconstruction
  - Delay until final histologic margin assessment complete
- **Adjuvant Therapy**
  - All adjuvant therapies should be discussed at a multidisciplinary tumor board
    - Postoperative adjuvant radiation therapy [47]
      - Local, low-risk positive margins
        - Nonsurgical candidates
      - Local, high-risk/very-high-risk
        - ≥6 cm primary tumor

- Positive margins
- Negative margins if extensive perineural, large, or named nerve involvement or poor prognostic features (see Table 12.1)
- Nonsurgical candidates
  - Lymph node basin after lymphadenectomy
    - Negative margins – 50–60 Gy over 5–6 weeks
    - Positive margins or extracapsular extension (ECE) – 60–66 Gy over 6–7 weeks
    - Trunk and extremities
      - Multiple involved lymph nodes
      - ECE (extracapsular extension)
    - Head and neck [64]
      - Consider if 1 + node ≤3 cm without ECE
      - ≥ 2 + nodes or 1 + >3 cm without ECE
      - Any node with ECE
      - Incomplete lymphadenectomy
  - Lymph node basin without lymphadenectomy (NCCN squamous cell carcinoma)
    - Positive regional lymph nodes but unresectable or medically inoperable – definitive 60–70 Gy over 6–7 weeks
    - Clinically negative but high-risk for metastases – 50 Gy over 5–7 weeks
  - Clinically at-risk nerves – 50–60 Gy over 5–6 weeks
- Systemic therapy
  - Systemic therapy with concurrent radiation therapy
    - Cisplatin – complete response rate 63% [61]
    - EGFR inhibitors
      - Cetuximab – RT vs. cetuximab + RT [10]
        - Disease control rate (DCR) = 14.9 months vs. 24.4 months, overall survival (OS) = 29.3 months vs. 49 months, progression-free survival (PFS) = 12.4 months vs. 17.1 months, objective response rate (ORR) = 64% vs. 74%
      - Erlotinib, gefitinib, and panitumumab
    - Cisplatin + 5-FU
    - Carboplatin ± paclitaxel
  - Systemic therapy alone (Table 12.5)
    - Cemiplimab-rwlc (first-line) [54, 55]
      - Locally advanced, recurrent, or metastatic disease
    - Pembrolizumab
      - KEYNOTE – 629 trial [34]
      - Locally advanced, recurrent, and metastatic disease

Table 12.5 Trials and responses to systemic treatments for locally advanced, recurrent, or metastatic cutaneous squamous cell carcinoma

Trial	Patients	Results
NCT02760498 [55]	Phase II, non-RCT Multicenter, open-label	1-year OS 93% 1-year PFS 58% ORR 44–53% PR 31–35% CR 13–17% DCR 79% DOR ≥ 6 months 68%
	78 patients Locally advanced cSCC Cemiplimab every 2 weeks up to 96 weeks	AEs Grades 3–4 44%
	59 patients Metastatic cSCC Cemiplimab every 2 weeks up to 96 weeks	1-year OS 81% 1-year PFS 53% ORR 47%, PR 40.7%, CR 6.8% DCR 61% AEs Grade ≥ 3 42%
NCT03565783 [26]	Phase II, non-RCT Single-center, open-label	1-year OS 95% 1-year DFS 89.5% 1 year DSS 95% ORR/PR 30% MPR 15%, pCR 55%
	20 patients Newly diagnosed or recurrent resectable cSCC head and neck stages III–IV Cemiplimab two cycles every three weeks + surgery	AEs Grades 1–2 35%, grade 3 5% N
KEYNOTE-629	Phase II, non-RCT Multicenter, open-label	Locally advanced cSCC 1-year OS 73.6% 1-year PFS 54.4% ORR 50%, PR 33.3%, CR 16.7% DCR 64.8% DOR ≥12 months 84.1%
	159 patients 54 locally advanced cSCC 105 recurrent/metastatic cSCC Pembrolizumab every 3 weeks up to 35 cycles	Recurrent/metastatic cSCC 1-year vs. 2-year OS 61% vs. 48.4% 1-yr PFS 36.4% ORR 35.2%, PR 24.8%, CR 16.7% DCR 52.4% DOR ≥12 months 77.8% AEs Grades 3–5 11.9%
NIVOSQUACS	Phase II, non-RCT Multicenter, open-label 31 patients Locally advanced and/or metastatic cSCC 7 prior systemic therapy 24 treatment naïve 11 with concomitant hematologic malignancies Nivolumab every two weeks ≤2 years	Overall Median OS not reached Median PFS 11.1 months ORR 61.3%, PR 38.7%, CR 22.6% DCR 64.5% Prior systemic therapy ORR 71.4% DCR 85% Concomitant hematologic malignancy Median OS and PFS 20.7 months and 10.9 months ORR 45.5% DCR 54.5% AEs Grade ≥ 3

(continued)

Table 12.5 (continued)

Trial	Patients	Results
Cetuximab [51]	Phase II, non-RCT Multicenter, open-label 36 patients Locally advanced or metastatic cSCC Evidence of mod-strong EGFR expression Cetuximab weekly up until 48 weeks	48-week OS 52% Median PFS 4.1 months ORR 28%, PR 22%, and CR 6% DCR 69% AEs Grades 3–4 64% Median age of study population 79 years
Panitumumab [27]	Phase II, non-RCT Single-center, open-label 16 patients Locally advanced, recurrent, or metastatic cSCC Panitumumab weekly until disease progression, toxicity, or nine total cycles	Median OS 11 months Median PFS 8 months ORR 31%, PR 18.8%, and CR 12.5% Median DOR 6 mo 6-wk DCR 69% AEs Grades 3–4 31%
NCT01198028 [30]	Phase II, non-RCT Single-center, open-label 39 patients Locoregional or metastatic cSCC without curative-intent therapy Erlotinib daily for 28-day cycles until disease progression	1-year and 3-year OS 53% and 19% Median PFS 4.7 months ORR/PR 10% DCR 72% Modest activity in incurable cSCC
NCT00054691 [87]	Phase II, non-RCT Single-center, open label 40 patients Locoregionally recurrent and/or metastatic cSCC not amenable to surgery or radiation Gefitinib daily until disease progression or toxicity	Median OS 12.9 months Median PFS 3.8 months ORR/PR 16% Median DOR 31.4 months AEs Grade 3 16% ORR did not meet targeted rate of 20%

- Nivolumab
    - NIVOSQUACS trial [43]
        - Locally advanced and metastatic cSCC
        - Included progressing or stable hematologic malignancies
- If ineligible for or progressed on immunotherapy
    - Carboplatin ± paclitaxel – if ineligible for immune checkpoint inhibitors
    - EGFR inhibitors
        - Cetuximab – Phase II trial [51]
            - Consider use in elderly patients (median age 79 years old)
        - Panitumumab – Phase II study [27]
            - Treatment option for incurable cSCC without local therapy options

- Erlotinib – Phase II trial [30]
  - Modest activity
- Gefitinib – Phase II trial [89]
  • Systemic chemotherapy
    - Data limited to case series and small retrospective studies
    - Cisplatin – ORR = 45%, CR = 22%, and DFS 14.6 months [79]
    - Can consider capecitabine, cisplatin + 5-FU, and carboplatin
• **Neoadjuvant Therapy**
  - Borderline resectable, unresectable, or high morbidity resections
  - Cemiplimab-rwlc
    • NCT03565783 Phase II trial [26]
      - Neoadjuvant immunotherapy safe and results in ~40% response rates
• **Management of Recurrence**
  - Local – see "Choice of therapy – local disease"
  - Regional – see "Regional lymph node examination," "choice of therapy – positive regional lymph nodes"
  - Distant metastases – multidisciplinary consultation
    • See "locally advanced unresectable, metastatic disease, or nonsurgical candidate"
    • Clinical trial

Basal Cell Skin Cancer

- **Introduction**
  - Basal cell cancer is the most common cancer worldwide.
  - Diagnosis is made by physical exam and confirmed via biopsy.
  - Although rare, locally advanced disease can be assessed with US, CT, and MRI.
  - Surgical excision is the current standard of care with a variety of modalities including topical therapies, radiotherapy, and systemic therapies.
- **Diagnosis**
  - History – enlarging, nonhealing skin lesions
  - Symptoms may include bleeding or pruritus or may be asymptomatic.
  - Physical exam findings concerning for regional metastatic disease (very rare)
    • Cervical, occipital, axillary, or inguinal lymphadenopathy
  - Risk factors [12]
    • Intense, intermittent sun exposure
    • Increasing age
    • Fair skin, red or blond hair, light eye color, inability to tan, and propensity to freckle
    • Recreational tanning/tanning beds
    • Immunosuppression

- HPV/HIV/AIDS
- Exposure to ionizing radiation
- Chemical exposure
  - Arsenic
- Personal history of skin cancer
- Family history of skin cancer
- Genetic syndromes [36]
  - Xeroderma pigmentosum
  - Oculocutaneous albinism
  - Muir-Torre syndrome
  - Fanconi anemia
  - Nevoid basal cell (Gorlin) syndrome
  - Bloom syndrome
  - Werner syndrome
  - Rombo syndrome
  - Bazex-Dupre-Chrisol syndrome
- Psoralen/PUVA for psoriasis
- Screening recommendations and total body skin exam
  - Immunosuppressed [97]
    - No skin cancer/field disease every 12 months
    - Field disease/one NMSC every 3–6 months
    - High-risk cSCC/multiple NMSC every 3 months
  - Xeroderma pigmentosum [46]
    - Every 3–6 months
  - Oculocutaneous albinism
    - Every 6–12 months
  - Muir-Torre syndrome
    - Annually
  - Fanconi anemia
    - Annually
  - Nevoid basal cell (Gorlin) syndrome [84]
    - Annual exams starting at age 10
    - Every 3–6 months after first BCC
  - Bloom syndrome
  - Werner syndrome
  - Rombo syndrome
    - Annual exams starting before age 10
  - Bazex-Dupre-Chrisol syndrome
    - Every 6–12 months before age 10
- Chemoprevention
  - No current recommendations although NCCN recognizes further clinical investigation is necessary for the following:
  - Solid organ transplant recipients
    - Nicotinamide did not lead to reduction in BCC incidence in SOTR at 12 months [3] (ONTRANS trial)

- Immunocompetent, high-risk of recurrence or metastases
  - Nicotinamide B3 and 500 mg BID
    - Phase III RCT 20% reduction in 12-month rate of new BCC [16] (ONTRAC trial)
  - Celecoxib
    - Phase III RCT = 56% relative risk reduction in BCC incidence at 11 months [24]
  - DFMO (α-difluoromethylornithine)
    - Phase III RCT = 30% relative risk reduction in BCC incidence at 4 years [5]
- Basal-cell nevus (Gorlin) syndrome
  - Vismodegib
    - NCT00957229 trial [74]
      - Basal-cell nevus syndrome with ≥10 surgically eligible BCCs
      - Daily Vismodegib for 3 months vs. placebo
      - Reduced incidence of new BCC lesions, size of existing lesions, and number of surgeries to remove BCC lesions
  - Adverse events lead to treatment interruption → tumor recurrence

- **Evaluation and Clinical Stage**
  - History and physical exam
    - History focusing on risk factors
    - Total body skin examination
      - Clinical exam findings consistent with BCC
        - Shiny
        - Pearly papule or nodule
        - Rolled borders and central clearing
        - Arborizing telangiectasias
        - Induration
        - Infiltrated plaque
      - Dermoscopy – diagnostic accuracy 95–99%
  - Biopsy and Pathology [12, 13]
    - Punch, shave, and excisional biopsy acceptable
    - Size and depth should be adequate to assess high-risk pathologic findings
    - Subtypes
      - Nodular, superficial, infundibulocystic, fibroepithelial, morpheaform, infiltrative, micronodular, and basosquamous
    - Clinically suspicious lesions for locoregional or metastatic disease
      - FNA, core needle biopsy, or excisional biopsy
    - Clinical imaging, if clinically concerning
    - CT with contrast to evaluate for bone disease or nodal involvement
    - MRI with contrast to assess for peripheral nerve involvement
  - Risk factors for recurrence – Table 12.6 (NCCN Basal cell Skin cancer 2024)

Table 12.6 Stratification of risk factors in local basal cell carcinoma for recurrence

Risk group	Low risk	High risk
H&P		
Location/size	Trunk, extremities <2 cm	Trunk, extremities ≥2 cm Head, neck, hands, feet, pretibial, and anogenital area (any size)
Borders	Well-defined	Poorly defined
Primary vs. recurrent	Primary	Recurrent
Immunosuppression	–	+
Site of prior RT	–	+
Pathology		
Subtype	Nodular and superficial	Aggressive growth pattern
Perineural involvement	–	+

Choice of Therapy [92]

- Local disease
  - Low-risk = Curettage and electrodessication, shave excision, standard excision, topical therapy, or definitive RT
  - High-risk = Mohs or PDEMA, standard excision, definitive RT, systemic therapy, or neoadjuvant vismodegib + PDEMA
- Positive margins following resection
  - Low-risk = Mohs or PDEMA, reexcision if feasible, RT for nonsurgical candidates
  - High-risk
    - Mohs or PDEMA as primary treatment = reresect, RT, or systemic therapy
    - Standard excision as primary treatment = Mohs or PDEMA, standard reexcision, multidisciplinary consultation, RT or systemic therapy (if unresectable)
- Locally advanced, unresectable, metastatic disease and nonsurgical candidates
  - Primary or recurrent nodal metastasis – multidisciplinary consultation
    - Surgery = Excision of primary tumor and regional lymph node dissection
    - RT
    - Systemic therapy = Hedgehog pathway inhibitors (HHI: vismodegib, sonidegib), cemiplimab-rwlc, clinical trial
  - Distant metastases – multidisciplinary consultation
    - Systemic therapy = HHI (vismodegib), cemiplimab-rwlc
    - RT or surgery for limited disease
    - Palliative and supportive care
- **Nonoperative Therapy**
  - Curettage and Electrodesiccation
    - Does not allow histologic margin assessment
    - A five-year recurrence rates 1.8–40% depending on high-risk pathology

- Contraindications as definitive therapy:
  - Areas of terminal hair growth – scalp, pubic or axillary regions, and beard area – due to potential follicular extension of tumor
  - If subcutaneous tissue reached requires surgical excision
  - Biopsy of lesion reveals high-risk pathologic features
- Consider on head, neck, and pretibial lesions < 6 mm depth if not candidate for Mohs or PDEMA
- Cryotherapy
  - Poorer cosmetic outcomes
  - A five-year recurrence rate 5–39% in prospective trials (NCCN 2023 basal cell skin cancer)
- Topical therapy
  - 5-FU
    - A five-year DFS 70.0% and cure rates up to 90% in superficial subtypes [38]
  - Imiquimod
    - Effective for superficial and nodular subtypes
    - 82.5% clinical success rate [7, 89]
- Photodynamic therapy [6]
  - Most evidence for superficial and nodular subtype
  - Optimal cosmetic outcomes compared to surgery or cryotherapy
  - Cure rates 60–100% (NCCN 2023 basal cell skin cancer)
- Radiation therapy
  - Primary lesion
    - 70–93 Gy for definitive conventional fractionation
    - 56–88 Gy for definitive hypofractionation
    - A five-year local control rate up to 95% [86]
    - A five-year recurrence rate 8.7% [66]
    - Efficacy dependent on stage, primary or recurrent, size, and histologic subtype
  - Lymph node basin
    - Clinically negative, at risk – 50 Gy over 5–7 weeks
    - Clinically positive – definitive 60–70 Gy over 6–7 weeks
- **Surgical Therapy**
  - Mohs vs. standard surgical excision
    - A five-year recurrence = primary lesions 2.5% vs. 4.1% and recurrent lesions 2.4% vs. 12.1% [57]
  - Mohs
    - Allows intraoperative analysis of 100% of excision margin via thin sequential excisions
    - Indications:
      - Low-risk lesions with positive margin following standard excision
    - High-risk lesions (first-line)
    - Unable to achieve negative margins with standard excision in high-risk lesions

- Significant tissue-sparing compared to standard excision (Muller et al. 2009; [83])
- PDEMA (see "surgical therapy – squamous cell carcinoma")
- Low-risk
  - Standard excision
    - 4 mm clinical margins
    - Cure rates up to 99% [70]
  - Postoperative margin assessment
    - Intraoperative frozen section
    - Permanent margin analysis with delayed tissue repair
- High risk
  - Standard excision
    - >4 mm clinical margins
    - No definitive margin recommendations due to high variability of high-risk lesions and lack of evidence
    - Key: Complete histologic margin assessment
  - Mohs or other PDEMA methods (preferred)
- Reconstruction
  - Delay reconstruction if significant tissue rearrangements required until negative histologic margins confirmed
  - Standard excision = linear repair, skin graft, or healing by secondary intention
  - Mohs = complex linear closure, skin flaps, skin grafts, and interpolation flaps or healing via secondary intention [9]
- **Adjuvant Therapy**
  - All adjuvant therapies should be discussed at a multidisciplinary tumor board
  - Adjuvant radiation therapy
    - 60–79 Gy for conventional fractionation
    - 56–70 Gy for hypofractionation
    - Local, low-risk positive margins
      - Nonsurgical candidates
    - Local, high-risk
      - Positive margins after Mohs or PDEMA
      - Positive margins after standard excision if further resection not feasible via Mohs or PDEMA
      - Negative margins but extensive perineural or large-nerve involvement [52]
        - 50–60 Gy over 5–6 weeks
    - Lymph node basin following lymphadenectomy
      - Negative margins, no ECE – 50–60 Gy over 5–6 weeks
      - Positive margins or ECE – 60–66 Gy over 6–7 weeks
  - Systemic therapy (Table 12.7)
    - Hedgehog pathway inhibitors (HHIs) (first line)
      - Vismodegib (first line)
        - Recurrence following surgery for locoregional or metastatic disease
        - Nonsurgical or radiation therapy candidates

Table 12.7 Hedgehog pathway inhibitor and immunotherapy trials for basal cell skin cancer

Trial	Patients	Results
ERIVANCE BCC	Phase II, non-RCT Multicenter 104 patients 71 locally advanced BCC 33 metastatic BCC Vismodegib daily	LaBCC 3-yr OS 79.4% PFS 12.9 months DOR 26.2 months ORR 60.3%, PR 28.6%, and CR 31.7% mBCC 3-yr OS 48.5% PFS 9.3 months DOR 14.8 months ORR/PR 48.5% AEs 100%, grade ≥ 3 55.4–56.3%
BOLT	Phase II, RCT Multicenter, double-blind 230 patients 194 laBCC: 66200 mg, 128,800 mg 36 mBCC: 13200 mg, 23,800 mg and 42 months analysis	LaBCC 200 mg: ORR 56%, PR 55%, CR 5%, DCR 91% DOR 26.1 months PFS 22.1 months 800 mg: ORR 46.1%, PR 44.5%, CR 1.6%, DCR 82% DOR 23.3 months, and PFS 24.9 months MBCC 200 mg: ORR/PR 8%, DCR 92% DOR 24 months, PFS 13.1 months 800 mg: ORR/PR 17%, DCR 91% DOR not estimable, PFS 11.1 months AEs 200 mg: 98%, grades 3–4 43% 800 mg: Grades 3–4 64%
NCT03132636 [73]	Phase II, non-RCT Multicenter, open-label 84 patients LaBCC or mBCC progressed or intolerant to HHI Cemiplimab every 3 weeks for 93 weeks	ORR 31%, PR 25%, CR 6% DCR 60% DOR 91% @ 6 months, 85% 12 months PFS 19 months 2-year OS 80% AEs 100%, grades 3–4 47%
VISMONEO	Phase II, non-RCT Multicenter, open-label 55 patients ≥1 facial BCC, inoperable or operable with functional or major aesthetic sequelae risk Vismodegib daily 4–10 months + surgery	80% had surgical downstaging ORR 70.9%, PR 45.5%, CR 25.5%, and Three-year recurrence 36.4% AEs 98.2%, grade ≥ 3 20%

(continued)

Table 12.7 (continued)

Trial	Patients	Results
NCT00957229 [74]	Phase II, RCT Multicenter, double-blind, placebo-controlled	
	41 patients Basal-cell nevus syndrome ≥10 surgically eligible BCCs Vismodegib vs. placebo over 3 months comparing new lesion development	Decreased surgically eligible BCCs 2 v 34 per year Crossover from placebo reduced new BCCs 0.4 v. 30 Noninterrupted treatment reduced new BCCs 0.6 vs. 1.7 Two patients developed resistance AEs 17% tolerated therapy for full 36 months

- ERIVANCE BCC trial [69]
  - Locally advanced BCC (laBCC) and metastatic BCC (mBCC)
  - Vismodegib daily until disease progression, unacceptable toxicity, or withdrawal from study
- Adverse events: significant and poorly tolerated
  - Treatment-emergent = muscle spasms, alopecia, taste loss, weight loss, decreased appetite, fatigue, nausea, and diarrhea
  - Serious – 25–32%
- Consider the development of drug resistance [22]
  - Sonidegib (second-line)
    - Recurrence following surgery or radiation therapy
    - Nonsurgical or radiation therapy in laBCC only, not mBCC
    - BOLT trial [53] [23]
      - laBCC and mBCC
      - Sonidegib daily at either dose of 200 mg or 800 mg
    - Adverse events: significant and poorly tolerated
    - Consider the development of drug resistance
- Immunotherapy
  - Cemiplimab-rwlc
    - Previous treatment with HHI or when HHI not appropriate
      - NCT03132636 trial [73]
      - laBCC or mBCC progressed on HHI/intolerant
      - Cemiplimab every 3 weeks for 93 weeks
- **Neoadjuvant Therapy**
  - Locally advanced disease where surgery associated with significant damage
  - VISMONEO [8]
    - Locally advanced facial lesions prior to curative intent surgery via PDEMA
    - Vismodegib daily 4–10 months prior to curative operation
    - Effective at surgical downstaging

- **Management of Recurrence**
  - Local – see "Choice of Therapy – local disease – high-risk"
  - Primary or recurrent nodal metastases – see "Choice of Therapy – Locally advanced, unresectable, metastatic disease, nonsurgical candidates – Primary or recurrent nodal metastasis"
  - Distant metastases – see "Choice of Therapy – Distant metastases"

Merkel Cell Carcinoma

- **Introduction**
  - Merkel cell carcinoma (MCC) is a rare, aggressive cutaneous neuroendocrine malignancy due to its potential for metastases
  - Diagnosis is often challenging clinically and requires confirmation via biopsy.
  - Locally advanced and metastatic disease can be assessed with US, CT, and MRI PET/CT.
  - Surgical resection is the cornerstone of management for localized disease.
  - Sentinel lymph node biopsy of draining lymph node basin is essential for prognostication.
  - Locally advanced, unresectable, and metastatic disease may be treated with a variety of radiation and systemic therapy including immunotherapy and rarely chemotherapy.
- **Diagnosis**
  - Lesions are usually asymptomatic.
  - History – painless, nontender, rapidly growing lesion
  - Physical exam findings concerning for metastatic disease
    - Cervical, occipital, axillary, or inguinal lymphadenopathy
  - Differential diagnosis
    - Cutaneous lymphoma
    - Melanoma
    - Ewing sarcoma
    - Neuroblastoma
    - Metastatic small cell lung cancer (SCLC)
  - Risk factors [95]
    - Ultraviolet light exposure
    - Merkel cell polyomavirus
    - Increasing age > 65 years old
    - Male sex
    - Fair skin
    - Immunosuppression – solid organ transplant
    - HIV
    - Chronic inflammatory disorders
    - Lymphoproliferative malignancies

- **Evaluation and Clinical Stage**
    - History and Physical Exam
        - History focusing on risk factors
        - Total body skin examination
            - Clinical exam findings consistent with MCC [18]
                - Variable signs, often misdiagnosed as benign lesion
                - Papule
                - Plaque
                - Cyst-like structures
                    - Dermoscopy is not definitive but can aid in decision to biopsy
                        - Polymorphous vascular pattern with architectural disruption
                        - Milky-red areas on white sheen
                        - Large-caliber arborizing vessels
                        - Sharply and poorly focused vessels
        - Lymph node examination
    - Biopsy and Pathology [29]
        - Shave, punch, incisional, or excisional biopsy acceptable
        - Histopathology
            - Dermal tumor with sheets and nests of crowded basaloid cells
            - "Salt and pepper" chromatin pattern, indistinct nucleoli, and scant cytoplasm
        - Immunohistochemistry critical to diagnostic confirmation
            - Cytokeratin 20 (CK2–) – diffuse cytoplasmic and paranuclear dot-like (sensitive stain)
            - Thyroid transcription factor 1 (TTF-1): – in MCC, + SCLC
            - Neuron-specific enolase (sensitive stain)
            - Synaptophysin
            - Chromogranin A – diffuse cytoplasmic (specific stain)
    - Merkel cell polyomavirus (MCPyV) oncoprotein antibodies [63]
        - Consider assessment of serum MCPyV oncoprotein antibodies within 3 months of treatment
            - Seropositive – Serial titers during surveillance to detect recurrence
            - Seronegative – Higher risk of recurrence, consider more intensive surveillance
    - Regional lymph node examination
        - US can be used as initial assessment of palpable regional lymph nodes
        - CT scan with contrast
            - Specific but not sensitive for nodal metastases
- FDG PET/CT
    - Increased sensitivity for detection of nodal disease compared to CT
    - Systemic imaging to evaluate metastatic disease
        - CT chest/abdomen/pelvis with contrast (can include head/neck as indicated)
            - Sensitive but not specific
        - FDG PET/CT skull to foot

- Often recommended due to high rate of occult metastases, 12–20%, in asymptomatic patients [72]
        - High sensitivity and specificity
    - MRI brain
        - Consider for patients suspicious for CNS metastases or those with widespread metastases
- Biopsy clinically suspicious lesions for locoregional or metastatic disease
    - FNA, core needle, or excisional biopsy
    - Multidisciplinary consultation
    - TNM Clinical and pathologic staging – Tables 12.8 and 12.9
    - AJCC Prognostic groups – Tables 12.10 and 12.11
- **Choice of Therapy**
    - Local disease
        - Standard excision preferred 1–2 cm margins, Mohs or PDEMA, or definitive RT
            - Margin + = reexcision preferred, RT alternative
            - Margin − and no adverse risk factors = consider observation
            - Margin − and adverse risk factors = adjuvant RT
        - Sentinel lymph node biopsy (SLNB)
            - Negative
                - Observation of nodal basin
                - Consider adjuvant RT to nodal basin for high-risk false negatives
            - Positive
                - See "Choice of Therapy – Positive regional lymph nodes"

Table 12.8 Clinical TNM Staging Classification of Merkel cell carcinoma (AJCC 8th edition)

T0	No evidence of primary tumor
Tis	In situ primary tumor
T1	≤2 cm
T2	>2 but ≤5 cm
T3	>5 cm
T4	Tumor invades fascia, muscle, cartilage, or bone
N0	No LN metastasis detected on clinical and/or radiologic exam
N1	Metastasis in regional LN(s)
N2	Intransit metastasis[a] without LN metastasis
N3	Intransit metastasis[a] with LN metastasis
M0	No distant metastasis on clinical and/or radiologic examination
M1	Distant metastasis detected on clinical and/or radiologic examination
M1a	Metastasis to distant skin, distant subcutaneous tissue, or distant LN(s)
M1b	Metastasis to the lung
M1c	Metastasis to all over visceral sites

[a]Discontinuous from primary tumor located between primary tumor and draining regional nodal basin or distal to the primary tumor

Table 12.9 Pathologic TNM staging classification of Merkel cell carcinoma (AJCC 8th edition)

T0	No evidence of primary tumor
Tis	In situ primary tumor
T1	≤2 cm
T2	>2 but ≤5 cm
T3	>5 cm
T4	Tumor invades the fascia, muscle, cartilage, or bone
N0	No regional LN metastasis detected on pathologic evaluation
N1	Metastasis in regional LN(s)
N1a(sn)	Clinically occult regional LN metastasis identified only by SLNB
N1a	Clinically occult regional LN metastasis following LN dissection
N1b	Clinically and/or radiologically detected regional LN metastasis, microscopically confirmed
N2	Intransit[a] metastasis without LN metastasis
N3	Intransit[a] metastasis with LN metastasis
M0	No distant metastasis detected on clinical and/or radiologic examination
M1	Distant metastasis microscopically confirmed
M1a	Metastasis to distant skin, distant subcutaneous tissue, or distant LN(s), microscopically confirmed
M1b	Metastasis to the lung, microscopically confirmed
M1c	Metastasis to all other distant sites, microscopically confirmed

[a]Discontinuous from primary tumor located between primary tumor and draining regional nodal basin or distal to the primary tumor

Table 12.10 Clinical prognostic stage groups for Merkel cell carcinoma (AJCC 8th edition)

	T	N	M
Stage 0	Tis	N0	M0
Stage I	T1	N0	M0
Stage IIA	T2–T3	N0	M0
Stage IIB	T4	N0	M0
Stage III	T0–T4	N1–N3	M0
Stage IV	T0–T4	Any N	M1

Table 12.11 Pathologic prognostic stage groups for Merkel cell carcinoma (AJCC 8th edition)

	T	N	M
Stage 0	Tis	N0	M0
Stage I	T1	N0	M0
Stage IIA	T2–T3	N0	M0
Stage IIB	T4	N0	M0
Stage IIIA	T1–T4	N1a(sn) or N1a	M0
	T0	N1b	M0
Stage IIIB	T1–T4	N1b-3	M0
Stabe IV	T0–T4	Any N	M1

- Positive regional lymph nodes
  - Excision of primary tumor +
    - Lymph node dissection + RT
    - Lymph node dissection or RT
    - Consider clinical trial for adjuvant therapy
  - Consider neoadjuvant immunotherapy prior to surgical excision for large locally advanced or clinical bulky nodal disease
- Locally advanced unresectable, metastatic disease, or nonsurgical candidate
  - RT, systemic therapy, clinical trial, and excision for limited metastases
- **Nonoperative Therapy**
  - Radiation therapy
    - Local disease, surgery refused, unresectable disease; MCC is very radiosensitive (NCCN Merkel Cell 2023)
      - 60–66 Gy for definitive dose
      - Schedule and fractionation to be determined by radiation oncologist
      - Median OS = 25 months, 5-year OS = 32%, 8-year OS = 25% for stage I/stage II [93]
    - Locoregional disease (NCCN Merkel Cell 2023)
      - Consider irradiation of intransit lymphatics of primary site close to nodal basin
      - Clinically node-negative, at risk for subclinical disease – 46–50 Gy
      - Clinically node-positive – 60–66 Gy
      - Median OS = 15 months, 5-year OS = 19%, 8-year OS = 16% [93]
- **Surgical Therapy**
  - Stage I/stage II: Median OS = 76 months, 5-year OS = 61%, 8-year OS = 42% [93]
  - Stage III: Median OS = 30 months, 5-year OS = 34%, 8-yearr OS = 21% [93]
  - Wide local excision (WLE)
    - 1–2-cm clinical margins to investing muscle fascia or pericranium
      - Sensitive areas such as the face, scalp, and ears may be unable to achieve 2-cm margins without significant morbidity
    - Consider feasibility of primary closure to expedite adjuvant radiation therapy
    - Margin size in stage I/stage II [4]
      - ≤1.0 cm: Median OS = 69 months
      - 1.1–2.0 cm: Median OS = 95 months
      - >2.0 cm: Median OS = 91 months
  - Mohs or PDE–A – See "Squamous cell carcinoma – Surgical therapy – Mohs/PDEMA"
    - Can be considered in select cases for margin control

- Similar rates of recurrence and survival
  - Stage I/stage II: Mohs vs. WLE [71]
  - Three-year overall survival = 65.1% vs. 68.1% ($p = 0.841$)
- Benefit: complete histologic margin assessment
- Sentinel lymph node biopsy
  - Indicated in all patients with clinically node-negative disease
    - SLN positivity 30–40% [33, 67]
  - Predictors of SLN positivity [48]
    - Primary site – head and neck
    - Presence of lymphovascular invasion, which portends worsened outcomes
    - Tumor size
    - Immunosuppression – history of chronic lymphocytic leukemia (CLL) and solid organ transplant
  - Positive SLN requires imaging to quantify regional and distant metastatic disease
  - False-negative rate up to 21% [32]
- Lymphadenectomy (LND)
  - Indications – Clinical node (+) and pathologic node (+) after SLNB
  - Provides optimal control of regional disease
  - Retrospective data – Increased DFS (28.5 months vs. 11.8 months) but no effects on overall survival [35]
- Reconstruction
  - Delay until negative histologic margins are verified and SLNB performed
  - Primary closure should be chosen, if possible, to allow for expeditious initiation of adjuvant radiation therapy

- **Adjuvant Therapy**
  - All adjuvant therapy should be discussed at a multidisciplinary tumor board
    - Postoperative adjuvant radiation therapy
      - Primary site – Negative resection margins – 50–56 Gy
        - Margin size in stage I/stage II with adjuvant radiation therapy [4]
          - ≤ 1.0 cm ($p = <0.001$)
            - + RT: Median OS = 84 months
            - − RT: Median OS = 56 months
          - 1.1–2.0 cm (p=0.046)
            - + RT: Median OS = 125 months
            - − RT: Median OS = 84 months
        - Stage I/stage II: A two-year recurrence-free survival in RT vs. observation [39]
          - Local = 89% vs. 36%
          - Regional = 84% vs. 43%
        - Stage I/stage II: guideline-concordant RT vs. observation [90]
          - A five-year OS = 75.7% vs. 68.2% ($p = <0.005$)
        - Adverse risk factors guiding preference for radiation
          - Primary tumor > 1 cm

- Chronic T-cell immunosuppression
- HIV
- CLL
- Solid organ transplant
- Head/neck primary site
- Lymphovascular invasion
- Primary site – Microscopically positive resection margins – 56–60 Gy
- Primary site – Grossly positive resection margins and further resection not possible – 60–66 Gy
- Lymph node basin without SLNB or LND
  - Clinically node-positive – 60–66 Gy
  - Clinically node –negative, but at risk for subclinical disease (See "Adverse risk factors) – 46–50 Gy
- Lymph node basin with SLNB without LND
  - SLN negative – observation (See "Adverse risk factors")
  - SLN positive – 50–56 Gy
    - Microscopic nodal disease = small metastatic foci, no ECE
  - A three-year OS observation vs. RT = 49.2% vs. 70.5% [19]
- Lymph node basin after LND – 60–66 Gy
  - Multiple involved nodes and/or ECE
  - A three-year OS LND vs. LND + RT = 52.9% vs. 79.5% [19]
- Systemic therapy (Table 12.12)
  - Regional disease
    - Clinical trial
    - Adjuvant chemotherapy not routinely recommended
  - Recurrent locally advanced or regional disease
    - Pembrolizumab – if curative surgery or curative RT are not feasible
    - Retifanlimab-dlwr – patient not amenable to surgery or RT
  - Disseminated metastatic disease
    - Clinical trial
    - Avelumab
      - JAVELIN Merkel 200 [20, 21, 40]
        - Chemotherapy-refractory metastatic MCC
        - Treatment-naïve metastatic MCC
        - Avelumab infusion every 2 weeks
    - Nivolumab
      - CheckMate 358 trial [77]
        - MCC with ≤ 2 prior therapies
        - Nivolumab every 2 weeks until disease progression or response
    - Pembrolizumab
      - KEYNOTE-017 [60]
        - Distant metastatic or recurrent locoregional MCC
        - Pembrolizumab every 3 weeks for ≤2 years
    - Retifanlimab-dlwr

Table 12.12 Immunotherapy trials and responses for Merkel cell carcinoma

Trial	Patients	Results
JAVELIN Merkel 200 [20, 21, 40]	Phase II non-RCT Multicenter, open-label	
	88 patients Metastatic chemo-refractory MCC Avelumab every 2 weeks	OS 12.6 months 5-year OS 26% ORR 31.8%, PR 22.7%, CR 9.1% AEs 70%, grade 3 5%
	116 patients Treatment-naïve metastatic MCC Avelumab every 2 eeks	OS 20.3 months PFS 4.1 months Response lasting ≥6 months 30.2% ORR 39.7%, PR 23.3%, CR 16.4% AEs 81%, grades 3–4 18.1% Response rates higher in those with MCPyV-negative tumors
CheckMate 358 (NCT02488759) [77, 78]	Phase I/phase II non-RCT Multicenter, open-label	
	25 patients MCC with ≤2 prior therapies Nivolumab every 2 weeks	3-month OS 92% 3-month PFS 82% ORR 68%, PR 55%, CR 14% AEs 68%, grades 3–4 20%
	39 patients Resectable stage IIA–IIIB MCC Nivolumab x2 doses + surgery	47.2% pCR, 15.4% MPR 87.9% had some radiographic tumor reduction 54.5% tumor reduction ≥30% RFS 12 and 24 months = 77.5% and 68.5% (+) MPR/pCR vs. (−) MPR/pCR 12 months 100% vs. 50% 24 months 88.9% vs. 50% OS 12 and 24 mo = 93.2% and 79.4% (+) MPR/pCR 12 months 100% 24 months 88.9% AEs 46.2%, grades 3–4 7.7% 3 patients did not undergo surgery
KEYNOTE-017 (NCT02267603)	Phase II non-RCT Multicenter, open-label 50 patients Unresectable MCC Pembrolizumab every 3 weeks for ≤2 years	3-year OS 59.4% (for responders = 89.5%), median OS not reached 3-year PFS 39.1%, median PFS 16.8 months ORR 58%, PR 28%, CR 30% AEs 98%, grade ≥ 3 30%
POD1UM-201 (NCT03599713)	Phase II non-RCT Multicenter, open-label 65 patients Chemotherapy-naïve metastatic or recurrent unresectable locoregional MCC Retifanlimab every 4 weeks for ≤2 years	ORR 46.2%, PR = 33.8%, CR 12.3% DCR 53.8% AEs 75.9%, grade ≥ 3 42.5%

- POD1UM-201 [31]
    - Metastatic or recurrent unresectable locoregional metastatic MCC
    - Retifanlimab every 4 weeks for ≤2 years
  - Cytotoxic chemotherapy (rare)
    - Overall response rates 40–60%
    - Median duration of response = 2–9 months
    - Cisplatin ± etoposide (most common)
    - Carboplatin ± etoposide (most common)
    - Cyclophosphamide, doxorubicin, and vincristine
    - Topotecan
- **Neoadjuvant Therapy** (Table 12.12)
  - CheckMate 358 trial – Nivolumab led to increased pCR (47.2%) and major pathologic response (15.4%) which was significantly associated with recurrence-free survival [78]
- **Management of Recurrence**
  - Local – Consider clinical trial
    - Systemic therapy ± RT ± surgical resection
  - Regional – Consider clinical trial
    - Systemic therapy ± RT ± surgical resection
  - Distant metastases – See "Choice of therapy – Locally advanced unresectable, metastatic disease, or nonsurgical candidate"

Dermatofibrosarcoma Protuberans

- **Introduction**
  - Dermatofibrosarcoma protuberans (DFSP) is rare cutaneous soft tissue sarcoma which is locally aggressive.
  - Diagnosis obtained via biopsy.
  - 5–10% of DFSPs have high-grade sarcomatous component and are considered an intermediate or high-grade sarcoma (DFSP-FS).
  - Metastases are rare (<5%) but local recurrences are common.
  - MRI can be used to assess degree of subcutaneous tissue involvement
  - >90% of DFSPs are caused by a translocation between chromosomes 17 and 22 causing a fusion protein transcript *PDGFB/COL1A1* with autocrine PDGFBR tyrosine kinase activation.
  - Surgical resection is the standard of care with options for radiotherapy as well targeted therapy for locally advanced or recurrent disease.
- **Diagnosis**
  - Symptoms may include ulceration, bleeding, and pain.
  - History – Small skin plaque that enlarges over months or years, becomes large, and protrudes as a skin nodule with fast growth

- Differential diagnosis
    - Dermatofibroma
    - Keloid
    - Lipoma
    - Abscess
- Risk factors
    - Male gender
    - African American race
    - Prior trauma or scar
- **Evaluation and Clinical Stage**
    - History and physical exam [85]
        - Total body skin examination
            - Pink, violaceous, or reddish-brown
            - Single lesion but possible satellite nodules
            - Irregular borders or fingerlike extensions
        - Regional lymph node evaluation
    - Biopsy and Pathology
        - Core needle, punch, or incisional biopsy to ensure sampling of subcutaneous tissue
        - Subtypes
            - Giant cell fibroblastoma, pigmented, atrophic, sclerosing, myxoid, myxoid, granular cell, and fibrosarcomatous transformation
        - Histopathology
            - Spindle cells with low mitotic activity arranged in storiform or fascicular pattern with minimal pleomorphism
            - DFSP-FS: herringbone pattern, increased cellularity, high pleomorphism, and mitotic rate >5/10 hpfs
                - Treat as true sarcoma
        - Immunohistochemistry
            - CD34+, vimentin+
            - Factor XIIIA-, desmin -, smooth muscle actin-, S100-, keratin-
        - Consider fluorescence in situ hybridization (FISH), and polymerase chain reaction (PCR) to detect t(17;22)(q22;q13) translocation for diagnostic confirmation
    - Clinical imaging
        - MRI
            - Preoperative planning
            - Determine extent of subcutaneous extension
- **Choice of Therapy** (NCCN DFSP)
    - Resectable disease
        - Mohs or PDEMA or wide local excision (WLE)
        - Positive margins + candidate for reresection
            - Mohs or PDEMA or WLE
        - Positive margins + noncandidate for reresection
            - Consider radiation therapy

- Borderline resectable disease
  - Consider neoadjuvant therapy
  - Mohs or PDEMA, WLE, and radiation therapy
- Unresectable or metastatic disease
  - Systemic targeted therapy, radiation therapy, and multidisciplinary consultation
- **Surgical Therapy**
  - No definitive resection margin, but goal is clear surgical margins
    - Classically margins of 2–3 cm
    - Relative risk reduction of 83% when resection margin ≥3 cm [15]
      - ≥3 cm margins = 3.9% recurrence
      - <3 cm margins = 23.1% recurrence
  - Mohs or PDEMA (first-line) – See "Squamous cell carcinoma – Surgical therapy – Mohs/PDEMA"
    - Preferred method to prevent missing small foci of tumor
    - Real-time histologic assessment of peripheral and deep margins limits overall tissue defect
    - Local recurrence rate [49]
      - DFSP + DFSP-FS = 1.5%
      - DFSP = 1.5%
  - Wide local excision
    - Inability to perform complete histologic assessment of margins
    - Local recurrence rate [49]
      - DFSP + DFPS-FS = 9.4%
      - DFSP = 8.1%
    - Median excision margin of 2 cm cm with total peripheral margin pathologic evaluation [25]
      - 0.9% recurrence rate at median follow-up of 64 months
  - Can consider combination for Mohs or PDEMA technique for peripheral margin clearance and WLE for deep margin clearance
    - 57 patients treated with staged Mohs of peripheral margin and WLE of deep margin and no recurrence at 3 years [14]
  - Reconstruction
    - Tissue rearrangement delayed until complete histologic margin assessment.
    - If concern for positive histologic margins, split thickness skin grafting is recommended to monitor for recurrence instead of tissue rearrangement.
- **Adjuvant Therapy**
  - All adjuvant therapies should be discussed at multidisciplinary tumor board.
    - Postoperative adjuvant radiation therapy (NCCN DFSP)
      - Positive margins or recurrence or metastasis
        - Indeterminate or positive margins – 50–60 Gy
        - Positive margins or gross tumor – up to 66 Gy
        - Recurrence rate after WLE + RT = 14.23% [17]
      - Negative margins
        - Consider if margins < 1 cm

- Recurrence rate after WLE + RT = 0% [17]
  - Disease-free recurrence: 86% at 10.5 years [88]
  - 5-year OS = 100% for RT for positive margin or possible local recurrence [11]
- Targeted therapy
  - Imatinib
    - Locally advanced or metastatic disease
    - Systematic review [59]
      - ORR = 60.5%, PR = 55.2%, CR 5.2%
      - DCR = 27.6%
- **Neoadjuvant Therapy**
  - Imatinib
    - Consider for unresectable or borderline resectable disease
    - Phase II nonrandomized trial (DeCOG) – 16 patients with advanced primary or locally recurrent disease received imatinib + surgery [82]
      - PR = 50%, CR = 7.1%, DCR = 35.7%, progressive disease 14.3%
      - No local recurrence at 6.4 years
- **Management of Recurrence**
  - Local – See "Choice of therapy – resectable and borderline resectable disease"
  - Metastasis – multidisciplinary consultation

Malignant Cutaneous Adnexal Tumors

- Rare, associated with germline mutations
- A ten-year overall survival and disease-specific survival, 54% and 97% [50]
- Eccrine and apocrine gland tumors
  - Porocarcinoma – head/neck and lower extremities in older patient
    - Tx: WLE, lymph node dissection for clinically positive LNs
  - Adenoid cystic carcinoma – Rx: WLE
  - Mucinous carcinoma and endocrine mucin-producing sweat gland carcinoma
    - Scalp, eyelids, and axilla
    - Endocrine mucin-producing sweat gland carcinoma can be precursor to mucinous carcinoma – on or near eyelid
  - Microcystic adnexal carcinoma occurs on central face
    - WLE/Mohs +/− RT
  - Digital papillary adenocarcinoma occurs on volar surface of digits of the hands and feet
    - Rx: WLE or digital amputation
  - Extramammary Paget disease
    - Primary cutaneous or secondary cutaneous involvement of GI or GU carcinoma
  - Cutaneous cribriform carcinoma – low-grade sweat gland carcinoma on upper and lower extremities
    - Surgical excision

- Cutaneous secretory carcinoma – low-grade sweat duct carcinoma
  - Surgical excision
- Follicular tumors
  - Trichoblastic carcinoma – Rx: WLE
  - Trichilemmal carcinoma – Sun-exposed surfaces of older adults
    - Rx: WLE/Mohs
  - Pilomatrix carcinoma – High-rate of local recurrence
    - Head and neck
    - Rx: WLE ≥2 cm or Mohs
  - Sebaceous carcinoma – head and neck, periocular
    - Rx: excision with PDEMA, nonsurgical candidate can receive RT or chemo; consider immunotherapy, +LNs require biopsy
- Cutaneous leiomyosarcoma
  - More indolent course compared to other soft tissue sarcoma and low rate of metastasis
  - Recurrence dependent on depth of invasion, higher if into subcutaneous tissue

References

1. Ad Hoc Task Force, Connolly SM, Baker DR, Coldiron BM, Fazio MJ, Storrs PA, Vidimos AT, Zalla MJ, Brewer JD, Smith Begolka W, Ratings Panel, Berger TG, Bigby M, Bolognia JL, Brodland DG, Collins S, Cronin TA Jr, Dahl MV, Grant-Kels JM, Hanke CW, Hruza GJ, James WD, Lober CW, McBurney EI, Norton SA, Roenigk RK, Wheeland RG, Wisco OJ. AAD/ACMS/ASDSA/ASMS 2012 appropriate use criteria for Mohs micrographic surgery: a report of the American Academy of Dermatology, American College of Mohs Surgery, American Society for Dermatologic Surgery Association, and the American Society for Mohs Surgery. J Am Acad Dermatol. 2012;67(4):531–50. https://doi.org/10.1016/j.jaad.2012.06.009. Epub 2012 Sep 5. Erratum in: J Am Acad Dermatol. 2015 Apr;72(4):748. PMID: 22959232.
2. Ahmed MM, Moore BA, Schmalbach CE. Utility of head and neck cutaneous squamous cell carcinoma sentinel node biopsy: a systematic review. Otolaryngol Head Neck Surg. 2014;150(2):180–7. https://doi.org/10.1177/0194599813511949. Epub 2013 Nov 7. PMID: 24201060.
3. Allen NC, Martin AJ, Snaidr VA, Eggins R, Chong AH, Fernandéz-Peñas P, Gin D, Sidhu S, Paddon VL, Banney LA, Lim A, Upjohn E, Schaider H, Ganhewa AD, Nguyen J, McKenzie CA, Prakash S, McLean C, Lochhead A, Ibbetson J, Dettrick A, Landgren A, Allnutt KJ, Allison C, Davenport RB, Mumford BP, Wong B, Stagg B, Tedman A, Gribbin H, Edwards HA, De Rosa N, Stewart T, Doolan BJ, Kok Y, Simpson K, Low ZM, Kovitwanichkanont T, Scolyer RA, Dhillon HM, Vardy JL, Chadban SJ, Bowen DG, Chen AC, Damian DL. Nicotinamide for skin-cancer chemoprevention in transplant recipients. N Engl J Med. 2023;388(9):804–12. https://doi.org/10.1056/NEJMoa2203086. PMID: 36856616.
4. Andruska N, Fischer-Valuck BW, Mahapatra L, Brenneman RJ, Gay HA, Thorstad WL, Fields RC, MacArthur KM, Baumann BC. Association between surgical margins larger than 1 cm and overall survival in patients with Merkel cell carcinoma. JAMA Dermatol. 2021;157(5):540–8. https://doi.org/10.1001/jamadermatol.2021.0247. PMID: 33760021; PMCID: PMC7992025.
5. Bailey HH, Kim K, Verma AK, Sielaff K, Larson PO, Snow S, Lenaghan T, Viner JL, Douglas J, Dreckschmidt NE, Hamielec M, Pomplun M, Sharata HH, Puchalsky D, Berg ER, Havighurst TC, Carbone PP. A randomized, double-blind, placebo-controlled phase 3 skin cancer prevention study of {alpha}-difluoromethylornithine in subjects with previous history

of skin cancer. Cancer Prev Res (Phila). 2010;3(1):35–47. https://doi.org/10.1158/1940-6207. CAPR-09-0096. PMID: 20051371; PMCID: PMC2804946
6. Basset-Seguin N, Ibbotson SH, Emtestam L, Tarstedt M, Morton C, Maroti M, Calzavara-Pinton P, Varma S, Roelandts R, Wolf P. Topical methyl aminolevulinate photodynamic therapy versus cryotherapy for superficial basal cell carcinoma: a 5 year randomized trial. Eur J Dermatol. 2008;18(5):547–53. https://doi.org/10.1684/ejd.2008.0472. Epub 2008 Aug 8. PMID: 18693158.
7. Bath-Hextall F, Ozolins M, Armstrong SJ, Colver GB, Perkins W, Miller PS, Williams HC. Surgery versus Imiquimod for Nodular Superficial basal cell carcinoma (SINS) study group. Surgical excision versus imiquimod 5% cream for nodular and superficial basal-cell carcinoma (SINS): a multicentre, non-inferiority, randomised controlled trial. Lancet Oncol. 2014;15(1):96–105. https://doi.org/10.1016/S1470-2045(13)70530-8. Epub 2013 Dec 11. PMID: 24332516.
8. Bertrand N, Guerreschi P, Basset-Seguin N, Saiag P, Dupuy A, Dalac-Rat S, Dziwniel V, Depoortère C, Duhamel A, Mortier L. Vismodegib in neoadjuvant treatment of locally advanced basal cell carcinoma: first results of a multicenter, open-label, phase 2 trial (VISMONEO study): Neoadjuvant Vismodegib in Locally Advanced Basal Cell Carcinoma. EClinicalMedicine. 2021;35:100844. https://doi.org/10.1016/j.eclinm.2021.100844. PMID: 33997740; PMCID: PMC8093898.
9. Bittner GC, Cerci FB, Kubo EM, Tolkachjov SN. Mohs micrographic surgery: a review of indications, technique, outcomes, and considerations. An Bras Dermatol. 2021;96(3):263–77. https://doi.org/10.1016/j.abd.2020.10.004. Epub 2021 Mar 24. PMID: 33849752; PMCID: PMC8178571
10. Bonner JA, Harari PM, Giralt J, Azarnia N, Shin DM, Cohen RB, Jones CU, Sur R, Raben D, Jassem J, Ove R, Kies MS, Baselga J, Youssoufian H, Amellal N, Rowinsky EK, Ang KK. Radiotherapy plus cetuximab for squamous-cell carcinoma of the head and neck. N Engl J Med. 2006;354(6):567–78. https://doi.org/10.1056/NEJMoa053422. PMID: 16467544.
11. Cai H, Wang Y, Wu J, Shi Y. Dermatofibrosarcoma protuberans: clinical diagnoses and treatment results of 260 cases in China. J Surg Oncol. 2012;105(2):142–8. https://doi.org/10.1002/jso.22000. Epub 2011 Aug 3. PMID: 21815146.
12. Cameron MC, Lee E, Hibler BP, Barker CA, Mori S, Cordova M, Nehal KS, Rossi AM. Basal cell carcinoma: Epidemiology; pathophysiology; clinical and histological subtypes; and disease associations. J Am Acad Dermatol. 2019a;80(2):303–17. https://doi.org/10.1016/j.jaad.2018.03.060. Epub 2018 May 18. Erratum in: J Am Acad Dermatol. 2021 Aug;85(2):535. PMID: 29782900.
13. Cameron MC, Lee E, Hibler BP, Giordano CN, Barker CA, Mori S, Cordova M, Nehal KS, Rossi AM. Basal cell carcinoma: Contemporary approaches to diagnosis, treatment, and prevention. J Am Acad Dermatol. 2019b;80(2):321–39. https://doi.org/10.1016/j.jaad.2018.02.083. Epub 2018 May 19. Erratum in: J Am Acad Dermatol. 2019 Jul;81(1):310. PMID: 29782901.
14. Chappell AG, Doe SC, Worley B, Yoo SS, Gerami P, Alam M, Buck DW 2nd, Kim JYS, Wayne JD. Multidisciplinary surgical treatment approach for dermatofibrosarcoma protuberans: an update. Arch Dermatol Res. 2021;313(5):367–72. https://doi.org/10.1007/s00403-020-02124-8. Epub 2020 Aug 7. PMID: 32770258.
15. Chen Y, Jiang G. Association between surgical excision margins and outcomes in patients with dermatofibrosarcoma protuberans: a meta-analysis. Dermatol Ther. 2021;34(4):e14954. https://doi.org/10.1111/dth.14954. Epub 2021 Apr 15. PMID: 33835635.
16. Chen AC, Martin AJ, Choy B, Fernández-Peñas P, Dalziell RA, McKenzie CA, Scolyer RA, Dhillon HM, Vardy JL, Kricker A, St George G, Chinniah N, Halliday GM, Damian DL. A Phase 3 randomized trial of nicotinamide for skin-cancer chemoprevention. N Engl J Med. 2015;373(17):1618–26. https://doi.org/10.1056/NEJMoa1506197. PMID: 26488693.
17. Chen YT, Tu WT, Lee WR, Huang YC. The efficacy of adjuvant radiotherapy in dermatofibrosarcoma protuberans: a systemic review and meta-analysis. J Eur Acad Dermatol Venereol. 2016;30(7):1107–14. https://doi.org/10.1111/jdv.13601. Epub 2016 Feb 16. PMID: 26879523.

18. Coggshall K, Tello TL, North JP, Yu SS. Merkel cell carcinoma: an update and review: pathogenesis, diagnosis, and staging. J Am Acad Dermatol. 2018;78(3):433–42. https://doi.org/10.1016/j.jaad.2017.12.001. Epub 2017 Dec 9. PMID: 29229574.
19. Cramer JD, Suresh K, Sridharan S. Completion lymph node dissection for merkel cell carcinoma. Am J Surg. 2020;220(4):982–6. https://doi.org/10.1016/j.amjsurg.2020.02.018. Epub 2020 Feb 15. PMID: 32087988.
20. D'Angelo SP, Bhatia S, Brohl AS, Hamid O, Mehnert JM, Terheyden P, Shih KC, Brownell I, Lebbé C, Lewis KD, Linette GP, Milella M, Xiong H, Guezel G, Nghiem PT. Avelumab in patients with previously treated metastatic Merkel cell carcinoma (JAVELIN Merkel 200): updated overall survival data after >5 years of follow-up. ESMO Open. 2021a;6(6):100290. https://doi.org/10.1016/j.esmoop.2021.100290. Epub 2021 Oct 26. PMID: 34715570; PMCID: PMC8564559.
21. D'Angelo SP, Lebbé C, Mortier L, Brohl AS, Fazio N, Grob JJ, Prinzi N, Hanna GJ, Hassel JC, Kiecker F, Georges S, Ellers-Lenz B, Shah P, Güzel G, Nghiem P. First-line avelumab in a cohort of 116 patients with metastatic Merkel cell carcinoma (JAVELIN Merkel 200): primary and biomarker analyses of a phase II study. J Immunother Cancer. 2021b;9(7):e002646. https://doi.org/10.1136/jitc-2021-002646. PMID: 34301810; PMCID: PMC8311489.
22. Danial C, Sarin KY, Oro AE, Chang AL. An investigator-initiated open-label trial of Sonidegib in advanced basal cell carcinoma patients resistant to Vismodegib. Clin Cancer Res. 2016;22(6):1325–9. https://doi.org/10.1158/1078-0432.CCR-15-1588. Epub 2015 Nov 6. PMID: 26546616; PMCID: PMC4794361
23. Dummer R, Guminksi A, Gutzmer R, Lear JT, Lewis KD, Chang ALS, Combemale P, Dirix L, Kaatz M, Kudchadkar R, Loquai C, Plummer R, Schulze HJ, Stratigos AJ, Trefzer U, Squittieri N, Migden MR. Long-term efficacy and safety of sonidegib in patients with advanced basal cell carcinoma: 42-month analysis of the phase II randomized, double-blind BOLT study. Br J Dermatol. 2020;182(6):1369–78. https://doi.org/10.1111/bjd.18552. Epub 2019 Dec 8. PMID: 31545507; PMCID: PMC7318253
24. Elmets CA, Viner JL, Pentland AP, Cantrell W, Lin HY, Bailey H, Kang S, Linden KG, Heffernan M, Duvic M, Richmond E, Elewski BE, Umar A, Bell W, Gordon GB. Chemoprevention of nonmelanoma skin cancer with celecoxib: a randomized, double-blind, placebo-controlled trial. J Natl Cancer Inst. 2010;102(24):1835–44. https://doi.org/10.1093/jnci/djq442. Epub 2010 Nov 29. PMID: 21115882; PMCID: PMC3001966
25. Farma JM, Ammori JB, Zager JS, Marzban SS, Bui MM, Bichakjian CK, Johnson TM, Lowe L, Sabel MS, Wong SL, Douglas Letson G, Messina JL, Cimmino VM, Sondak VK. Dermatofibrosarcoma protuberans: how wide should we resect? Ann Surg Oncol. 2010;17(8):2112–8. https://doi.org/10.1245/s10434-010-1046-8. Epub 2010 Mar 31. PMID: 20354798.
26. Ferrarotto R, Amit M, Nagarajan P, Rubin ML, Yuan Y, Bell D, El-Naggar AK, Johnson JM, Morrison WH, Rosenthal DI, Glisson BS, Johnson FM, Lu C, Mott FE, Esmaeli B, Diaz EM Jr, Gidley PW, Goepfert RP, Lewis CM, Weber RS, Wargo JA, Basu S, Duan F, Yadav SS, Sharma P, Allison JP, Myers JN, Gross ND. Pilot Phase II Trial of Neoadjuvant Immunotherapy in Locoregionally Advanced, Resectable cutaneous squamous cell carcinoma of the head and neck. Clin Cancer Res. 2021;27(16):4557–65. https://doi.org/10.1158/1078-0432.CCR-21-0585. Epub 2021 Jun 29. Erratum in: Clin Cancer Res. 2022 Apr 14;28(8):1735. PMID: 34187851; PMCID: PMC8711237.
27. Foote MC, McGrath M, Guminski A, Hughes BGM, Meakin J, Thomson D, Zarate D, Simpson F, Porceddu SV. Phase II study of single-agent panitumumab in patients with incurable cutaneous squamous cell carcinoma. Ann Oncol. 2014;25(10):2047–52. https://doi.org/10.1093/annonc/mdu368. Epub 2014 Aug 4. PMID: 25091317.
28. Fukushima S, Masuguchi S, Igata T, Harada M, Aoi J, Miyashita A, Nakahara S, Inoue Y, Jinnin M, Shiraishi S, Yamashita Y, Ishihara T, Ihn H. Evaluation of sentinel node biopsy for cutaneous squamous cell carcinoma. J Dermatol. 2014;41(6):539–41. https://doi.org/10.1111/1346-8138.12508. PMID: 24909214.

29. Gauci ML, Aristei C, Becker JC, Blom A, Bataille V, Dreno B, Del Marmol V, Forsea AM, Fargnoli MC, Grob JJ, Gomes F, Hauschild A, Hoeller C, Harwood C, Kelleners-Smeets N, Kaufmann R, Lallas A, Malvehy J, Moreno-Ramirez D, Peris K, Pellacani G, Saiag P, Stratigos AJ, Vieira R, Zalaudek I, van Akkooi ACJ, Lorigan P, Garbe C, Lebbé C, European Dermatology Forum (EDF), the European Association of Dermato-Oncology (EADO) and the European Organization for Research and Treatment of Cancer (EORTC). Diagnosis and treatment of Merkel cell carcinoma: European consensus-based interdisciplinary guideline – update 2022. Eur J Cancer. 2022;171:203–31. https://doi.org/10.1016/j.ejca.2022.03.043. Epub 2022 Jun 19. PMID: 35732101.
30. Gold KA, Kies MS, William WN Jr, Johnson FM, Lee JJ, Glisson BS. Erlotinib in the treatment of recurrent or metastatic cutaneous squamous cell carcinoma: a single-arm phase 2 clinical trial. Cancer. 2018;124(10):2169–73. https://doi.org/10.1002/cncr.31346. Epub 2018 Mar 26. PMID: 29579331; PMCID: PMC5935588
31. Grignani G, Rutkowski P, Lebbe C, et al. 545 A phase 2 study of retifanlimab in patients with advanced or metastatic merkel cell carcinoma (MCC) (POD1UM-201). J Immunother Cancer. 2021;9:A574–5.
32. Gunaratne DA, Howle JR, Veness MJ. Sentinel lymph node biopsy in Merkel cell carcinoma: a 15-year institutional experience and statistical analysis of 721 reported cases. Br J Dermatol. 2016;174(2):273–81. https://doi.org/10.1111/bjd.14240. Epub 2015 Dec 19. PMID: 26480031.
33. Gupta SG, Wang LC, Peñas PF, Gellenthin M, Lee SJ, Nghiem P. Sentinel lymph node biopsy for evaluation and treatment of patients with Merkel cell carcinoma: the Dana-Farber experience and meta-analysis of the literature. Arch Dermatol. 2006;142(6):685–90. https://doi.org/10.1001/archderm.142.6.685. PMID: 16785370.
34. Hughes BGM, Munoz-Couselo E, Mortier L, Bratland Å, Gutzmer R, Roshdy O, González Mendoza R, Schachter J, Arance A, Grange F, Meyer N, Joshi A, Billan S, Zhang P, Gumuscu B, Swaby RF, Grob JJ. Pembrolizumab for locally advanced and recurrent/metastatic cutaneous squamous cell carcinoma (KEYNOTE-629 study): an open-label, nonrandomized, multicenter, phase II trial. Ann Oncol. 2021;32(10):1276–85. https://doi.org/10.1016/j.annonc.2021.07.008. Epub 2021 Jul 20. Erratum in: Ann Oncol. 2022 Aug;33(8):853. PMID: 34293460.
35. Jabbour J, Cumming R, Scolyer RA, Hruby G, Thompson JF, Lee S. Merkel cell carcinoma: assessing the effect of wide local excision, lymph node dissection, and radiotherapy on recurrence and survival in early-stage disease–results from a review of 82 consecutive cases diagnosed between 1992 and 2004. Ann Surg Oncol. 2007;14(6):1943–52. https://doi.org/10.1245/s10434-006-9327-y. Epub 2007 Mar 14. PMID: 17356954.
36. Jaju PD, Ransohoff KJ, Tang JY, Sarin KY. Familial skin cancer syndromes: increased risk of nonmelanotic skin cancers and extracutaneous tumors. J Am Acad Dermatol. 2016;74(3):437–51. https://doi.org/10.1016/j.jaad.2015.08.073.
37. Jambusaria-Pahlajani A, Kanetsky PA, Karia PS, Hwang WT, Gelfand JM, Whalen FM, Elenitsas R, Xu X, Schmults CD. Evaluation of AJCC tumor staging for cutaneous squamous cell carcinoma and a proposed alternative tumor staging system. JAMA Dermatol. 2013;149(4):402–10. https://doi.org/10.1001/jamadermatol.2013.2456. PMID: 23325457.
38. Jansen MHE, Mosterd K, Arits AHMM, Roozeboom MH, Sommer A, Essers BAB, van Pelt HPA, Quaedvlieg PJF, Steijlen PM, Nelemans PJ, Kelleners-Smeets NWJ. Five-year results of a randomized controlled trial comparing effectiveness of photodynamic therapy, topical Imiquimod, and topical 5-fluorouracil in patients with superficial basal cell carcinoma. J Invest Dermatol. 2018;138(3):527–33. https://doi.org/10.1016/j.jid.2017.09.033. Epub 2017 Oct 16. PMID: 29045820.
39. Kang SH, Haydu LE, Goh RY, Fogarty GB. Radiotherapy is associated with significant improvement in local and regional control in Merkel cell carcinoma. Radiat Oncol. 2012;7:171. https://doi.org/10.1186/1748-717X-7-171. PMID: 23075308; PMCID: PMC3494567.
40. Kaufman HL, Russell J, Hamid O, Bhatia S, Terheyden P, D'Angelo SP, Shih KC, Lebbé C, Linette GP, Milella M, Brownell I, Lewis KD, Lorch JH, Chin K, Mahnke L, von Heydebreck A, Cuillerot JM, Nghiem P. Avelumab in patients with chemotherapy-refractory metastatic

Merkel cell carcinoma: a multicentre, single-group, open-label, phase 2 trial. Lancet Oncol. 2016;17(10):1374–85. https://doi.org/10.1016/S1470-2045(16)30364-3. Epub 2016 Sep 1. PMID: 27592805; PMCID: PMC5587154.

41. Krausz AE, Ji-Xu A, Smile T, Koyfman S, Schmults CD, Ruiz ES. A systematic review of primary, adjuvant, and salvage radiation therapy for cutaneous squamous cell carcinoma. Dermatologic Surg. 2021;47(5):587–92. https://doi.org/10.1097/DSS.0000000000002965. PMID: 33577212.

42. Kwon S, Dong ZM, Wu PC. Sentinel lymph node biopsy for high-risk cutaneous squamous cell carcinoma: clinical experience and review of literature. World J Surg Oncol. 2011;9:80. https://doi.org/10.1186/1477-7819-9-80. PMID: 21771334; PMCID: PMC3156743.

43. Lang R, Welponer T, Richtig E, Wolf I, Hoeller C, Hafner C, Nguyen VA, Kofler J, Barta M, Koelblinger P, Hitzl W, Emberger M, Laimer M. Nivolumab for locally advanced and metastatic cutaneous squamous cell carcinoma (NIVOSQUACS study)-Phase II data covering impact of concomitant haematological malignancies. J Eur Acad Dermatol Venereol. 2023; https://doi.org/10.1111/jdv.19218. Epub ahead of print. PMID: 37210651.

44. Lansbury L, Leonardi-Bee J, Perkins W, Goodacre T, Tweed JA, Bath-Hextall FJ. Interventions for non-metastatic squamous cell carcinoma of the skin. Cochrane Database Syst Rev. 2010;14(4):CD007869. https://doi.org/10.1002/14651858.CD007869.pub2. PMID: 20393962.

45. Lansbury L, Bath-Hextall F, Perkins W, Stanton W, Leonardi-Bee J. Interventions for non-metastatic squamous cell carcinoma of the skin: systematic review and pooled analysis of observational studies. BMJ. 2013;347:f6153. https://doi.org/10.1136/bmj.f6153. PMID: 24191270; PMCID: PMC3816607.

46. Leung AKC, Barankin B, Lam JM, Leong KF, Hon KL. Xeroderma pigmentosum: an updated review. Drugs Context. 2022;11:2022-2-5. https://doi.org/10.7573/dic.2022-2-5.

47. Likhacheva A, Awan M, Barker CA, Bhatnagar A, Bradfield L, Brady MS, Buzurovic I, Geiger JL, Parvathaneni U, Zaky S, Devlin PM. Definitive and postoperative radiation therapy for basal and squamous cell cancers of the skin: executive summary of an American Society for Radiation Oncology Clinical Practice Guideline. Pract Radiat Oncol. 2020;10(1):8–20. https://doi.org/10.1016/j.prro.2019.10.014. Epub 2019 Dec 9. PMID: 31831330.

48. Maloney NJ, Aasi SZ, Kibbi N, Hirotsu KE, Zaba LC. Online risk calculator and nomogram for predicting sentinel lymph node positivity in Merkel cell carcinoma. J Am Acad Dermatol. 2023;89(3):621–3. https://doi.org/10.1016/j.jaad.2023.05.042. Epub 2023 May 26. PMID: 37244414.

49. Martin ECS, Vyas KS, Batbold S, Erwin PJ, Brewer JD. Dermatofibrosarcoma protuberans recurrence after wide local excision versus mohs micrographic surgery: a systematic review and meta-analysis. Dermatol Surg. 2022;48(5):479–85. https://doi.org/10.1097/DSS.0000000000003411. Epub 2022 Mar 30. Erratum in: Dermatol Surg. 2023;49(2):221. PMID: 35353755.

50. Martinez SR, Barr KL, Canter RJ. Rare tumors through the looking glass: an examination of malignant cutaneous adnexal tumors. Arch Dermatol. 2011;147(9):1058–62. https://doi.org/10.1001/archdermatol.2011.229. PMID: 21931043.

51. Maubec E, Petrow P, Scheer-Senyarich I, Duvillard P, Lacroix L, Gelly J, Certain A, Duval X, Crickx B, Buffard V, Basset-Seguin N, Saez P, Duval-Modeste AB, Adamski H, Mansard S, Grange F, Dompmartin A, Faivre S, Mentré F, Avril MF. Phase II study of cetuximab as first-line single-drug therapy in patients with unresectable squamous cell carcinoma of the skin. J Clin Oncol. 2011;29(25):3419–26. https://doi.org/10.1200/JCO.2010.34.1735. Epub 2011 Aug 1. PMID: 21810686.

52. Mendenhall WM, Ferlito A, Takes RP, Bradford CR, Corry J, Fagan JJ, Rinaldo A, Strojan P, Rodrigo JP. Cutaneous head and neck basal and squamous cell carcinomas with perineural invasion. Oral Oncol. 2012;48(10):918–22. https://doi.org/10.1016/j.oraloncology.2012.02.015. Epub 2012 Mar 15. PMID: 22425152.

53. Migden MR, Guminski A, Gutzmer R, Dirix L, Lewis KD, Combemale P, Herd RM, Kudchadkar R, Trefzer U, Gogov S, Pallaud C, Yi T, Mone M, Kaatz M, Loquai C, Stratigos AJ, Schulze HJ, Plummer R, Chang AL, Cornélis F, Lear JT, Sellami D, Dummer R. Treatment

with two different doses of sonidegib in patients with locally advanced or metastatic basal cell carcinoma (BOLT): a multicentre, randomised, double-blind phase 2 trial. Lancet Oncol. 2015;16(6):716–28. https://doi.org/10.1016/S1470-2045(15)70100-2. Epub 2015 May 14. PMID: 25981810.
54. Migden MR, Rischin D, Schmults CD, Guminski A, Hauschild A, Lewis KD, Chung CH, Hernandez-Aya L, Lim AM, Chang ALS, Rabinowits G, Thai AA, Dunn LA, Hughes BGM, Khushalani NI, Modi B, Schadendorf D, Gao B, Seebach F, Li S, Li J, Mathias M, Booth J, Mohan K, Stankevich E, Babiker HM, Brana I, Gil-Martin M, Homsi J, Johnson ML, Moreno V, Niu J, Owonikoko TK, Papadopoulos KP, Yancopoulos GD, Lowy I, Fury MG. PD-1 blockade with Cemiplimab in advanced cutaneous squamous-cell carcinoma. N Engl J Med. 2018;379(4):341–51. https://doi.org/10.1056/NEJMoa1805131. Epub 2018 Jun 4. PMID: 29863979.
55. Migden MR, Khushalani NI, Chang ALS, Lewis KD, Schmults CD, Hernandez-Aya L, Meier F, Schadendorf D, Guminski A, Hauschild A, Wong DJ, Daniels GA, Berking C, Jankovic V, Stankevich E, Booth J, Li S, Weinreich DM, Yancopoulos GD, Lowy I, Fury MG, Rischin D. Cemiplimab in locally advanced cutaneous squamous cell carcinoma: results from an open-label, phase 2, single-arm trial. Lancet Oncol. 2020;21(2):294–305. https://doi.org/10.1016/S1470-2045(19)30728-4. Epub 2020 Jan 14. PMID: 31952975; PMCID: PMC7771329.
56. Möhrle M, Breuninger H. Die Muffin-Technik–eine Alternative zur Mohs' Chirurgie [The Muffin technique–an alternative to Mohs' micrographic surgery]. J Dtsch Dermatol Ges. 2006;4(12):1080–4. https://doi.org/10.1111/j.1610-0387.2006.06152.x. German. PMID: 17176417.
57. Mosterd K, Krekels GA, Nieman FH, Ostertag JU, Essers BA, Dirksen CD, Steijlen PM, Vermeulen A, Neumann H, Kelleners-Smeets NW. Surgical excision versus Mohs' micrographic surgery for primary and recurrent basal-cell carcinoma of the face: a prospective randomised controlled trial with 5-years' follow-up. Lancet Oncol. 2008;9(12):1149–56. https://doi.org/10.1016/S1470-2045(08)70260-2. Epub 2008 Nov 17. PMID: 19010733.
58. Navarrete-Dechent C, Veness MJ, Droppelmann N, Uribe P. High-risk cutaneous squamous cell carcinoma and the emerging role of sentinel lymph node biopsy: a literature review. J Am Acad Dermatol. 2015;73(1):127–37. https://doi.org/10.1016/j.jaad.2015.03.039. PMID: 26089049.
59. Navarrete-Dechent C, Mori S, Barker CA, Dickson MA, Nehal KS. Imatinib treatment for locally advanced or metastatic dermatofibrosarcoma protuberans: a systematic review. JAMA Dermatol. 2019;155(3):361–9. https://doi.org/10.1001/jamadermatol.2018.4940. PMID: 30601909; PMCID: PMC8909640.
60. Nghiem P, Bhatia S, Lipson EJ, Sharfman WH, Kudchadkar RR, Brohl AS, Friedlander PA, Daud A, Kluger HM, Reddy SA, Boulmay BC, Riker A, Burgess MA, Hanks BA, Olencki T, Kendra K, Church C, Akaike T, Ramchurren N, Shinohara MM, Salim B, Taube JM, Jensen E, Kalabis M, Fling SP, Homet Moreno B, Sharon E, Cheever MA, Topalian SL. Three-year survival, correlates and salvage therapies in patients receiving first-line pembrolizumab for advanced Merkel cell carcinoma. J Immunother Cancer. 2021;9(4):e002478. https://doi.org/10.1136/jitc-2021-002478. PMID: 33879601; PMCID: PMC8061836.
61. Nottage MK, Lin C, Hughes BG, Kenny L, Smith DD, Houston K, Francesconi A. Prospective study of definitive chemoradiation in locally or regionally advanced squamous cell carcinoma of the skin. Head Neck. 2017;39(4):679–83. https://doi.org/10.1002/hed.24662. Epub 2016 Dec 29. PMID: 28032670.
62. Paoli J, Cogrel O, van der Geer S, Krekels G, de Leeuw J, Moehrle M, Ostertag J, Rios Buceta L, Sheth N, Lauchli S. ESMS position document on the use of Mohs micrographic surgery and other micrographic surgery techniques in Europe; 2019
63. Paulson KG, Lewis CW, Redman MW, Simonson WT, Lisberg A, Ritter D, Morishima C, Hutchinson K, Mudgistratova L, Blom A, Iyer J, Moshiri AS, Tarabadkar ES, Carter JJ, Bhatia S, Kawasumi M, Galloway DA, Wener MH, Nghiem P. Viral oncoprotein antibodies as a marker for recurrence of Merkel cell carcinoma: a prospective validation study.

Cancer. 2017;123(8):1464–74. https://doi.org/10.1002/cncr.30475. Epub 2016 Dec 7. PMID: 27925665; PMCID: PMC5384867
64. Porceddu SV, Daniels C, Yom SS, Liu H, Waldron J, Gregoire V, Moore A, Veness M, Yao M, Johansen J, Mehanna H, Rischin D, Le QT. Head and Neck Cancer International Group (HNCIG) consensus guidelines for the delivery of postoperative radiation therapy in complex Cutaneous Squamous Cell Carcinoma of the Head and Neck (cSCCHN). Int J Radiat Oncol Biol Phys. 2020;107(4):641–51. https://doi.org/10.1016/j.ijrobp.2020.03.024. Epub 2020 Apr 11. PMID: 32289475.
65. Que SKT, Zwald FO, Schmults CD. Cutaneous squamous cell carcinoma: incidence, risk factors, diagnosis, and staging. J Am Acad Dermatol. 2018;78(2):237–47. https://doi.org/10.1016/j.jaad.2017.08.059. PMID: 29332704.
66. Rowe DE, Carroll RJ, Day CL Jr. Long-term recurrence rates in previously untreated (primary) basal cell carcinoma: implications for patient follow-up. J Dermatol Surg Oncol. 1989;15(3):315–28. https://doi.org/10.1111/j.1524-4725.1989.tb03166.x. PMID: 2646336.
67. Santamaria-Barria JA, Boland GM, Yeap BY, Nardi V, Dias-Santagata D, Cusack JC Jr. Merkel cell carcinoma: 30-year experience from a single institution. Ann Surg Oncol. 2013;20(4):1365–73. https://doi.org/10.1245/s10434-012-2779-3. Epub 2012 Dec 1. PMID: 23208132.
68. Schmitt AR, Brewer JD, Bordeaux JS, Baum CL. Staging for cutaneous squamous cell carcinoma as a predictor of sentinel lymph node biopsy results: meta-analysis of American Joint Committee on Cancer criteria and a proposed alternative system. JAMA Dermatol. 2014;150(1):19–24. https://doi.org/10.1001/jamadermatol.2013.6675. PMID: 24226651.
69. Sekulic A, Migden MR, Basset-Seguin N, Garbe C, Gesierich A, Lao CD, Miller C, Mortier L, Murrell DF, Hamid O, Quevedo JF, Hou J, McKenna E, Dimier N, Williams S, Schadendorf D, Hauschild A, ERIVANCE BCC Investigators. Long-term safety and efficacy of vismodegib in patients with advanced basal cell carcinoma: final update of the pivotal ERIVANCE BCC study. BMC Cancer. 2017;17(1):332. https://doi.org/10.1186/s12885-017-3286-5. Erratum in: BMC Cancer. 2019 Apr 18;19(1):366. PMID: 28511673; PMCID: PMC5433030.
70. Silverman MK, Kopf AW, Bart RS, Grin CM, Levenstein MS. Recurrence rates of treated basal cell carcinomas. Part 3: surgical excision. J Dermatol Surg Oncol. 1992;18(6):471–6. https://doi.org/10.1111/j.1524-4725.1992.tb03307.x. PMID: 1592998.
71. Singh B, Qureshi MM, Truong MT, Sahni D. Demographics and outcomes of stage I and II Merkel cell carcinoma treated with Mohs micrographic surgery compared with wide local excision in the National Cancer Database. J Am Acad Dermatol. 2018;79(1):126–134.e3. https://doi.org/10.1016/j.jaad.2018.01.041. Epub 2018 Feb 3. PMID: 29408552.
72. Singh N, Alexander NA, Lachance K, Lewis CW, McEvoy A, Akaike G, Byrd D, Behnia S, Bhatia S, Paulson KG, Nghiem P. Clinical benefit of baseline imaging in Merkel cell carcinoma: analysis of 584 patients. J Am Acad Dermatol. 2021;84(2):330–9. https://doi.org/10.1016/j.jaad.2020.07.065. Epub 2020 Jul 21. PMID: 32707254; PMCID: PMC7854967.
73. Stratigos AJ, Sekulic A, Peris K, Bechter O, Prey S, Kaatz M, Lewis KD, Basset-Seguin N, Chang ALS, Dalle S, Orland AF, Licitra L, Robert C, Ulrich C, Hauschild A, Migden MR, Dummer R, Li S, Yoo SY, Mohan K, Coates E, Jankovic V, Fiaschi N, Okoye E, Bassukas ID, Loquai C, De Giorgi V, Eroglu Z, Gutzmer R, Ulrich J, Puig S, Seebach F, Thurston G, Weinreich DM, Yancopoulos GD, Lowy I, Bowler T, Fury MG. Cemiplimab in locally advanced basal cell carcinoma after hedgehog inhibitor therapy: an open-label, multi-centre, single-arm, phase 2 trial. Lancet Oncol. 2021;22(6):848–57. https://doi.org/10.1016/S1470-2045(21)00126-1. Epub 2021 May 14. PMID: 34000246.
74. Tang JY, Ally MS, Chanana AM, Mackay-Wiggan JM, Aszterbaum M, Lindgren JA, Ulerio G, Rezaee MR, Gildengorin G, Marji J, Clark C, Bickers DR, Epstein EH Jr. Inhibition of the hedgehog pathway in patients with basal-cell nevus syndrome: final results from the multicentre, randomised, double-blind, placebo-controlled, phase 2 trial. Lancet Oncol. 2016;17(12):1720–31. https://doi.org/10.1016/S1470-2045(16)30566-6. Epub 2016 Nov 10. PMID: 27838224.

75. Thompson AK, Kelley BF, Prokop LJ, Murad MH, Baum CL. Risk factors for cutaneous squamous cell carcinoma outcomes: a systematic review and meta-analysis. JAMA Dermatol. 2017;152(4):419–28.
76. Thomson J, Hogan S, Leonardi-Bee J, Williams HC, Bath-Hextall FJ. Interventions for basal cell carcinoma of the skin. Cochrane Database Syst Rev. 2020;11(11):CD003412. https://doi.org/10.1002/14651858.CD003412.pub3. PMID: 33202063; PMCID: PMC8164471
77. Topalian SL, Bhatia S, Hollebecque A, Awada A, De Boer JP, Kudchadkar RR, Goncalves A, Delord J-P, Martens UM, Picazo JML, Oaknin A, Spanos WC, Aljumaily R, Sharfman WH, Rao S, Soumaoro I, Cao A, Nghiem P, Schadendorf D. Abstract CT074: Non-comparative, open-label, multiple cohort, phase 1/2 study to evaluate nivolumab (NIVO) in patients with virus-associated tumors (CheckMate 358): Efficacy and safety in Merkel cell carcinoma (MCC). Cancer Res. 2017;77(13_Supplement):CT074. https://doi.org/10.1158/1538-7445.AM2017-CT074.
78. Topalian SL, Bhatia S, Amin A, Kudchadkar RR, Sharfman WH, Lebbé C, Delord JP, Dunn LA, Shinohara MM, Kulikauskas R, Chung CH, Martens UM, Ferris RL, Stein JE, Engle EL, Devriese LA, Lao CD, Gu J, Li B, Chen T, Barrows A, Horvath A, Taube JM, Nghiem P. Neoadjuvant Nivolumab for patients with Resectable Merkel cell carcinoma in the CheckMate 358 trial. J Clin Oncol. 2020;38(22):2476–87. https://doi.org/10.1200/JCO.20.00201. Epub 2020 Apr 23. PMID: 32324435; PMCID: PMC7392746
79. Trodello C, Pepper JP, Wong M, Wysong A. Cisplatin and Cetuximab treatment for metastatic cutaneous squamous cell carcinoma: a systematic review. Dermatologic Surg. 2017;43(1):40–9. https://doi.org/10.1097/DSS.0000000000000799. PMID: 27618393.
80. Tromovitch TA, Stegeman SJ. Microscopically controlled excision of skin tumors. Arch Dermatol. 1974;110(2):231–2. PMID: 4853214.
81. Tschetter AJ, Campoli MR, Zitelli JA, Brodland DG. Long-term clinical outcomes of patients with invasive cutaneous squamous cell carcinoma treated with Mohs micrographic surgery: a 5-year, multicenter, prospective cohort study. J Am Acad Dermatol. 2020;82(1):139–48. https://doi.org/10.1016/j.jaad.2019.06.1303. Epub 2019 Jul 3. PMID: 31279037.
82. Ugurel S, Mentzel T, Utikal J, Helmbold P, Mohr P, Pföhler C, Schiller M, Hauschild A, Hein R, Kämpgen E, Kellner I, Leverkus M, Becker JC, Ströbel P, Schadendorf D. Neoadjuvant imatinib in advanced primary or locally recurrent dermatofibrosarcoma protuberans: a multicenter phase II DeCOG trial with long-term follow-up. Clin Cancer Res. 2014;20(2):499–510. https://doi.org/10.1158/1078-0432.CCR-13-1411. Epub 2013 Oct 30. PMID: 24173542.
83. van Kester MS, Goeman JJ, Genders RE. Tissue-sparing properties of Mohs micrographic surgery for infiltrative basal cell carcinoma. J Am Acad Dermatol. 2019;80(6):1700–3. https://doi.org/10.1016/j.jaad.2019.01.057. Epub 2019 Jan 31. PMID: 30710602.
84. Verkouteren BJA, Cosgun B, Reinders MGHC, Kessler PAWK, Vermeulen RJ, Klaassens M, Lambrechts S, van Rheenen JR, van Geel M, Vreeburg M, Mosterd K. A guideline for the clinical management of basal cell naevus syndrome (Gorlin-Goltz syndrome). Br J Dermatol. 2022;186(2):215–26. https://doi.org/10.1111/bjd.20700. Epub 2021 Nov 8. PMID: 34375441; PMCID: PMC9298899
85. Vitiello GA, Lee AY, Berman RS. Dermatofibrosarcoma protuberans: what is this? Surg Clin North Am. 2022;102(4):657–65. https://doi.org/10.1016/j.suc.2022.05.004. PMID: 35952694.
86. Wilder RB, Kittelson JM, Shimm DS. Basal cell carcinoma treated with radiation therapy. Cancer. 1991;68(10):2134–7. https://doi.org/10.1002/1097-0142(19911115)68:10<2134::aid-cncr2820681008>3.0.co;2-m. PMID: 1913451.
87. William WN Jr, Feng L, Ferrarotto R, Ginsberg L, Kies M, Lippman S, Glisson B, Kim ES. Gefitinib for patients with incurable cutaneous squamous cell carcinoma: a single-arm phase II clinical trial. J Am Acad Dermatol. 2017;77(6):1110–1113.e2. https://doi.org/10.1016/j.jaad.2017.07.048. Epub 2017 Sep 28. PMID: 28964539; PMCID: PMC5685879.
88. Williams N, Morris CG, Kirwan JM, Dagan R, Mendenhall WM. Radiotherapy for dermatofibrosarcoma protuberans. Am J Clin Oncol. 2014;37(5):430–2. https://doi.org/10.1097/COC.0b013e31827dee86. PMID: 23388563.

89. Williams HC, Bath-Hextall F, Ozolins M, Armstrong SJ, Colver GB, Perkins W, Miller PSJ. Surgery versus Imiquimod for nodular and superficial basal cell carcinoma (SINS) study group. Surgery versus 5% Imiquimod for nodular and superficial basal cell carcinoma: 5-year results of the SINS randomized controlled trial. J Invest Dermatol. 2017;137(3):614–9. https://doi.org/10.1016/j.jid.2016.10.019. Epub 2016 Dec 5. PMID: 27932240.
90. Wong WG, Stahl K, Olecki EJ, Holguin RP, Pameijer C, Shen C. Survival benefit of guideline-concordant postoperative radiation for local Merkel cell carcinoma. J Surg Res. 2021;266:168–79. https://doi.org/10.1016/j.jss.2021.03.062. Epub 2021 May 17. PMID: 34015514.
91. Work Group, Invited Reviewers, Kim JYS, Kozlow JH, Mittal B, Moyer J, Olenecki T, Rodgers P. Guidelines of care for the management of cutaneous squamous cell carcinoma. J Am Acad Dermatol. 2018a;78(3):560–78. https://doi.org/10.1016/j.jaad.2017.10.007. Epub 2018 Jan 10. PMID: 29331386; PMCID: PMC6652228.
92. Work Group, Invited Reviewers, Kim JYS, Kozlow JH, Mittal B, Moyer J, Olencki T, Rodgers P. Guidelines of care for the management of basal cell carcinoma. J Am Acad Dermatol. 2018b;78(3):540–59. https://doi.org/10.1016/j.jaad.2017.10.006. Epub 2018 Jan 10. PMID: 29331385.
93. Wright GP, Holtzman MP. Surgical resection improves median overall survival with marginal improvement in long-term survival when compared with definitive radiotherapy in Merkel cell carcinoma: a propensity score matched analysis of the National Cancer Database. Am J Surg. 2018;215(3):384–7. https://doi.org/10.1016/j.amjsurg.2017.10.045. Epub 2017 Nov 11. PMID: 29157891.
94. Wysong A. Squamous-cell carcinoma of the skin. N Engl J Med. 2023;388(24):2262–73. https://doi.org/10.1056/NEJMra2206348. PMID: 37314707.
95. Xue Y, Thakuria M. Merkel Cell Carcinoma Review. Hematol Oncol Clin North Am. 2019;33(1):39–52. https://doi.org/10.1016/j.hoc.2018.08.002. PMID: 30497676.
96. Yan F, Tillman BN, Nijhawan RI, Srivastava D, Sher DJ, Avkshtol V, Homsi J, Bishop JA, Wynings EM, Lee R, Myers LL, Day AT. High-risk cutaneous squamous cell carcinoma of the head and neck: a clinical review. Ann Surg Oncol. 2021;28(13):9009–30. https://doi.org/10.1245/s10434-021-10108-9. Epub 2021 Jun 30. PMID: 34195900.
97. Zwald FO, Brown M. Skin cancer in solid organ transplant recipients: advances in therapy and management: part II. Management of skin cancer in solid organ transplant recipients. J Am Acad Dermatol. 2011;65(2):263 79. https://doi.org/10.1016/j.jaad.2010.11.063.

Pancreatic Cancer

Michael Sestito, Britney Niemann, and Brian A. Boone

Introduction

- Pancreatic adenocarcinoma (PDAC) is a systemic disease
- Requires BOTH systemic therapy and surgical removal for best chance of cure or cancer control
- Tenth most common cancer in the United States
- Fourth leading cause of cancer-related death
- Five-year survival in United States is 10–12% [1–3]
- 80% of patients have metastatic or unresectable disease at diagnosis
- Genetic progression from pancreatic intraepithelial neoplasia to invasive ductal adenocarcinoma [4, 5] involves these mutations, among others:
  - *KRAS* (90–95%)
  - *CDKN2A* (80%)
  - *P53* (80%)/*SMAD4* (50–55%)

Diagnostic Workup

- Imaging [6, 7]
  - Multiphase contrast-enhanced CT
    - Arterial, pancreatic parenchymal, and portal venous phases

---

M. Sestito · B. Niemann
Department of Surgery, West Virginia University, Morgantown, WV, USA
e-mail: michael.sestito@hsc.wvu.edu; britney.neimann@hsc.wvu.edu

B. A. Boone (✉)
Department of Surgery, West Virginia University, Morgantown, WV, USA

Department of Microbiology, Immunology and Cell Biology, West Virginia University, Morgantown, WV, USA
e-mail: brian.boone@hsc.wvu.edu

- Pancreatic parenchymal phase – acquired after the arterial phase and before the portal venous phase to optimize the visual contrast of enhanced pancreatic parenchyma and hypoattenuating tumor
- Portal venous phase – liver metastases may appear as hypoattenuating lesions
  - MRI of abdomen with contrast
    - Equally sensitive and specific for staging as CT
    - Cost and availability limit use
    - Primarily used to evaluate isoattenuating pancreatic and liver lesions
  - EUS
    - Primarily used to obtain a biopsy sample via FNA
    - Complementary to CT and MRI for staging, should not be primary staging modality
  - PET-CT
    - Evaluate for metastatic disease when high risk or suspected (nonspecific liver abnormality, high Ca 19-9, etc.)
- CA 19-9
  - Sialylated Lewis A blood group antigen
  - Baseline level is a prognostic biomarker
  - Prognosis also associated with response after systemic therapy and surgical resection [8]
  - Not useful if Lewis blood group negative (5–10% of population)
  - Nonspecific – may be elevated by other malignancies and benign biliary disease (e.g., cholangitis, biliary obstruction)
  - Should recheck if obtained in the setting of jaundice or hyperbilirubinemia once those conditions have resolved (such as after biliary stent)
  - Low PPV – should not be used for cancer screening (0.9%) [9]
  - NCCN recommends measurement of CA 19-9 at baseline, after neoadjuvant therapy, prior to adjuvant therapy, and for surveillance [10]
  - CA 19-9 >500 units/mL suggests occult metastatic disease - supports neoadjuvant therapy even in resectable disease [11]
  - >50% decrease in CA 19-9 after neoadjuvant therapy associated with improved R0 resection rate and overall survival in borderline resectable [12]
  - Change in CA 19-9 is useful in evaluating benefit of treatment [13]
  - Prognostic marker for postresection survival:
    - In resectable disease, median survival after operation is higher if CA 19-9 level <180 U/mL [14]
    - Low CA 19-9 associated with longer DFS after adjuvant therapy (26 months vs 16.7 months) [15]
- Tumor biopsy and biliary brushing
  - Pathologic diagnosis is required prior to administration of neoadjuvant therapy.
  - If original biopsy not definitive, repeat biopsy should not delay attempt at surgical removal if resectable disease and cancer is highly suspected.

- Pathologic confirmation preferred when higher-risk patient for operation or imaging suggests alternate diagnosis such as chronic pancreatitis or autoimmune pancreatitis.
- Biopsies should target lesions that provide highest stage of disease (suspected metastatic lesions).
- EUS-FNA (preferred modality) – sensitivity 90.8% and specificity 96.5% [16]
  - Biopsies prone to sampling error.
  - Pancreatic tumors are densely fibrotic with relatively sparse tumor cell clusters.
- ERCP biliary brushings – sensitivity 40–60%, specificity >98% [17]
  - May be performed if in need of concurrent biliary decompression
  - Not used for diagnosis alone without biliary obstruction due to the risk of pancreatitis and inferior sensitivity
- Percutaneous CT- or US-guided biopsy – rarely performed for pancreatic tissue sampling
• Genetic Testing
  - Genetic basis of inherited predisposition not known in most cases.
  - Eighty percent of patients with family history of pancreatic cancer have no known genetic cause [18].
  - One first-degree relative with pancreatic cancer raises risk 4.6-fold.
  - Two affected first-degree relatives raise the risk 6.4-fold [19].
  - NCCN guidelines recommend genetic testing of hereditary cancer syndromes for *any* patient with confirmed pancreatic cancer:
    - Targeted treatment options may be available.
    - Genetic counseling recommended when testing positive [10] (Table 13.1).
• Staging Laparoscopy
  - Not universally accepted – reasonable in select patients
  - Consider prior to neoadjuvant treatment in high-risk patients (suspicious imaging for abdominal metastatic disease or markedly elevated CA19-9)
  - May increase accuracy of resectability status [20]

Table 13.1 Genetic syndromes associated with PDAC [10]

Genetic mutation	Syndrome	Cumulative risk	Risk relative to general population
STK11	Peutz-Jeghers Syndrome	11–36% by age 70	130-fold increase
PRSS1, SPINK1, and CFTR	Familial pancreatitis	40–50% by age 75	25–85-fold increase
CDKN2A	Familial atypical mole and multiple melanoma syndrome	14% by age 70	>40-fold increase
BRCA1/BRCA2	Hereditary breast and ovarian cancer	1.5% (female), 2–4% (male)	Tenfold increase
MLH1, MSH2, and MSH6	Lynch syndrome	4% by age 70	Tenfold increase

Assessment of Primary Tumor [6, 10, 21, 22]

- First determine presence or absence of metastatic disease.
- Primary tumor resection status – resectable, borderline, or locally advanced unresectable.
    - Table 13.2 – NCCN definition of resectable and borderline resectable
        - More extensive disease than outlined in the table indicates locally advanced/unresectable disease.
        - Other published standards for resection status may vary (MD Anderson Cancer Center [22] and Society for Surgery of the Alimentary Tract [21]).
- CT PPV for locally advanced unresectable (89–100%); PPV for resectable is 45–79%.

Table 13.2 Resectability status of pancreatic cancer

	Resectable	Borderline
Venous[a]		
SMV or Portal Vein	≤ 180° contact *without* contour irregularity. No involvement of first jejunal vein branches draining SMV	≤ 180° contact *with* contour irregularity or thrombosis. >180° contact
IVC	----	Any contact
Arterial		
Celiac Axis	----	≤ 180° contact
SMA	----	≤ 180° contact
Common Hepatic	----	Contact allowing for safe and complete resection and reconstruction[b]
Variant anatomy	----	Any contact with variant anatomy

Created in BioRender. Henderson, E. (2024) BioRender.com/m85s584
[a]Must be able to resect and reconstruct
[b]Without extension to celiac axis or the hepatic artery bifurcation

Neoadjuvant Treatment

- First define as resectable, borderline, or locally advanced to be clear about goal of preoperative therapy.
- Histologic confirmation of disease is required prior to initiation of chemotherapy, not necessarily required in a surgery first approach.
- Neoadjuvant therapy for resectable disease:
  - Increasingly used at select institutions
  - Data less clear to support role in this population
  - Not recommended by NCCN guidelines except with clinical trial or high-risk patient (large primary tumor, markedly elevated CA19-9, highly symptomatic, bulky lymph nodes) [10]
  - Advantages:
    - Surgical complications and difficult postoperative recovery can delay or preclude receipt of systemic treatment in up to 40% of patients [23].
    - Early treatment of occult metastatic disease [24]
    - Evaluate histopathologic response to preoperative treatment [25]
    - Opportunity to change therapy if lack of response [26]
    - Possible decrease in tumor size, increased likelihood of R0 resection, and reduction in number positive nodes [27, 28].
  - Disadvantages
    - Inability to operate on the primary tumor if progression to unresectable.
    - Chemotherapy-related complications result in surgical delay.
- PREOPANC trial – phase III randomized trial, $n = 246$ [29]
  - Resectable AND borderline resectable randomized to surgery and adjuvant chemotherapy ($n = 127$) or neoadjuvant chemotherapy and chemoradiation ($n = 119$)
  - Median OS – 15.7 months for neoadjuvant group vs 14.3 months for adjuvant group ($p = 0.025$)
  - R0 resection rate – 72% vs 43% ($p < 0.001$)
  - Of patients who underwent resection, neoadjuvant survival 33.7 months vs 17.3 months ($p = 0.029$)
- Preferred Regimens:
  - FOLFIRINOX or gemcitabine + albumin-bound paclitaxel
  - FOLFIRINOX or gemcitabine + cisplatin (BRCA 1/BRCA 2 or PALB2 mutations)
- Radiologic response after neoadjuvant therapy may not correlate with pathologic response [6].
- Timing of surgery: 4–8 weeks following neoadjuvant completion

Surgical Technical Approach

Obstructive Jaundice

- May proceed with operation in setting of jaundice and resectable tumor
  - Total bilirubin < ~8–10 mg/dL.
  - Preoperative biliary drainage may increase rate of serious complications [30].
  - Preoperative biliary decompression is indicated if cholangitis, coagulopathy, severe bilirubin elevation, and anticipated delay in surgery.
- Preoperative biliary stenting is needed prior to neoadjuvant therapy.
- Self-expanding metal stent (SEMS) is preferred over plastic stents – improved patency rate and less migration [31]

Pancreatoduodenectomy (Whipple) [10]

- Careful review of preoperative imaging to evaluate for aberrant anatomy, particularly replaced right hepatic artery
- Intraoperative staging to assess for liver or peritoneal metastases
- Six steps of pancreatoduodenectomy (resection) [32] (order of steps may vary)
  1. Entry into lesser sac, separation of colon, and mesentery from duodenum and identification of infrapancreatic superior mesenteric vein (SMV)
     (a) May require mobilization of right colon and hepatic flexure.
     (b) Some surgeons ligate right gastroepiploic vein at this stage.
  2. Extended Kocher maneuver – elevate lymphatic and fatty tissue anterior to the IVC and extend dissection to left renal vein
  3. Division of distal stomach or first portion of duodenum if pylorus preservation
  4. Dissection of porta hepatis:
     (a) Remove hepatic artery node and ligate right gastric artery.
     (b) Clamp gastroduodenal artery (GDA) before division to check for celiac stenosis and retrograde flow – if found may abort case or consider arterial bypass.
     (c) Expose suprapancreatic portal vein (PV).
     (d) Cholecystectomy and divide common hepatic duct – manual palpation to check for replaced right hepatic artery posterior to bile duct.
     (e) Create tunnel under the neck of pancreas overlying PV/SMV confluence.
  5. Division of jejunum and all attachments at ligament of Treitz followed by ligation of jejunal mesentery and duodenal mesentery to near level of pancreas head
  6. Division of pancreas neck and retroperitoneal dissection – identify and preserve first jejunal branch when dividing connective tissue between uncinate process and lateral border of SMA (this is most common positive margin due to tumor spread along perineural autonomic plexus) [33, 34] (Table 13.3).

Table 13.3 Representative images demonstrating tumor involvement with vasculature

	Schematic	Representative image
Venous*		
Contour irregularity		
SMV thrombus		
Encasement and impingement of PV		
Arterial		
SMA abutment with tumor		
Variant anatomy: CHA arising from SMA with tumor abutment		

Created in BioRender. Henderson (2024) BioRender.com/m85s584

- Reconstruction
  - Pancreaticojejunostomy:
    - Common approach to outer layer – transpancreatic horizontal mattress sutures placed 1–2 cm from the cut edge of the pancreas followed by seromuscular bite of jejunum and then passing needle back through pancreas.
    - Consider a probe or stent in duct to prevent occlusion during outer layer sutures.
    - Interrupted duct-to-mucosa layer between pancreatic duct and small enterotomy.
    - Return to the outer layer by completing more seromuscular jejunal bites to bring bowel wall over anterior surface of pancreas [35, 36].
  - Hepaticojejunostomy – single layer with *absorbable* suture, running or interrupted
  - Gastrojejunostomy (GJ) or duodenojejunostomy – stapled or handsewn for GJ
  - Drain(s) around HJ and PJ

Vein Resection

- Not a contraindication to resection especially after neoadjuvant therapy
- Comparable outcomes including long-term survival to surgery without vein resection [37, 38]
- Classified by ISGPS:
  - *Partial* resection with direct closure or patch venoplasty (types 1 and 2)
  - *Segmental* resection with primary venous anastomosis or interposition conduit (types 3 and 4) [39] (Fig. 13.1)
- Postoperative imaging changes after venous resection may be confused for recurrent disease [40].

Arterial Resection

- Generally considered locally advanced unresectable; few advocates for its use [41, 42]
- Increased perioperative mortality [OR 5.04; $p < 0.0001$] and poor survival at one year (49%) [43]

Distal pancreatectomy with en bloc celiac axis resection (DP-CAR); modified Appleby procedure:

- Operation involves division of celiac artery – common hepatic artery flow maintained by retrograde flow-through GDA.
- Contraindications include tumor involvement of GDA or base of celiac at aorta.
- Outcomes superior at high-volume centers [44].

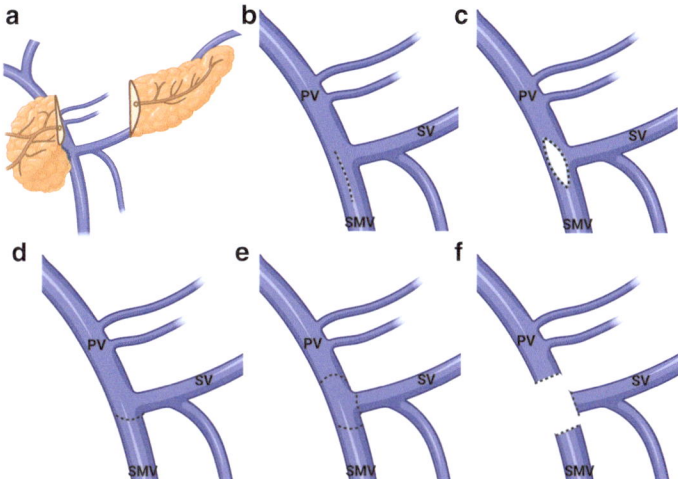

Fig. 13.1 (**a**) Head of pancreas mass invading portal vein. (**b, c**) Partial resection with direct closure and patch venoplasty (types 1 and 2). (**d–f**) Segmental resection with primary venous anastomosis (type 3) and interposition graft with vein and synthetic graft (type 4). PV, portal vein; SV, splenic vein; and SMV, superior mesenteric vein; (Graphics illustrated by Emily Henderson and created with BioRender.com)

- Complications (overall rate 40%) include chyle leak (16%), gastric, or liver ischemia
- Median overall survival 19 months [45, 46].

Intraoperative Radiation (IORT)

- Has been used for patients with borderline resectable disease to treat close or positive margins [47]
- Delivered prior to reconstruction to avoid radiation to anastomotic structures
- Dose of radiation varies from 10 to 20 Gy depending on resection status and field geometry

Other Considerations

- Elderly patients with poor performance status have worse outcomes [48].
- Reasonable alternative to surgical resection in high-risk patients without metastatic disease is a stereotactic body radiation therapy (SBRT). [49]
- Lymphadenectomy [50] (Table 13.4)
- Pancreaticoduodenectomy – stations 5, 6, 8a, 12b1, 12b2, 12c 13a, 13b, 14a right lateral side, 14b right lateral side, 17a, and 17b.

Table 13.4 Pancreatic cancer TMN staging (AJCC 8th edition) [90]

T stage—primary tumor	
Tx	Tumor cannot be assessed
T0	No evidence of primary tumor
Tis	Carcinoma in situ
T1	Tumor ≤2 cm in greatest dimension
T1a	Tumor ≤0.5 cm in greatest dimension
T1b	Tumor >0.5 cm and < 1.0 cm in greatest dimension
T1c	Tumor 1–2 cm in greatest dimension
T2	Tumor >2 cm and ≤ 4 cm in greatest dimension
T3	Tumor >4 cm in greatest dimension
T4	Tumor involves the celiac axis, superior mesenteric artery, and/or common hepatic artery
N stage—regional lymph nodes	
Nx	Regional lymph nodes cannot be assessed
N0	No regional LN metastases
N1	Cancer in 1–3 LNs
N2	Cancer in ≥4 LNs
M stage—distant metastasis	
M0	No distant metastasis
M1	Distant metastasis

- Distal subtotal pancreatectomy – stations 9, 10, 11, and 18.
- Adequate staging requires ≥15 nodes.
- No benefit to extended lymphadenectomy [51].

Complications After Operation

- Outcomes superior for pancreaticoduodenectomy with high-volume surgeon and hospital [52]
- 30–40% complication rate for Whipple [53]
- Delayed gastric emptying – 15–20% [54] – incidence unaffected by classic vs pylorus-preserving pancreaticoduodenectomy [55]
- Pancreatic leak or fistula – at least 10% (wide range reported)
  - Drain output of any measurable volume on or after postoperative day 3 with amylase >3 times upper limit of normal [56–58]
    - Grade A – biochemical leak only without clinical impact, can be discharged with a drain, but removed <21 days postoperatively
    - Grade B – change in management such as NPO with TPN, often discharged with drains and possibly antibiotics or somatostatin analogues, may require drainage for extended period (>21 days)
    - Grade C – significant clinical deterioration requiring intensive care unit, may have sepsis and organ dysfunction, may require interventions such as percutaneous drainage, and attempted repair of leak or completion pancreatectomy
    - High-output fistula = more than 200 ml/day

- Risk factors for leak = soft pancreatic parenchyma, small pancreatic duct (<4mm), nonpancreatic adenocarcinoma indication for surgery, high BMI, and arterial vascular disease [59]
- Endocrine and Exocrine Insufficiency
  - Risk of new-onset diabetes following pancreaticoduodenectomy – 12–20% [60]
  - Exocrine insufficiency requiring supplementation – up to 36% [61]
- Hemorrhage [62]
  - Early – within 1–2 weeks of operation
    - Most worrisome cause is gastroduodenal artery bleed or pseudoaneurysm, most often in setting of pancreatic leak.
    - May present as gastrointestinal bleed due to blood entry into bowel through anastomotic dehiscence.
    - Obtain urgent CT angiogram or straight to angiography if unstable.
    - Intervention most commonly coiling or covered metal stent.
  - Bleeding anastomosis, gastritis, or marginal ulceration also possible
  - Late (>2 months, may occur many years later) – most common cause is marginal ulcer at gastrojejunostomy anastomosis, treated with endoscopy interventions and proton pump inhibitors

Adjuvant Therapy

- Consider restaging imaging and repeat CA 19-9 level before initiation [10].
- Superior outcomes if initiation within 12 weeks of resection.
- Completion of six total months associated with improved survival [63, 64].
- Total therapy goal is six months when perioperative (pre and post) strategy used (e.g., 2 months neoadjuvant + 4 months adjuvant) [65]
- Regimens:
  - No neoadjuvant therapy:
    - Modified FOLFIRINOX – patients with optimal performance status
    - Gemcitabine + capecitabine vs gemcitabine + *nab*-paclitaxel – unable to tolerate FOLFIRINOX or less fit patients
  - Following neoadjuvant therapy – tailored based on response to neoadjuvant therapy.
  - Chemoradiation is also an option in the adjuvant setting [66].
  - Benefit of adjuvant chemotherapy greater after R0 resection [67].

Landmark Trials:

ESPAC-1: [68]
- Compared chemoradiation (5-FU, 20 Gy) vs chemotherapy (5-FU) vs both vs observation. $N = 541$

- A five-year survival significantly less in chemoradiotherapy than other groups (10% vs 20%; p= 0.05)
- A five-year survival significantly more in chemotherapy group (21% vs 8%; p <0.009)
- Takeaway: chemotherapy as opposed to chemoradiation provided overall survival benefit in adjuvant setting (Table 13.5)

CONKO-001: [69]
- Compared chemotherapy (gemcitabine x6 cycles for 6 months) vs observation group. N= 354
- DFS significantly improved in treatment group, 13.4 vs 6.9 months, p <0.001
- OS benefit seen on subsequent five- and ten-year analyses with 20.7% vs 10.4% and 12.2% vs 7.7%, respectively.
- Takeaway: established use of gemcitabine as adjuvant therapy in pancreatic cancer

ESPAC-3: [70]
- Compared 5-FU/leucovorin chemotherapy vs gemcitabine chemotherapy after curative surgery. $N = 1088$
- OS similar between treatment arms (5-FU/leucovorin – 23.0 months vs gemcitabine 23.6 months, $p = 0.39$).
- 14% receiving 5-FU/leucovorin group had serious adverse events compared to 7.5% of gemcitabine group (p<0.001), better overall compliance in the gemcitabine group.
- Takeaway: Gemcitabine has key advantages over 5-FU/leucovorin including reduced side effects and risk of serious adverse events.

ESPAC-4: [71]
- Compared gemcitabine and capecitabine vs gemcitabine monotherapy after curative surgery. $N = 732$
- OS for gemcitabine plus capecitabine group was 28.0 months vs 25.5 months ($p = 0.032$) in gemcitabine monotherapy group.
- Takeaway: established combination treatment as standard adjuvant regimen over gemcitabine alone.

PRODIGE 24: [72]
- Compared adjuvant mFOLFIRINOX vs gemcitabine therapy. $N = 493$
- Eligibility included WHO performance 0–1, CA 19-9 <189 U/mL, and R0 or R1 resection.
- DFS 21.6 months in mFOLFIRINOX group vs 12.8 months in gemcitabine group (HR 0.58; p <0.001). OS 54.4 months in the mFOLFIRINOX group vs 35.0 months in the gemcitabine group (HR 0.64; $p = 0.03$).
- Grade 3 or 4 adverse events were seen more frequently with mFOLFIRINOX therapy group (75.9%) than in gemcitabine therapy group (52.9%).

- Takeaway: mFOLFIRINOX is the current standard of care in the adjuvant setting.

APACT: [73]
- Compared gemcitabine plus *nab*-paclitaxel vs gemcitabine monotherapy. $N = 866$
- Eligibility included ECOG 1-0, CA 19-9 <100 U/mL, and R0 or R1 resection.
- DFS (primary end point) with no significant difference in either group – 19.4 vs 18.8 months HR 0.88, $P = 0.18$.
- OS 40.5 and 36.2 months favoring the combined gemcitabine plus *nab*-paclitaxel (HR 0.82, $P = 0.045$).
- Takeaway: gemcitabine plus *nab*-paclitaxel is used for adjuvant therapy; however, it is probably inferior to mFOLFIRINOX.

Management Unresectable/Metastatic

- Goals of chemotherapy in this population are cancer control and prolonged survival [10, 74].
- Therapy choice based on performance status, symptom burden, and comorbidities:
  - ECOG score 0–1 – multiple-agent therapy preferred
  - ECOG score of 2 – single-agent therapy preferred
- First-line regimens: [75]
  - FOLFIRINOX or gemcitabine + albumin-bound paclitaxel
  - FOLFIRINOX or gemcitabine + cisplatin (*BRCA 1/2* or *PALB2* mutations)
- Special treatment populations
  - Genetic testing performed soon after diagnosis – targeted therapy may be available for specific subpopulations [76]
  - Germline *BRCA 1/2* or *PALB2* pathogenic variants
    - Mutations that sensitize cells to therapeutics that either further damage DNA (platinum-based chemotherapy) or prevent other mechanisms of repair (poly(ADP-ribose) polymerase [PARP] inhibitors).
    - Exceptional response rates when compared to population data [77, 78].
    - PARP inhibitors may be used for maintenance after chemotherapy [77, 79].
  - Patients with microsatellite unstable tumors
    - <2% of patients presenting with advanced disease [80].
    - Immunotherapy has impressive objective and durable response rates in those who progress on first-line treatment regimens [80, 81].
  - Pembrolizumab approved as a second-line treatment strategy [76].
- Chemoradiation or short-beam radiation therapy can potentially maintain local control while offering patients systemic therapy holiday [74, 82, 83] [84].
- Aggressive treatment of pain and other cancer-related symptoms: [85]
  - Radiation for bleeding or painful tumors
  - EUS- or IR-guided celiac block for intractable pain

Landmark Trials to Know:
- Single-agent 5-fluorouracil (5-FU) was standard of care for unresectable/metastatic disease until the 1990s.
- Single-agent gemcitabine found to be superior to 5-FU with overall survival advantage (5.6 vs 4.4 months, $p < 0.003$) and QOL [86].

ACCORD 11: [87]
- Compared FOLFIRINOX vs gemcitabine monotherapy. $N = 342$
- Chemotherapy naïve, performance status 0 or 1, and serum bilirubin <1.5 times upper limit of normal
- FOLFIRINOX – found to have superior overall survival (11.1 months vs 6.8 months; HR 0.57, $p < 0.001$), progression-free survival (6.4 months vs 3.3 months; HR 0.47; $p < 0.001$), and QOL compared to gemcitabine.
- Grade 3 or 4 adverse events occurred more often in FOLFIRINOX group.
- Takeaway: FOLFIRINOX has survival advantage in metastatic disease but with greater toxicity than gemcitabine.

MPACT: [88]
- Compared gemcitabine plus *nab*-paclitaxel to gemcitabine monotherapy. $N = 861$
- Gemcitabine plus nab-paclitaxel found to be superior to single-agent gemcitabine, with improvement in overall survival (8.5 vs 6.7 months [HR 0.72, 0.62–0.83; $p < 0.001$]) and progression-free survival (5.5 months vs 3.7 months [HR 0.69; 0.58–0.82]) with a response rate of 23% vs 7%.
- Take away: OS, PFS and response rate was higher with combination gemcitabine and *nab*-paclitaxel.

GEMCAP: [89]
- Compared gemcitabine plus capecitabine vs gemcitabine monotherapy. $N = 533$
- Gemcitabine with capecitabine found to have improved response rate 19.1% vs 12.4% ($p = 0.034$) and improved progression-free survival (HR, 0.78; 0.66–0.93; $p = 0.020$)

Table 13.5 Landmark trials evaluating chemotherapy and/or chemoradiation in the neoadjuvant, adjuvant, and unresectable setting

Trial	Patients	Results	Takeaway point
Neoadjuvant			
PREOPANC [29]	246 patients Resectable and borderline resectable adenocarcinoma Surgery and adjuvant chemotherapy vs neoadjuvant chemotherapy/chemoradiation	OS 15.7 vs 14.3 months (HR 0.73; $p = 0.025$) If underwent resection, neoadjuvant survival 33.7 months vs 17.3 months (HR 0.47; $p = 0.029$) R0 resection rate was 72% vs 43% ($p < 0.001$)	Neoadjuvant chemoradiation has many benefits over adjuvant gemcitabine alone, including long-term survival and R0 resection rate

(continued)

Table 13.5 (continued)

Trial	Patients	Results	Takeaway point
Adjuvant			
ESPAC-1 [68]	541 patients Chemoradiation (5-FU, 20 Gy) vs chemotherapy (5-FU) vs both vs observation	A five-year survival less in chemoradiotherapy groups than all others 10% vs 20% ($p = 0.05$) A five-year survival significantly more in chemotherapy group 21% vs 8% ($p < 0.009$)	Chemotherapy as opposed to chemoradiation provided OS benefit in adjuvant setting
CONKO-001 [69]	354 patients Gemcitabine six cycles for six months vs observation	DFS 13.4 vs 6.9 months in gemcitabine group ($p < 0.001$) OS at 5 and 10 years were 20.7% vs 10.4% and 12.2% vs 7.7%, respectively	Established use of gemcitabine as adjuvant therapy in pancreatic cancer
ESPAC-3 [70]	1088 patients 5-FU/leucovorin chemotherapy vs gemcitabine chemotherapy after curative resection	OS with no difference 23.0 vs 23.6 months ($p = 0.39$) 14% serious adverse events with 5-FU/leucovorin vs 7.5% gemcitabine ($p < 0.001$)	Gemcitabine has key advantages over 5-FU/leucovorin including reduced side effects and serious adverse events
ESPAC-4 [71]	732 patients Gemcitabine and capecitabine vs gemcitabine monotherapy after curative resection	OS for combination 28.0 vs 25.5 months ($p = 0.032$)	Established combination treatment as standard adjuvant regimen over gemcitabine monotherapy
PRODIGE 24 [72]	493 patients Modified FOLFIRINOX vs gemcitabine Eligibility: WHO performance 0 or 1, CA19–9 < 189 u/mL, and R0 or R1 resection	DFS 21.6 months in mFOLFIRINOX vs 12.8 months in Gemcitabine group ($p < 0.001$) OS 54.4 vs 35.0 months ($p = 0.03$) Grade 3 or 4 adverse events 75.9% vs 52.9%	Survival is significantly improved with mFOLFIRINOX over gemcitabine but with greater toxicity
APACT [73]	866 patients Gemcitabine and *nab*-Paclitaxel vs gemcitabine monotherapy Eligibility: ECOG 1–0, CA 19-9 < 100 U/mL, and R0 or R1 resection	DFS no difference 19.4 vs 18.8 months ($p = 0.18$) OS 40.5 vs 36.2 ($p = 0.045$) months favoring combination therapy	Combination gemcitabine plus *nab*-paclitaxel has improved survival over gemcitabine monotherapy

(continued)

Table 13.5 (continued)

Trial	Patients	Results	Takeaway point
Metastatic disease			
Accord 11 [87]	342 patients FOLFIRINOX vs gemcitabine monotherapy Eligibility: Performance status 0 or 1 and serum bilirubin <1.5 times upper limit of normal	OS 11.1 months FOLFIRINOX vs 6.8 months ($p < 0.001$) PFS 6.4 vs 3.3 months ($p < 0.001$) Grade 3 or 4 adverse events more frequent in FOLFIRINOX group	FOLFIRINOX has survival advantage over gemcitabine but with greater toxicity
MPACT [88]	861 patients Gemcitabine and *nab*-paclitaxel vs gemcitabine monotherapy	Combination therapy showed improved OS 8.5 vs 6.7 months ($p < 0.001$), PFS 5.5 vs 3.7 months and response rate 23% vs 7%	Combination Gemcitabine plus *nab*-paclitaxel has better survival and response rate than gemcitabine monotherapy
GEMCAP [89]	533 patients Gemcitabine and capecitabine vs gemcitabine monotherapy	Combination therapy has improved response rate 19.1% vs 12.4% ($p = 0.034$) and PFS (HR 0.78, $p = 0.02$)	

Pancreatic cancer by numbers

Question	Answer
% metastatic/unresectable at diagnosis	80–85%
Overall survival in those who undergo R0 resection and complete neoadjuvant/adjuvant therapy	40–54 months [72, 73]
% who have familial pancreatic cancer syndrome	5–10%
% reduction of OS if R1 resection	25%
Overall morbidity after pancreaticoduodenectomy	30–40%

References

1. Sung H, Ferlay J, Siegel RL, et al. Global Cancer Statistics 2020: GLOBOCAN estimates of incidence and mortality worldwide for 36 cancers in 185 countries. CA Cancer J Clin. 2021;71(3):209–49. https://doi.org/10.3322/caac.21660.
2. Cronin KA, Scott S, Firth AU, et al. Annual report to the nation on the status of cancer, part 1: National cancer statistics. Cancer. 2022;128(24):4251–84. https://doi.org/10.1002/cncr.34479.
3. statistics SEAiwfSc. Surveillance Research Program, National Cancer Institute. 2023. Accessed 12 July 2023. https://seer.cancer.gov/statistics-network/explorer/
4. Wilentz RE, Iacobuzio-Donahue CA, Argani P, et al. Loss of expression of Dpc4 in pancreatic intraepithelial neoplasia: evidence that DPC4 inactivation occurs late in neoplastic progression. Cancer Res. 2000;60(7):2002–6.
5. Bailey P, Chang DK, Nones K, et al. Genomic analyses identify molecular subtypes of pancreatic cancer. Nature. 2016;531(7592):47–52. https://doi.org/10.1038/nature16965.
6. Al-Hawary MM, Francis IR, Chari ST, et al. Pancreatic ductal adenocarcinoma radiology reporting template: consensus statement of the society of abdominal radiology and the

american pancreatic association. Gastroenterology. 2014;146(1):291–304.e1. https://doi.org/10.1053/j.gastro.2013.11.004.
7. Bipat S, Phoa SS, van Delden OM, et al. Ultrasonography, computed tomography and magnetic resonance imaging for diagnosis and determining resectability of pancreatic adenocarcinoma: a meta-analysis. J Comput Assist Tomogr. 2005;29(4):438–45. https://doi.org/10.1097/01.rct.0000164513.23407.b3.
8. Tempero MA, Uchida E, Takasaki H, Burnett DA, Steplewski Z, Pour PM. Relationship of carbohydrate antigen 19-9 and Lewis antigens in pancreatic cancer. Cancer Res. 1987;47(20):5501–3.
9. Kim JE, Lee KT, Lee JK, Paik SW, Rhee JC, Choi KW. Clinical usefulness of carbohydrate antigen 19-9 as a screening test for pancreatic cancer in an asymptomatic population. J Gastroenterol Hepatol. 2004;19(2):182–6. https://doi.org/10.1111/j.1440-1746.2004.03219.x.
10. Network NCC. Pancreatic Adenocarcinoma (Version 2.2023).
11. Khorana AA, Mangu PB, Berlin J, et al. Potentially curable pancreatic cancer: American Society of Clinical Oncology Clinical Practice Guideline. J Clin Oncol. 2016;34(21):2541–56. https://doi.org/10.1200/jco.2016.67.5553.
12. Boone BA, Steve J, Zenati MS, et al. Serum CA 19-9 response to neoadjuvant therapy is associated with outcome in pancreatic adenocarcinoma. Ann Surg Oncol. 2014;21(13):4351–8. https://doi.org/10.1245/s10434-014-3842-z.
13. Bauer TM, El-Rayes BF, Li X, et al. Carbohydrate antigen 19-9 is a prognostic and predictive biomarker in patients with advanced pancreatic cancer who receive gemcitabine-containing chemotherapy: a pooled analysis of 6 prospective trials. Cancer. 2013;119(2):285–92. https://doi.org/10.1002/cncr.27734.
14. Berger AC, Garcia M Jr, Hoffman JP, et al. Postresection CA 19-9 predicts overall survival in patients with pancreatic cancer treated with adjuvant chemoradiation: a prospective validation by RTOG 9704. J Clin Oncol. 2008;26(36):5918–22. https://doi.org/10.1200/jco.2008.18.6288.
15. Humphris JL, Chang DK, Johns AL, et al. The prognostic and predictive value of serum CA19.9 in pancreatic cancer. Ann Oncol. 2012;23(7):1713–22. https://doi.org/10.1093/annonc/mdr561.
16. Banafea O, Mghanga FP, Zhao J, Zhao R, Zhu L. Endoscopic ultrasonography with fine-needle aspiration for histological diagnosis of solid pancreatic masses: a meta-analysis of diagnostic accuracy studies. BMC Gastroenterol. 2016;16(1):108. https://doi.org/10.1186/s12876-016-0519-z.
17. Korc P, Sherman S. ERCP tissue sampling. Gastrointest Endosc. 2016;84(4):557–71. https://doi.org/10.1016/j.gie.2016.04.039.
18. Hruban RH, Canto MI, Goggins M, Schulick R, Klein AP. Update on familial pancreatic cancer. Adv Surg. 2010;44:293–311. https://doi.org/10.1016/j.yasu.2010.05.011.
19. Klein AP, Brune KA, Petersen GM, et al. Prospective risk of pancreatic cancer in familial pancreatic cancer kindreds. Cancer Res. 2004;64(7):2634–8. https://doi.org/10.1158/0008-5472.can-03-3823.
20. Allen VB, Gurusamy KS, Takwoingi Y, Kalia A, Davidson BR. Diagnostic accuracy of laparoscopy following computed tomography (CT) scanning for assessing the resectability with curative intent in pancreatic and periampullary cancer. Cochrane Database Syst Rev. 2016;7(7):Cd009323. https://doi.org/10.1002/14651858.CD009323.pub3.
21. Callery MP, Chang KJ, Fishman EK, Talamonti MS, William Traverso L, Linehan DC. Pretreatment assessment of resectable and borderline resectable pancreatic cancer: expert consensus statement. Ann Surg Oncol. 2009;16(7):1727–33. https://doi.org/10.1245/s10434-009-0408-6.
22. Varadhachary GR, Tamm EP, Abbruzzese JL, et al. Borderline resectable pancreatic cancer: definitions, management, and role of preoperative therapy. Ann Surg Oncol. 2006;13(8):1035–46. https://doi.org/10.1245/aso.2006.08.011.
23. Merkow RP, Bilimoria KY, Tomlinson JS, et al. Postoperative complications reduce adjuvant chemotherapy use in resectable pancreatic cancer. Ann Surg. 2014;260(2):372–7. https://doi.org/10.1097/sla.0000000000000378.

24. Tuveson DA, Neoptolemos JP. Understanding metastasis in pancreatic cancer: a call for new clinical approaches. Cell. 2012;148(1–2):21–3. https://doi.org/10.1016/j.cell.2011.12.021.
25. Chatterjee D, Katz MH, Rashid A, et al. Histologic grading of the extent of residual carcinoma following neoadjuvant chemoradiation in pancreatic ductal adenocarcinoma: a predictor for patient outcome. Cancer. 2012;118(12):3182–90. https://doi.org/10.1002/cncr.26651.
26. AlMasri S, Zenati M, Hammad A, et al. Adaptive dynamic therapy and survivorship for operable pancreatic cancer. JAMA Netw Open. 2022;5(6):e2218355. https://doi.org/10.1001/jamanetworkopen.2022.18355.
27. Pingpank JF, Hoffman JP, Ross EA, et al. Effect of preoperative chemoradiotherapy on surgical margin status of resected adenocarcinoma of the head of the pancreas. J Gastrointest Surg. 2001;5(2):121–30. https://doi.org/10.1016/s1091-255x(01)80023-8.
28. Gillen S, Schuster T, Meyer Zum Büschenfelde C, Friess H, Kleeff J. Preoperative/neoadjuvant therapy in pancreatic cancer: a systematic review and meta-analysis of response and resection percentages. PLoS Med. 2010;7(4):e1000267. https://doi.org/10.1371/journal.pmed.1000267.
29. Versteijne E, Suker M, Groothuis K, et al. Preoperative chemoradiotherapy versus immediate surgery for resectable and borderline resectable pancreatic cancer: results of the Dutch randomized Phase III PREOPANC trial. J Clin Oncol. 2020;38(16):1763–73. https://doi.org/10.1200/jco.19.02274.
30. van der Gaag NA, Rauws EA, van Eijck CH, et al. Preoperative biliary drainage for cancer of the head of the pancreas. N Engl J Med. 2010;362(2):129–37. https://doi.org/10.1056/NEJMoa0903230.
31. Mullen JT, Lee JH, Gomez HF, et al. Pancreaticoduodenectomy after placement of endobiliary metal stents. J Gastrointest Surg. 2005;9(8):1094–104.; discussion 1104-5. https://doi.org/10.1016/j.gassur.2005.08.006.
32. Yen TWF, Abdalla EK, Pisters PWT, Evans DB. Chapter 18: Pancreaticoduodenectomy. In: Pancreatic cancer. 1st ed. Jones & Bartlett Learning; 2005. p. 265–85.
33. Huang JJ, Yeo CJ, Sohn TA, et al. Quality of life and outcomes after pancreaticoduodenectomy. Ann Surg. 2000;231(6):890–8. https://doi.org/10.1097/00000658-200006000-00014.
34. Raut CP, Tseng JF, Sun CC, et al. Impact of resection status on pattern of failure and survival after pancreaticoduodenectomy for pancreatic adenocarcinoma. Ann Surg. 2007;246(1):52–60. https://doi.org/10.1097/01.sla.0000259391.84304.2b.
35. Grobmyer SR, Kooby D, Blumgart LH, Hochwald SN. Novel pancreaticojejunostomy with a low rate of anastomotic failure-related complications. J Am Coll Surg. 2010;210(1):54–9. https://doi.org/10.1016/j.jamcollsurg.2009.09.020.
36. Behrns KE. Surgery of the liver and biliary tract. 3rd ed. Saunders Co Ltd; 2000.
37. Kelly KJ, Winslow E, Kooby D, et al. Vein involvement during pancreaticoduodenectomy: is there a need for redefinition of "borderline resectable disease"? J Gastrointest Surg. 2013;17(7):1209–17; discussion 1217. https://doi.org/10.1007/s11605-013-2178-5.
38. Riediger H, Makowiec F, Fischer E, Adam U, Hopt UT. Postoperative morbidity and long-term survival after pancreaticoduodenectomy with superior mesenterico-portal vein resection. J Gastrointest Surg. 2006;10(8):1106–15. https://doi.org/10.1016/j.gassur.2006.04.002.
39. Bockhorn M, Uzunoglu FG, Adham M, et al. Borderline resectable pancreatic cancer: a consensus statement by the International Study Group of Pancreatic Surgery (ISGPS). Surgery. 2014;155(6):977–88. https://doi.org/10.1016/j.surg.2014.02.001.
40. Javed AA, Bleich K, Bagante F, et al. Pancreaticoduodenectomy with venous resection and reconstruction: current surgical techniques and associated postoperative imaging findings. Abdom Radiol (NY). 2018;43(5):1193–203. https://doi.org/10.1007/s00261-017-1290-5.
41. Christians KK, Pilgrim CH, Tsai S, et al. Arterial resection at the time of pancreatectomy for cancer. Surgery. 2014;155(5):919–26. https://doi.org/10.1016/j.surg.2014.01.003.
42. Jegatheeswaran S, Baltatzis M, Jamdar S, Siriwardena AK. Superior mesenteric artery (SMA) resection during pancreatectomy for malignant disease of the pancreas: a systematic review. HPB (Oxford). 2017;19(6):483–90. https://doi.org/10.1016/j.hpb.2017.02.437.
43. Mollberg N, Rahbari NN, Koch M, et al. Arterial resection during pancreatectomy for pancreatic cancer: a systematic review and meta-analysis. Ann Surg. 2011;254(6):882–93. https://doi.org/10.1097/SLA.0b013e31823ac299.

44. Klompmaker S, Peters NA, van Hilst J, et al. Outcomes and risk score for distal pancreatectomy with celiac axis resection (DP-CAR): an international multicenter analysis. Ann Surg Oncol. 2019;26(3):772–81. https://doi.org/10.1245/s10434-018-07101-0.
45. Schmocker RK, Wright MJ, Ding D, et al. An aggressive approach to locally confined pancreatic cancer: defining surgical and oncologic outcomes unique to pancreatectomy with celiac axis resection (DP-CAR). Ann Surg Oncol. 2021;28(6):3125–34. https://doi.org/10.1245/s10434-020-09201-2.
46. Peters NA, Javed AA, Cameron JL, et al. Modified Appleby procedure for pancreatic adenocarcinoma: does improved Neoadjuvant therapy warrant such an aggressive approach? Ann Surg Oncol. 2016;23(11):3757–64. https://doi.org/10.1245/s10434-016-5303-3.
47. Calvo FA, Asencio JM, Roeder F, et al. ESTRO IORT Task Force/ACROP recommendations for intraoperative radiation therapy in borderline-resected pancreatic cancer. Clin Transl Radiat Oncol. 2020;23:91–9. https://doi.org/10.1016/j.ctro.2020.05.005.
48. Hsu CC, Wolfgang CL, Laheru DA, et al. Early mortality risk score: identification of poor outcomes following upfront surgery for resectable pancreatic cancer. J Gastrointest Surg. 2012;16(4):753–61. https://doi.org/10.1007/s11605-011-1811-4.
49. Rosati LM, Herman JM. Role of stereotactic body radiotherapy in the treatment of elderly and poor performance status patients with pancreatic cancer. J Oncol Pract. 2017;13(3):157–66. https://doi.org/10.1200/jop.2016.020628.
50. Tol JA, Gouma DJ, Bassi C, et al. Definition of a standard lymphadenectomy in surgery for pancreatic ductal adenocarcinoma: a consensus statement by the International Study Group on Pancreatic Surgery (ISGPS). Surgery. 2014;156(3):591–600. https://doi.org/10.1016/j.surg.2014.06.016.
51. Yeo CJ, Cameron JL, Lillemoe KD, et al. Pancreaticoduodenectomy with or without distal gastrectomy and extended retroperitoneal lymphadenectomy for periampullary adenocarcinoma, part 2: randomized controlled trial evaluating survival, morbidity, and mortality. Ann Surg. 2002;236(3):355–66. https://doi.org/10.1097/00000658-200209000-00012; discussion 366-8
52. Hata T, Motoi F, Ishida M, et al. Effect of hospital volume on surgical outcomes after pancreaticoduodenectomy: a systematic review and meta-analysis. Ann Surg. 2016;263(4):664–72. https://doi.org/10.1097/sla.0000000000001437.
53. Kneuertz PJ, Pitt HA, Bilimoria KY, et al. Risk of morbidity and mortality following hepato-pancreato-biliary surgery. J Gastrointest Surg. 2012;16(9):1727–35. https://doi.org/10.1007/s11605-012-1938-y.
54. Traverso LW, Hashimoto Y. Delayed gastric emptying: the state of the highest level of evidence. J Hepato-Biliary-Pancreat Surg. 2008;15(3):262–9. https://doi.org/10.1007/s00534-007-1304-8.
55. Horstmann O, Markus PM, Ghadimi MB, Becker H. Pylorus preservation has no impact on delayed gastric emptying after pancreatic head resection. Pancreas. 2004;28(1):69–74. https://doi.org/10.1097/00006676-200401000-00011.
56. Bassi C, Dervenis C, Butturini G, et al. Postoperative pancreatic fistula: an international study group (ISGPF) definition. Surgery. 2005;138(1):8–13. https://doi.org/10.1016/j.surg.2005.05.001.
57. Bassi C, Marchegiani G, Dervenis C, et al. The 2016 update of the International Study Group (ISGPS) definition and grading of postoperative pancreatic fistula: 11 Years After. Surgery. 2017;161(3):584–91. https://doi.org/10.1016/j.surg.2016.11.014.
58. Butturini G, Daskalaki D, Molinari E, Scopelliti F, Casarotto A, Bassi C. Pancreatic fistula: definition and current problems. J Hepato-Biliary-Pancreat Surg. 2008;15(3):247–51. https://doi.org/10.1007/s00534-007-1301-y.
59. Lermite E, Pessaux P, Brehant O, et al. Risk factors of pancreatic fistula and delayed gastric emptying after pancreaticoduodenectomy with pancreaticogastrostomy. J Am Coll Surg. 2007;204(4):588–96. https://doi.org/10.1016/j.jamcollsurg.2007.01.018.
60. Scholten L, Mungroop TH, Haijtink SAL, et al. New-onset diabetes after pancreatoduodenectomy: a systematic review and meta-analysis. Surgery. 2018;164:6. https://doi.org/10.1016/j.surg.2018.01.024.

61. Kusakabe J, Anderson B, Liu J, et al. Long-term endocrine and exocrine insufficiency after pancreatectomy. J Gastrointest Surg. 2019;23(8):1604–13. https://doi.org/10.1007/s11605-018-04084-x.
62. Magge D, Zenati M, Lutfi W, et al. Robotic pancreatoduodenectomy at an experienced institution is not associated with an increased risk of post-pancreatic hemorrhage. HPB (Oxford). 2018;20(5):448–55. https://doi.org/10.1016/j.hpb.2017.11.005.
63. Khorana AA, Mangu PB, Berlin J, et al. Potentially curable pancreatic cancer: American Society of Clinical Oncology Clinical Practice Guideline Update. J Clin Oncol. 2017;35(20):2324–8. https://doi.org/10.1200/jco.2017.72.4948.
64. Valle JW, Palmer D, Jackson R, et al. Optimal duration and timing of adjuvant chemotherapy after definitive surgery for ductal adenocarcinoma of the pancreas: ongoing lessons from the ESPAC-3 study. J Clin Oncol. 2014;32(6):504–12. https://doi.org/10.1200/jco.2013.50.7657.
65. Epelboym I, Zenati MS, Hamad A, et al. Analysis of perioperative chemotherapy in resected pancreatic cancer: identifying the number and sequence of chemotherapy cycles needed to optimize survival. Ann Surg Oncol. 2017;24(9):2744–51. https://doi.org/10.1245/s10434-017-5975-3.
66. Stocken DD, Büchler MW, Dervenis C, et al. Meta-analysis of randomised adjuvant therapy trials for pancreatic cancer. Br J Cancer. 2005;92(8):1372–81. https://doi.org/10.1038/sj.bjc.6602513.
67. Neoptolemos JP, Stocken DD, Dunn JA, et al. Influence of resection margins on survival for patients with pancreatic cancer treated by adjuvant chemoradiation and/or chemotherapy in the ESPAC-1 randomized controlled trial. Ann Surg. 2001;234(6):758–68. https://doi.org/10.1097/00000658-200112000-00007.
68. Neoptolemos JP, Stocken DD, Friess H, et al. A randomized trial of chemoradiotherapy and chemotherapy after resection of pancreatic cancer. N Engl J Med. 2004;350(12):1200–10. https://doi.org/10.1056/NEJMoa032295.
69. Oettle H, Post S, Neuhaus P, et al. Adjuvant chemotherapy with gemcitabine vs observation in patients undergoing curative-intent resection of pancreatic cancer: a randomized controlled trial. JAMA. 2007;297(3):267–77. https://doi.org/10.1001/jama.297.3.267.
70. Neoptolemos JP, Stocken DD, Bassi C, et al. Adjuvant chemotherapy with fluorouracil plus folinic acid vs gemcitabine following pancreatic cancer resection: a randomized controlled trial. JAMA. 2010;304(10):1073–81. https://doi.org/10.1001/jama.2010.1275.
71. Neoptolemos JP, Palmer DH, Ghaneh P, et al. Comparison of adjuvant gemcitabine and capecitabine with gemcitabine monotherapy in patients with resected pancreatic cancer (ESPAC-4): a multicentre, open-label, randomised, Phase 3 trial. Lancet. 2017;389(10073):1011–24. https://doi.org/10.1016/s0140-6736(16)32409-6.
72. Conroy T, Hammel P, Hebbar M, et al. FOLFIRINOX or gemcitabine as adjuvant therapy for pancreatic cancer. N Engl J Med. 2018;379(25):2395–406. https://doi.org/10.1056/NEJMoa1809775.
73. Tempero MA, Pelzer U, O'Reilly EM, et al. Adjuvant nab-Paclitaxel + gemcitabine in resected pancreatic ductal adenocarcinoma: results from a randomized, open-label, Phase III trial. J Clin Oncol. 2023;41(11):2007–19. https://doi.org/10.1200/jco.22.01134.
74. Balaban EP, Mangu PB, Khorana AA, et al. Locally advanced, unresectable pancreatic cancer: American Society of Clinical Oncology Clinical Practice Guideline. J Clin Oncol. 2016;34(22):2654–68. https://doi.org/10.1200/jco.2016.67.5561.
75. Sultana A, Smith CT, Cunningham D, Starling N, Neoptolemos JP, Ghaneh P. Meta-analyses of chemotherapy for locally advanced and metastatic pancreatic cancer. J Clin Oncol. 2007;25(18):2607–15. https://doi.org/10.1200/jco.2006.09.2551.
76. Sohal DPS, Kennedy EB, Cinar P, et al. Metastatic pancreatic cancer: ASCO guideline update. J Clin Oncol. 2020;38(27):3217–30. https://doi.org/10.1200/jco.20.01364.
77. Golan T, Hammel P, Reni M, et al. Maintenance olaparib for germline BRCA-mutated metastatic pancreatic cancer. N Engl J Med. 2019;381(4):317–27. https://doi.org/10.1056/NEJMoa1903387.

78. O'Reilly EM, Lee JW, Zalupski M, et al. Randomized, multicenter, Phase II trial of gemcitabine and Cisplatin with or without Veliparib in patients with pancreas adenocarcinoma and a Germline BRCA/PALB2 mutation. J Clin Oncol. 2020;38(13):1378–88. https://doi.org/10.1200/jco.19.02931.
79. Kindler HL, Hammel P, Reni M, et al. Overall survival results from the POLO trial: a Phase III study of active maintenance olaparib versus placebo for germline BRCA-mutated metastatic pancreatic cancer. J Clin Oncol. 2022;40(34):3929–39. https://doi.org/10.1200/jco.21.01604.
80. Le DT, Durham JN, Smith KN, et al. Mismatch repair deficiency predicts response of solid tumors to PD-1 blockade. Science. 2017;357(6349):409–13. https://doi.org/10.1126/science.aan6733.
81. Marabelle A, Le DT, Ascierto PA, et al. Efficacy of pembrolizumab in patients with noncolorectal high microsatellite instability/mismatch repair-deficient cancer: results from the Phase II KEYNOTE-158 study. J Clin Oncol. 2020;38(1):1–10. https://doi.org/10.1200/jco.19.02105.
82. Mahadevan A, Miksad R, Goldstein M, et al. Induction gemcitabine and stereotactic body radiotherapy for locally advanced nonmetastatic pancreas cancer. Int J Radiat Oncol Biol Phys. 2011;81(4):e615–22. https://doi.org/10.1016/j.ijrobp.2011.04.045.
83. Schellenberg D, Kim J, Christman-Skieller C, et al. Single-fraction stereotactic body radiation therapy and sequential gemcitabine for the treatment of locally advanced pancreatic cancer. Int J Radiat Oncol Biol Phys. 2011;81(1):181–8. https://doi.org/10.1016/j.ijrobp.2010.05.006.
84. Yip D, Karapetis C, Strickland A, Steer CB, Goldstein D. Chemotherapy and radiotherapy for inoperable advanced pancreatic cancer. Cochrane Database Syst Rev. 2006:3, Cd002093. https://doi.org/10.1002/14651858.CD002093.pub2.
85. Morganti AG, Trodella L, Valentini V, et al. Pain relief with short-term irradiation in locally advanced carcinoma of the pancreas. J Palliat Care. 2003;19(4):258–62.
86. Burris HA 3rd, Moore MJ, Andersen J, et al. Improvements in survival and clinical benefit with gemcitabine as first-line therapy for patients with advanced pancreas cancer: a randomized trial. J Clin Oncol. 1997;15(6):2403–13. https://doi.org/10.1200/jco.1997.15.6.2403.
87. Conroy T, Desseigne F, Ychou M, et al. FOLFIRINOX versus gemcitabine for metastatic pancreatic cancer. N Engl J Med. 2011;364(19):1817–25. https://doi.org/10.1056/NEJMoa1011923.
88. Von Hoff DD, Ervin T, Arena FP, et al. Increased survival in pancreatic cancer with nab-paclitaxel plus gemcitabine. N Engl J Med. 2013;369(18):1691–703. https://doi.org/10.1056/NEJMoa1304369.
89. Cunningham D, Chau I, Stocken DD, et al. Phase III randomized comparison of gemcitabine versus gemcitabine plus capecitabine in patients with advanced pancreatic cancer. J Clin Oncol. 2009;27(33):5513–8. https://doi.org/10.1200/jco.2009.24.2446.
90. Amin MB, Edge SB, Greene FL, et al. AJCC cancer staging manual. 8th ed. Springer; 2017. p. 1032.

Palliative Interventions

14

Sarah Mitchem, Frances Salisbury, Barbara Diane Gillis, Laura J. Ostapenko, and Katherine A. Hill

What Is Palliative Care?

The term "palliative care" was introduced by a surgeon, Dr. Balfour Mount, in 1975 [1].

The goal of palliative care is to preserve *quality of life* and treat suffering.

- To weigh not only longevity, but to consider survival together with comfort and function [2]
  - Twin obligations: relief of suffering and cure of disease [3]
- Recognized as important by many national and international organizations, including the American College of Surgeons [4]

S. Mitchem
Department of Obstetrics and Gynecology, Charleston Area Medical Center, Charleston, WV, USA
e-mail: sarah.n.mitchem@vandaliahealth.org

F. Salisbury
Department of Obstetrics and Gynecology, West Virginia University, Morgantown, WV, USA
e-mail: frances.salisbury@hsc.wvu.edu

B. D. Gillis
Department of Surgery, University of Louisville School of Medicine, Louisville, KY, USA
e-mail: bdgill05@louisville.edu

L. J. Ostapenko
Department of Anesthesiology and Perioperative Medicine, MaineHealth-Maine Medical Center, Portland, ME, USA
e-mail: laura.ostapenko@mainehealth.org

K. A. Hill (✉)
Department of Surgery, Division of General Surgery, Department of Medicine, Division of Geriatrics, Palliative Medicine & Hospice, West Virginia University, Morgantown, WV, USA
e-mail: katherine.hill2@hsc.wvu.edu

© The Author(s), under exclusive license to Springer Nature Switzerland AG 2025
C. Schmidt, M. G. Kledzik (eds.), *Complex General Surgical Oncology*,
https://doi.org/10.1007/978-3-031-88954-7_14

- Members of the Society of Surgical Oncology estimate that 21% of their surgeries are palliative in nature (determined by tumor still evident postoperatively and poor prognosis, with a goal of symptom relief) [5]

Opportunities and roles for palliative care [6, 7]:

1. Symptom management
2. Advance care planning
3. Goals of care clarification and challenging communication
4. Hospice transition

Studies show that palliative care is often underutilized or not addressed until late in a patient's course [2, 6]. In contrast, early palliative care has been associated with improved quality of life *and* longer survival [8].

Barriers to involving palliative care clinicians or discussing a palliative approach:

- Lack of training in this area – in 2015, only 60% of surgical oncology fellowships included formal training in aspects of palliative care [9]
- Uncertainty about prognosis [10, 11]
- Emotional stress, fear of damaging patient-provider relationship [12]
    - However, studies show that the physician-patient relationship is actually *strengthened* by discussion of prognosis [13].
- Systemic barriers – referring physician expectations, urgency, or time constraints [14, 15]
- Bias or stigma associated with the label "palliative care." Some institutions have substituted "supportive care" [16].
- Patients who identify as underrepresented minorities have been shown to be less likely to receive palliative care services [17].

Palliative care includes skills that each individual physician (including surgical oncologists) can practice and develop, and it also often includes involvement of an interdisciplinary team [6]:

- Physicians
- Nurses
- Nutritionists
- Counselors
- Chaplains and clergy
- Social workers
- Others

When considering a palliative approach – ask for help and engage the team.

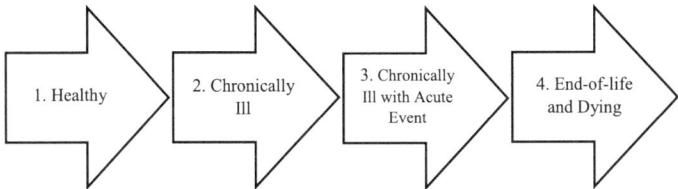

Fig. 14.1 Phases of illness

Surgical oncologists see patients through many phases of cancer treatment and with varying prognoses. For the purposes of this chapter, the overall health of a surgical oncology patient may fall into four categories (Fig. 14.1):

In general, surgical oncology patients may benefit from considering palliative interventions in any of these categories but particularly #2, 3, and 4.

Chronically Ill

Most patients undergoing cancer treatment can be considered chronically ill. Cancer itself, as well as its treatments, can lead to symptoms that significantly impact quality of life. These symptoms can be difficult to manage and are one opportunity to provide a palliative approach. Some of the most common symptoms for cancer patients include pain, nausea, anorexia/loss of appetite, and fatigue. The patient early in their cancer course also provides an opportunity to provide palliative support by doing advance care planning.

Pain

- Type of pain: nociceptive (visceral vs. somatic) and neuropathic
- Remember that pain is multifactorial, for example, the concept of "total pain" (Fig. 14.2) and cannot always be fully addressed by physical analgesia [18, 19].
- Treat pain in step-wise fashion (Fig. 14.3) and use multimodal approach
- Opioids – short-acting opioids include morphine, hydrocodone, oxycodone, oxymorphone, and fentanyl:
  - Conversions between formulations are complex and imprecise:
    - Calculate total oral morphine equivalents (OME) and refer to a conversion chart [21].
  - If taking short-acting opioids around the clock for pain that is expected to be long-term and constant, consider initiating long-acting scheduled opioid in addition (morphine extended-release, oxycodone extended-release, oxymorphone extended-release, fentanyl transdermal).

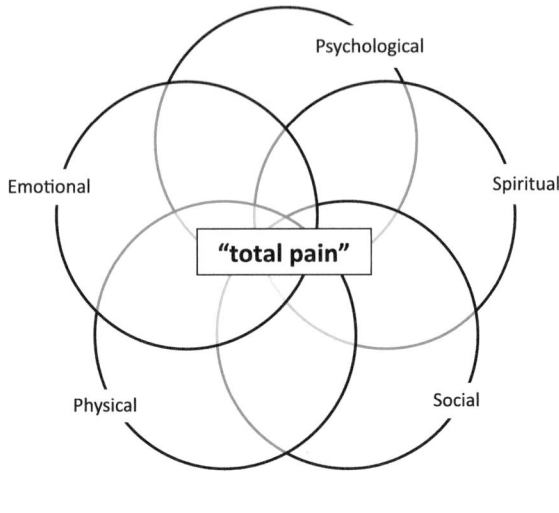

Fig. 14.2 Total pain

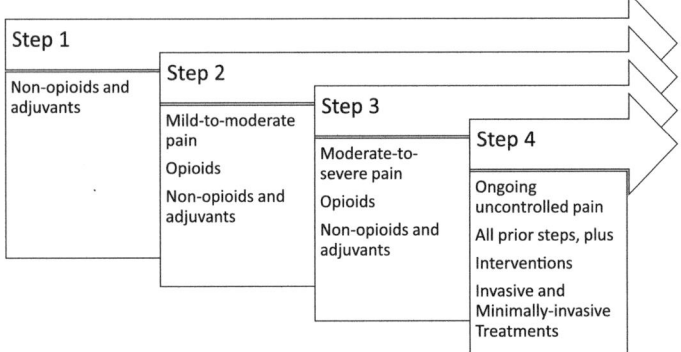

Fig. 14.3 WHO Analgesic Ladder [20]

- If initiating long-acting medications, consider referral to palliative care or pain specialist.
- Patients on prior long-acting opioid therapy should have this continued in the perioperative period – either with home regimen or converted to IV if unable to take oral medications [2].
- Adverse and Side Effects
  - Always screen for opioid misuse before initiating opioids: [22]
    - Risk factors for opioid misuse: personal or family history of alcohol, tobacco, or substance use disorder, age < 35 years old, concomitant psychiatric disease (particularly if uncontrolled)
    - Check state registries (PDMP) for prescription history
    - Routine urine drug screening to ensure results as expected
  - Opioid-induced constipation [23]
    - Tolerance never develops.

- Prevention is easier than treatment.
- Docusate typically ineffective.
- Multimodal regimen: sennosides (motility) + polyethylene glycol (osmotic)
 – Nausea, sedation, and confusion [23]
    - Alternate opioid forms can be tolerated differently by individuals.
    - Tolerance to these effects often develop with time (a few doses or days).
    - Add a PRN antiemetic.
    - Respiratory depression is rare; tolerance develops quickly – "start low and go slow" [23]
 – Neurotoxicity – myoclonus and seizure
    - Avoid morphine in renal impairment due to accumulation of neurologically active metabolites.
- Nonopioids and Adjuncts
 – Scheduled acetaminophen as adjunct to potentiate opioid effect.
 – NSAIDS – consider comorbidities (renal function, anticoagulation, bleeding diathesis or history of bleeding events), and if permissible with cancer therapy regimen [24]
 – Steroids (short-term) if pain from bony metastases or liver capsular stretch
 – Neuropathic pain agents: antiepileptics (gabapentin, pregabalin) or SNRIs (duloxetine, venlafaxine)
 – Others: ketamine, methadone, and buprenorphine (consider palliative care or pain specialist referral) [2, 20, 24]
 – Cannabinoids – moderate quality evidence for neuropathic and cancer pain [25–27]
- Interventional pain management (consider anesthesiology or interventional pain referral)
 – Local and regional anesthetics and nerve blocks
 – Physical therapy, massage, and acupuncture
 – Transcutaneous electrical nerve stimulation (TENS)
 – Behavioral treatments
 – Cancer-directed therapies such as chemotherapy, immunotherapy, hormonal therapy, and external beam radiation (discussed later in chapter) [2, 20, 28, 29]

Nausea

Chronic GI symptoms, both during and after cancer treatments, are common and significantly impact function and quality of life [30].

In treatment, consider (and treat if possible) the *underlying cause* and mechanism (Fig. 14.4) [31, 32].

Nausea mechanisms:

- *Not* mutually exclusive; rather, most etiologies arise due to more than one of these.
- Most medications affect more than one receptor and/or nausea pathway as well.

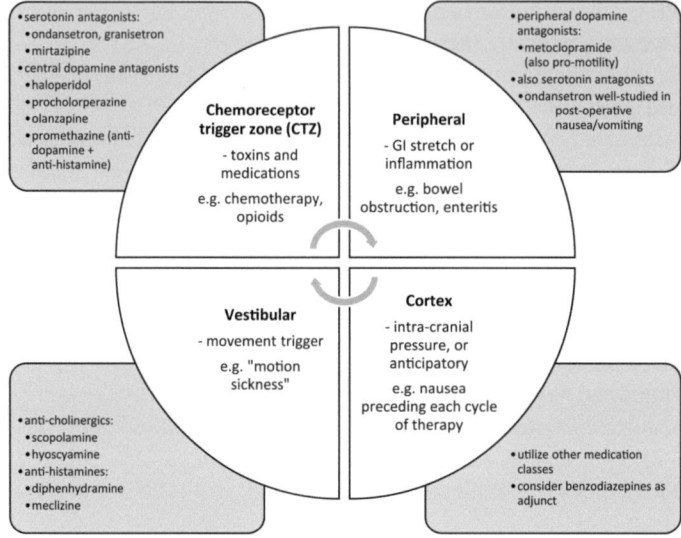

Fig. 14.4 Mechanisms and treatment of nausea

Nausea treatment pearls [31, 32]:

- Most medications affect multiple receptors; mechanism-based treatment is not an absolute rule – if one agent is not effective, try another.
- Avoid dopamine antagonists in patients with Parkinson's disease.
- Use caution if QTc >500 – most antiemetics are QT-prolonging.
- Anticholinergics have highest risk for delirium, particularly in elderly.

Adjuncts: cannabinoids, inhaled isopropyl alcohol [33], ginger, and acupuncture

Appetite and Weight Loss

- Common among patients with cancer.
- Screen for inadequately treated symptoms (nausea, constipation, pain)
- Consider intestinal dysmotility due to disease.
- Refer to a registered dietician for nutritional assessment and counseling on non-pharmacologic strategies.

Cancer Anorexia-Cachexia Syndrome [2, 34]

- Definition – Reduced appetite + weight loss (multiple eligibility criteria)
- Clinical diagnosis
- In context of advanced malignancy
  - Poor prognosis – typically <3 months

- Caused by neuroendocrine alterations:
- Systemic phenomenon
- Cytokine and hormonal mediators causing increased cellular oxidative stress
  - Calorie supplementation does not benefit: [35]
- Refocus on hunger and thirst and not on weight gain and caloric intake.
  - Consider discussion of prognosis and goals.

When to provide artificial enteral nutrition? Who will benefit from gastrostomy tube placement (Fig. 14.5)? [36–40]

What about parenteral nutrition (PN)? Who benefits? Guidelines and criteria include the following: [41, 42]

- Patients with a nonfunctioning GI tract as the primary problem, rather than cachexia itself.
- Death would occur from starvation or malnutrition soon than from disease progression alone.
- Life expectancy sufficient for adequate trial of PN (several months).
- Life prolongation is consistent with their goals/values.
- They are informed and accepting of the risks.
- The patient or caregiver, and their home environment can safely accommodate PN administration.
- The patient or caregiver can comply with close laboratory monitoring.
- Frequent reassessments of PN appropriateness and benefit

Appetite stimulants [2, 43–47]

- May affect appetite:
  - Few (if any) reliably increase strength.
  - Weight gain is typically water or fat rather than muscle mass.
  - No demonstrated effects on survival.
- FDA-approved agents include megestrol acetate and dronabinol:
  - Megestrol can increase risk for thrombotic events – use caution.

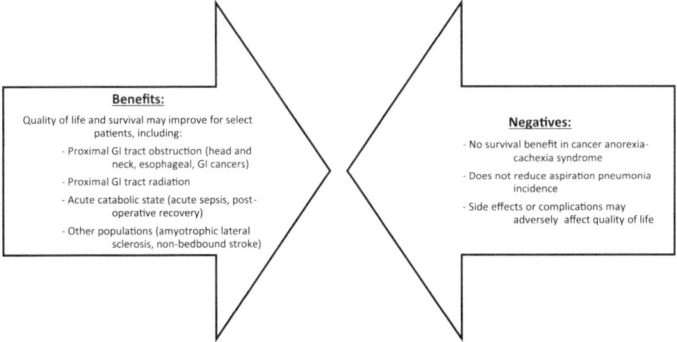

Fig. 14.5 Benefits and negatives of artificial enteral nutrition

- Other options: steroids (short-term), mirtazapine, olanzapine, and other cannabinoids.
- Screen for other symptoms (such as nausea, mood disorder, or sleep disturbance) in considering choice of medication.
- Per American Society of Clinical Oncology (ASCO) Guidelines:
- *Evidence remains insufficient to strongly endorse any pharmacologic agent to improve cancer cachexia outcomes; clinicians may choose not to offer medications for the treatment of cancer cachexia.*

Fatigue

- Fatigue and low energy levels are common [48] – may exceed pain as most prevalent symptom in cancer patients [49]
- Multifactorial: disease effects, treatment effects, sleep disturbances, psychologic and emotional effects

Treatments: [2, 50]

- Nonpharmacologic – sleep hygiene, anticipatory guidance and counseling patients and families, relaxation techniques, "batching" activities such as visits from friends and family, and exercise
- Pharmacologic:
  - Steroids (short-term)
  - Stimulants (methylphenidate, may suppress appetite, dose BID in morning and at noon to preserve sleep drive; modafinil)
  - Treat concomitant depression

Cancer-Directed Therapies

- Surgical, pharmacologic (chemotherapy, immunotherapy, hormonal therapy), radiation
- Ensure that patients understand the palliative vs. curative intent of their treatments.
  - Often misunderstood by patients [51]
  - Discussing intent and prognosis improves patient prognostic awareness and physician-patient relationship [52].
  - Weigh benefits (life prolongation, symptom benefit) vs. risks and side effects.

Palliative Radiation [53, 54]

- Localized tumor burden reduction without systemic side effects
- Often daily, schedule can be shortened when for palliative (rather than curative) intent

- *Pain*
  - Isolated bone mets can cause "incident"-type pain and be difficult to control.
  - Consider single-fraction radiation therapy for analgesia [55].
  - Any radiation can lead to pain flare within days after treatment (30–40% patients) [56]
    - Dexamethasone or NSAIDs can help or prevent.
  - Pain relief can continue to improve for up to 4 weeks after completion
- *Bleeding* – GI, head and neck, bladder, and gynecologic cancers
- *Mass Effect* – vascular, GI, or biliary obstruction
- *CNS* – often utilized for epidural (+/− spinal cord compression) or brain metastases
- Side effects – pain flare and inflammation of tissues in field (e.g., mucositis, skin burn)

Advance Care Planning

- Definition: communication between patient and healthcare team to prospectively identify a surrogate, clarify values, and develop individualized care plans near the end of life [57]
- *Advance directives* – legal documents that vary by jurisdiction:
  - Living wills
  - Medical power of attorney
  - Power of attorney for healthcare
- Recognize *caregiver burden* (common) [58] – advance care planning may help
- *When should you do advance care planning?* (Fig. 14.6)
- Patients want these discussions *early* in disease course [60]
- Assess the patient's *capacity*
  - Decision-making capacity has *four criteria:*
    1. The patient can indicate his or her treatment choice.
    2. The patient understands the relevant information being conveyed.

Fig. 14.6 "Surprise question" [59]

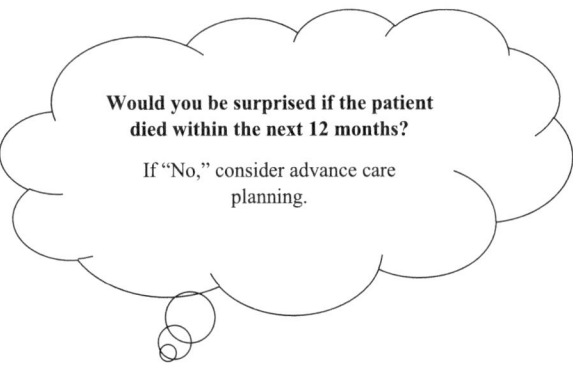

3. The patient acknowledges his or her medical condition, options, and likely outcomes.
  4. The patient can reason about treatment options.
  – Even if a patient has capacity, a patient may prefer to share or delegate decision-making [61].
- Avoid jargon.
- Example phrases:
  – "I'd like to spend some time talking to you about the future course of your illness so that I have a clear understanding of your wishes"
  – "Have you given any thought to how you wish to be cared for, if your illness worsens?" [57]
  – *"Who would you trust us to talk to if you were so sick that we could not talk to you?"*
  – *"Have you talked to ____ about what is most important should you get sicker?"*
- Patients may not want to, or be able to, discuss preferences at the time – consider revisiting the discussion at a future encounter.

How to find an advance directive form:

- Search by state (see Resources at the end of the chapter)
- May include POLST (Portable Medical Orders)
  – Many states have registries.
  – Copy for medical record.
  – Patients should be given the original.

Chronically Ill with Acute Event

Often cancer patients will face one or more acute changes in their health throughout their course. Sometimes this is an acute exacerbation of symptoms, a hospitalization, a complication of treatment, or a surgery itself. In these situations, a palliative approach might include effectively delivering this news and forming a plan based on their goals and priorities. Some specific acute changes faced by cancer patients and their surgeons include events such as malignant bowel obstruction or malignant ascites – palliative symptom management in these situations includes both medical and surgical or procedural options.

Delivering Serious News

- What is considered a "difficult conversation"?
  – Emotional information is presented, discussed, and processed.
  – Highly consequential decisions are made – impact future function, survival, etc.

- Shared decision-making between the patient and healthcare provider is the intent.
- For surgical oncologists, this can include conveying diagnostic information, surgical planning, intraoperative findings, or postoperative complications, among others.
• In oncology as well as palliative medicine, multiple structured communication tools have been developed to aid in shared decision-making [62–65].
  - SPIKES
  - Serious Illness Conversation Guide
  - REMAP
• Most communication frameworks share *four key steps* (Fig. 14.7):
• One example is REMAP, which is a mnemonic including five steps (Fig. 14.8) [63].
  - Reframe the Information, Expect Emotion, Map Patient Values, Align with Values, and Propose a Plan

Best Case: Worst Case (Fig. 14.9) [66]

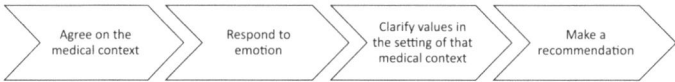

Fig. 14.7 Communication framework key steps

		Definition	Example
R	Reframe	Assess the patient's understanding and provide new information. Place details into a bigger picture – give a "headline."	"What have the doctors told you so far? ...That's correct, your colonoscopy found a cancer in your large intestine. Unfortunately, your other tests show that it has spread to other organs. This means doing a surgery won't help your cancer overall, and we should talk about other cancer treatments."
E	Expect Emotion	Look for verbal or nonverbal emotional responses. Attending to emotion often needs to occur multiple times in a conversation.	"This is so unexpected. Nobody could blame you for being overwhelmed and afraid. I wish there was an operation we could do to take it all out."
M	Map values	Step back to explore the patient's values before discussing choices – what matters most, and what concerns are there for the future?	"I wonder, hearing this news, what you are thinking now? What's most important to you? What are you worried about? Have you ever seen family or friends go through cancer treatments?"
A	Align	Verbally reflect back what you hear from the patient, sometimes this includes contradiction or ambivalence. Use reflections to hypothesize what the patient means.	"It sounds like you're willing to go through a lot of medical care, to get more time with your grandkids and family. I also hear you saying that your physical independence is very important, and you wouldn't ever want to live in a nursing home."
P	Propose a Plan	Make a recommendation based on patient values. Choose the options that you believe have the best chance to attain the patient's goals.	"Could I make a recommendation? I think given what you've told me, we should get you to a medical oncologist to discuss starting systemic treatment as soon as possible. If we reach a time when you become weaker, or need help with basic care, then you and your family should ask for another conversation, to re-evaluate whether more treatment makes sense for you."

Fig. 14.8 REMAP framework for difficult conversations

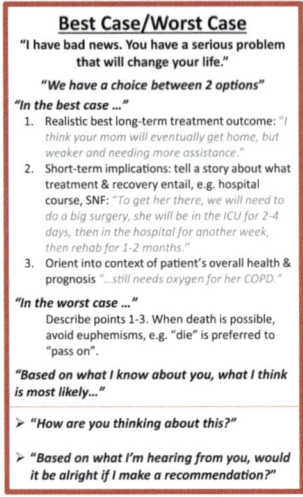 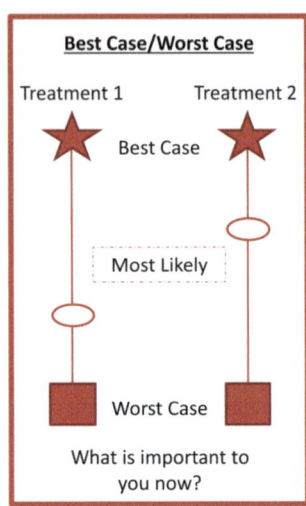

Fig. 14.9 Best case/worst case framework. (Used with permission by author)

- Tool developed by surgeons for presenting the medical context, that is, the "Reframe."
- Can be helpful when there are two options, that is, surgery and no surgery.
- Utilizes a drawn graphic aid that patients can take with them.
- See Resources at the end of the chapter for more information.

Malignant Obstruction [2, 67–69]

- Most common in GI or gynecologic cancers
- High morbidity and mortality when urgent surgery is performed and high reobstruction rate
- Overall indicator of limited prognosis (typically months)
- Variable proportion of bowel obstructions (3–48%) in patients with previously diagnosed malignancy are due to benign causes – always consider surgery
- *Surgical* management:
  - Resection – may lengthen survival, highest complication risk [70]
  - Bypass
  - Fecal diversion/ostomy
  - Venting gastrostomy – very effective for symptom relief [71]
- *Procedural/Interventional* Management:
  - Nasogastric decompression – typically not long term
  - Endoscopic stenting (GI, biliary, respiratory)
  - Radiation
  - Endoscopic laser

- *Medical* management:
  - Reduce gastric secretions – PPI.
  - Metoclopramide – for partial obstruction, can cause cramping, and do not give in complete obstruction.
  - Antisecretory medications, for example, glycopyrrolate.
  - Octreotide for high-volume output.
  - Dexamethasone 4–8 mg per day.
  - If parenteral nutrition not recommended or aligned with patient goals, stopping caloric supplementation often reduces GI tract secretions.

Malignant Ascites [72, 73]

- Cause of pain, pressure, nausea, bloating, and constipation

Medical management

- Typically does not respond to diuretics
  - Patients with concurrent portal hypertension may respond.

Paracentesis

- Immediate relief of symptoms for up to 90% of patients.
- Pigtail catheters can be considered in short-term situations.

Tunneled drainage catheter

- Patients who require frequent paracenteses
- Limited prognosis but life expectancy of at least one month is recommended
- Can by drained repeatedly, as needed, in the home
- FDA approved for this indication
- Performed usually by interventional radiology clinician

For low-grade cancers and patients with longer survival, hyperthermic intraperitoneal chemotherapy (HIPEC) is associated with high rates of ascites control [74].

End of Life and Dying

Cancer patients sometimes reach a point at which their disease progresses despite therapy, and therefore (or for any other medical reason) their time is very short. In these scenarios, palliative care may become the predominant strategy or even the only treatment plan available to them.

Indicators That Prognosis Is Short [2, 75, 76]

Weeks to Months

- Cancer anorexia-cachexia syndrome
- Malignant obstruction
- Hypercalcemia of malignancy
- Malignant pericardial effusion
- Malignant ascites
- Spinal cord compression
- Confusion, altered mentation, and multiple brain metastases

Days to weeks

- Bed-bound state
- Decreased desire for food or fluids
- Decreased urine output
- Increased sleep
- Difficulty with oral secretions – "death rattle"
- Open-mouthed breathing and flattened nasolabial folds
- Delirium
- Incontinence
- Change in respiratory pattern and apneic pauses
- Mottling or cool extremities

Hospice [77–79]

- What is hospice?
  - Philosophy
    - Transition to focus on symptoms and quality of life, maximizing time out of the hospital, rather than life prolongation or disease-directed therapy.
    - The word "hospice" is scary and emotional for many.
    - The family is the unit of care.
  - Medicare Benefit
    - If <65 years old, most insurances will have a hospice benefit modelled after the Medicare benefit but will need to be verified by social work/care management.
  - Hospice team consists of nurse, physician, social worker, chaplain, and sometimes others (aid, volunteer, therapist).
- Who can enroll in hospice care?
  - Eligibility – prognosis of 6 months or less "if the illness runs its normal course."
    - Certified by two physicians – typically referring physician and the hospice medical director

- Patient or surrogate must elect to enroll in hospice.
- Limited code status is *not* required.
- Not required to be certain they will die within 6 months, just more likely than not
  - Patients can be recertified indefinitely if they remain eligible, that is, continue to have a prognosis of 6 months or less.
- Where can hospice occur?
  - Home
  - Nursing homes
  - Inpatient hospice facility – hospice house or hospital
- What do they provide?
  - Medications for symptoms and those related to the hospice diagnosis
  - Equipment and supplies
  - Visits from hospice nurse, typically 2–3 times per week
  - On-call number for as-needed visits available 24 h
  - Bereavement support for families for up to 13 months after patient's death
  - Inpatient level of care if symptoms unable to be controlled in less-acute setting
  - Respite care up to 5 days
- What do they *not* provide?
  - Daily around-the-clock custodial care – in the home, this is done by family, friends, or privately hired caregivers.
  - They do not cover nursing home room and board costs.
  - Curative treatment.
  - Medications not related to the hospice diagnosis.
  - Hospice is not "giving up," does not "stop all care," and does not give medications that hasten death.
- Special cases: dialysis, tube feeding, parenteral nutrition, radiation, blood transfusions, and inotropes
  - Case by case and hospice-specific

Counseling for Families [75]

"How long do they have?" [76]

- Confirm that patient, and/or all individuals present, are ready and want a prognostic estimate.
  - Ask whether specific goal or milestone in mind.
- Present information in a range (days to weeks, short months, months to short years, etc.).
- Allow silence and attend to emotion.

"Have we made the right decision?" "Are they suffering?"

- Reiterate patient goals.
- Discuss symptom management.

- Offer spiritual, psychological, social support – therapeutic presence.

"Are they hungry/thirsty/starving?":

- Patients at end of life do not experience hunger/thirst [80].
- Reiterate that the disease is leading to end of life, not starvation.

"Can they hear me?" [81]

- Yes – evidence demonstrates that hearing persists at end of life.
- Encourage families to talk to their loved one and to each other.
- Familiar voices can bring symptom relief and calm to their dying loved one.

Palliative Care Resources

- Fast Facts – www.mypcnow.org
- CaringInfo Advance Directives – www.caringinfo.org/planning/advance-directives/by-state/
- POLST (Portable Medical Orders) – www.polst.org
- The Patient Preferences Project (Best Case/Worst Case) – www.patientpreferences.org
- VitalTalk – www.vitaltalk.org
- Ariadne Labs (Serious Illness Care Program) – www.ariadnelabs.org/serious-illness-care
- Hospice Care Overview and FAQs – www.nhpco.org/
- *Gone from My Sight: The Dying Experience* by Barbara Karnes, RN – www.bkbooks.com

References

1. Williams MA, Wheeler MS. Palliative care: what is it? Home Healthc Nurse. 2001;19(9):550–6; quiz 557. https://doi.org/10.1097/00004045-200109000-00013.
2. Dunn GPMR, Weissman D, editors. Surgical palliative care: a resident's guide. American College of Surgeons, Cunniff-Dixon Foundation; 2009.
3. Cassel EJ. The nature of suffering and the goals of medicine. N Engl J Med. 1982;306(11):639–45. https://doi.org/10.1056/nejm198203183061104.
4. Dunn GP. Surgery, palliative care, and the American College of Surgeons. Ann Palliat Med. 2015;4(1):5–9. https://doi.org/10.3978/j.issn.2224-5820.2015.01.03.
5. McCahill LE, Krouse R, Chu D, et al. Indications and use of palliative surgery-results of Society of Surgical Oncology survey. Ann Surg Oncol. 2002;9(1):104–12. https://doi.org/10.1245/aso.2002.9.1.104.
6. Ferrell BR, Twaddle ML, Melnick A, Meier DE. National Consensus Project Clinical Practice Guidelines for Quality Palliative Care Guidelines, 4th edition. J Palliat Med. 2018;21(12):1684–9. https://doi.org/10.1089/jpm.2018.0431.
7. Kelley AS, Meier DE. Palliative care–a shifting paradigm. N Engl J Med. 2010;363(8):781–2. https://doi.org/10.1056/NEJMe1004139.

8. Temel JS, Greer JA, Muzikansky A, et al. Early palliative care for patients with metastatic non-small-cell lung cancer. N Engl J Med. 2010;363(8):733–42. https://doi.org/10.1056/NEJMoa1000678.
9. Larrieux G, Wachi BI, Miura JT, et al. Palliative care training in surgical oncology and hepatobiliary fellowships: a National Survey of program directors. Ann Surg Oncol. 2015;22(Suppl 3):S1181–6. https://doi.org/10.1245/s10434-015-4805-8.
10. Christakis NA, Iwashyna TJ. Attitude and self-reported practice regarding prognostication in a national sample of internists. Arch Intern Med. 1998;158(21):2389–95. https://doi.org/10.1001/archinte.158.21.2389.
11. Christakis NA, Lamont EB. Extent and determinants of error in doctors' prognoses in terminally ill patients: prospective cohort study. BMJ. 2000;320(7233):469–72. https://doi.org/10.1136/bmj.320.7233.469.
12. Ptacek JT, McIntosh EG. Physician challenges in communicating bad news. J Behav Med. 2009;32(4):380–7. https://doi.org/10.1007/s10865-009-9213-8.
13. Fenton JJ, Duberstein PR, Kravitz RL, et al. Impact of prognostic discussions on the patient-physician relationship: prospective cohort study. J Clin Oncol. 2018;36(3):225–30. https://doi.org/10.1200/JCO.2017.75.6288.
14. Suwanabol PA, Kanters AE, Reichstein AC, et al. Characterizing the role of U.S. surgeons in the provision of palliative care: a systematic review and mixed-methods meta-synthesis. J Pain Symptom Manag. 2018;55(4):1196–1215.e5. https://doi.org/10.1016/j.jpainsymman.2017.11.031.
15. Zimmermann CJ, Taylor LJ, Tucholka JL, et al. The association between factors promoting nonbeneficial surgery and moral distress: a National Survey of surgeons. Ann Surg. 2022;276(1):94–100. https://doi.org/10.1097/SLA.0000000000004554.
16. Fadul N, Elsayem A, Palmer JL, et al. Supportive versus palliative care: what's in a name?: a survey of medical oncologists and midlevel providers at a comprehensive cancer center. Cancer. 2009;115(9):2013–21. https://doi.org/10.1002/cncr.24206.
17. Giap F, Ma SJ, Oladeru OT, et al. Palliative care utilization and racial and ethnic disparities among women with de novo metastatic breast cancer in the United States. Breast Cancer Res Treat. 2023;200(3):347–54. https://doi.org/10.1007/s10549-023-06963-7.
18. Clark D. 'Total pain', disciplinary power and the body in the work of Cicely Saunders, 1958–1967. Soc Sci Med. 1999;49(6):727–36. https://doi.org/10.1016/s0277-9536(99)00098-2.
19. Saunders C. The evolution of palliative care. J R Soc Med. 2001;94(9):430–2. https://doi.org/10.1177/014107680109400904.
20. Anekar AA, Hendrix JM, Cascella M. WHO Analgesic Ladder. StatPearls. StatPearls Publishing. Copyright © 2023, StatPearls Publishing LLC.; 2023.
21. McPherson MLM. Demystifying opioid conversion calculations: a guide for effective dosing. 2nd ed. American Society of Health-System Pharmacists; 2018.
22. Katz NP, Adams EH, Benneyan JC, et al. Foundations of opioid risk management. Clin J Pain. 2007;23(2):103–18. https://doi.org/10.1097/01.ajp.0000210953.86255.8f.
23. Chau DL, Walker V, Pai L, Cho LM. Opiates and elderly: use and side effects. Clin Interv Aging. 2008;3(2):273–8. https://doi.org/10.2147/cia.s1847.
24. Wood H, Dickman A, Star A, Boland JW. Updates in palliative care – overview and recent advancements in the pharmacological management of cancer pain. Clin Med (Lond). 2018;18(1):17–22. https://doi.org/10.7861/clinmedicine.18-1-17.
25. Busse JW, Vankrunkelsven P, Zeng L, et al. Medical cannabis or cannabinoids for chronic pain: a clinical practice guideline. BMJ. 2021;374:n2040. https://doi.org/10.1136/bmj.n2040.
26. Wang L, Hong PJ, May C, et al. Medical cannabis or cannabinoids for chronic non-cancer and cancer related pain: a systematic review and meta-analysis of randomised clinical trials. BMJ. 2021;374:n1034. https://doi.org/10.1136/bmj.n1034.
27. Whiting PF, Wolff RF, Deshpande S, et al. Cannabinoids for medical use: a systematic review and meta-analysis. JAMA. 2015;313(24):2456–73. https://doi.org/10.1001/jama.2015.6358.

28. Coelho A, Parola V, Cardoso D, Bravo ME, Apóstolo J. Use of non-pharmacological interventions for comforting patients in palliative care: a scoping review. JBI Database System Rev Implement Rep. 2017;15(7):1867–904. https://doi.org/10.11124/JBISRIR-2016-003204.
29. Guenther M, Görlich D, Bernhardt F, et al. Virtual reality reduces pain in palliative care-A feasibility trial. BMC Palliat Care. 2022;21(1):169. https://doi.org/10.1186/s12904-022-01058-4.
30. Han CJ, Reding KW, Kalady MF, Yung R, Greenlee H, Paskett ED. Factors associated with long-term gastrointestinal symptoms in colorectal cancer survivors in the women's health initiatives (WHI study). PLoS One. 2023;18(5):e0286058. https://doi.org/10.1371/journal.pone.0286058.
31. Wood GJ, Shega JW, Lynch B, Von Roenn JH. Management of intractable nausea and vomiting in patients at the end of life: "I was feeling nauseous all of the time ... nothing was working". JAMA. 2007;298(10):1196–207. https://doi.org/10.1001/jama.298.10.1196.
32. Kamell A, Marks S, Hallenbeck J. Fast facts and concepts #05. Nausea and Vomiting: Common Etiologies and Management. 2021.
33. Beadle KL, Helbling AR, Love SL, April MD, Hunter CJ. Isopropyl alcohol nasal inhalation for nausea in the emergency department: a randomized controlled trial. Ann Emerg Med. 2016;68(1):1–9.e1. https://doi.org/10.1016/j.annemergmed.2015.09.031.
34. Fearon K, Strasser F, Anker SD, et al. Definition and classification of cancer cachexia: an international consensus. Lancet Oncol. 2011;12(5):489–95. https://doi.org/10.1016/S1470-2045(10)70218-7.
35. Amano K, Maeda I, Ishiki H, et al. Effects of enteral nutrition and parenteral nutrition on survival in patients with advanced cancer cachexia: analysis of a multicenter prospective cohort study. Clin Nutr. 2021;40(3):1168–75. https://doi.org/10.1016/j.clnu.2020.07.027.
36. Rabeneck L, McCullough LB, Wray NP. Ethically justified, clinically comprehensive guidelines for percutaneous endoscopic gastrostomy tube placement. Lancet. 1997;349(9050):496–8. https://doi.org/10.1016/S0140-6736(96)07369-2.
37. Hallenbeck J. Tube feed or not tube feed? J Palliat Med. 2002;5(6):909–10. https://doi.org/10.1089/10966210260499104.
38. DeLegge MH, McClave SA, DiSario JA, et al. Ethical and medicolegal aspects of PEG-tube placement and provision of artificial nutritional therapy. Gastrointest Endosc. 2005;62(6):952–9. https://doi.org/10.1016/j.gie.2005.08.024.
39. Good P, Richard R, Syrmis W, Jenkins-Marsh S, Stephens J. Medically assisted nutrition for adult palliative care patients. Cochrane Database Syst Rev. 2014;2014(4):CD006274. https://doi.org/10.1002/14651858.CD006274.pub3.
40. Orrevall Y, Tishelman C, Permert J, Lundström S. A national observational study of the prevalence and use of enteral tube feeding, parenteral nutrition and intravenous glucose in cancer patients enrolled in specialized palliative care. Nutrients. 2013;5(1):267–82. https://doi.org/10.3390/nu5010267.
41. Pironi L, Boeykens K, Bozzetti F, et al. ESPEN practical guideline: Home parenteral nutrition. Clin Nutr. 2023;42(3):411–30. https://doi.org/10.1016/j.clnu.2022.12.003.
42. Mirhosseini M, Fainsinger R. Parenteral nutrition in patients with advanced cancer #190. J Palliat Med. 2009;12(3):260–1. https://doi.org/10.1089/jpm.2009.9660.
43. Salacz ME. Megestrol acetate for cancer anorexia/cachexia #100. J Palliat Med. 2006;9(3):803–4.
44. Wilner LS, Arnold RM. Cannabinoids in the treatment of symptoms in cancer and AIDS #93. J Palliat Med. 2006;9(3):802–4. https://doi.org/10.1089/jpm.2006.9.802.
45. Khoo SY, Quinlan N. Mirtazapine: a drug with many palliative uses #314. J Palliat Med. 2016;19(10):1116–7. https://doi.org/10.1089/jpm.2016.0222.
46. Felton M, Weinberg R, Pruskowski J. Olanzapine for nausea, delirium, anxiety, insomnia, and cachexia #315. J Palliat Med. 2016;19(11):1224–5. https://doi.org/10.1089/jpm.2016.0220.
47. Roeland EJ, Bohlke K, Baracos VE, et al. Management of Cancer Cachexia: ASCO guideline. J Clin Oncol. 2020;38(21):2438–53. https://doi.org/10.1200/jco.20.00611.

48. Kim HJ, Malone PS. Roles of biological and psychosocial factors in experiencing a psychoneurological symptom cluster in cancer patients. Eur J Oncol Nurs. 2019;42:97–102. https://doi.org/10.1016/j.ejon.2019.08.005.
49. Morrow GR, Shelke AR, Roscoe JA, Hickok JT, Mustian K. Management of cancer-related fatigue. Cancer Investig. 2005;23(3):229–39. https://doi.org/10.1081/cnv-200055960.
50. Chow R, Bruera E, Sanatani M, et al. Cancer-related fatigue-pharmacological interventions: systematic review and network meta-analysis. BMJ Support Palliat Care. 2021; https://doi.org/10.1136/bmjspcare-2021-003244.
51. Ghandourh WA. Palliative care in cancer: managing patients' expectations. J Med Radiat Sci. 2016;63(4):242–57. https://doi.org/10.1002/jmrs.188.
52. George LS, Prigerson HG, Epstein AS, et al. Palliative chemotherapy or radiation and prognostic understanding among advanced cancer patients: the role of perceived treatment intent. J Palliat Med. 2020;23(1):33–9. https://doi.org/10.1089/jpm.2018.0651.
53. Rutter C, Weissman DE. Radiation for palliation–part 1. J Palliat Med. 2004;7(6):865–6. https://doi.org/10.1089/jpm.2004.7.865.
54. Rutter C, Weissman DE. Radiation for palliation–part 2. J Palliat Med. 2004;7(6):866–7.
55. Fischberg D, Bull J, Casarett D, et al. Five things physicians and patients should question in hospice and palliative medicine. J Pain Symptom Manag. 2013;45(3):595–605. https://doi.org/10.1016/j.jpainsymman.2012.12.002.
56. Chow E, Meyer RM, Ding K, et al. Dexamethasone in the prophylaxis of radiation-induced pain flare after palliative radiotherapy for bone metastases: a double-blind, randomised placebo-controlled, phase 3 trial. Lancet Oncol. 2015;16(15):1463–72. https://doi.org/10.1016/S1470-2045(15)00199-0.
57. Davison S. Advance Care Planning in Chronic Illness #162. https://www.mypcnow.org/fast-fact/advance-care-planning-in-chronic-illness/
58. Litzelman K, Berghoff A, Stevens J, Kwekkeboom K. Predictors of psychoneurological symptoms in cancer caregivers over time: role of caregiving burden, stress, and patient symptoms. Support Care Cancer. 2023;31(5):274. https://doi.org/10.1007/s00520-023-07741-3.
59. Moss AH, Lunney JR, Culp S, et al. Prognostic significance of the "surprise" question in cancer patients. J Palliat Med. 2010;13(7):837–40. https://doi.org/10.1089/jpm.2010.0018.
60. Johnston SC, Pfeifer MP, McNutt R. The discussion about advance directives. Patient and physician opinions regarding when and how it should be conducted. End of Life Study Group. Arch Intern Med. 1995;155(10):1025–30. https://doi.org/10.1001/archinte.155.10.1025.
61. Chow WB, Rosenthal RA, Merkow RP, et al. Optimal preoperative assessment of the geriatric surgical patient: a best practices guideline from the American College of Surgeons National Surgical Quality Improvement Program and the American Geriatrics Society. J Am Coll Surg. 2012;215(4):453–66. https://doi.org/10.1016/j.jamcollsurg.2012.06.017.
62. Baile WF, Buckman R, Lenzi R, Glober G, Beale EA, Kudelka AP. SPIKES-A six-step protocol for delivering bad news: application to the patient with cancer. Oncologist. 2000;5(4):302–11. https://doi.org/10.1634/theoncologist.5-4-302.
63. Childers JW, Back AL, Tulsky JA, Arnold RM. REMAP: a framework for goals of care conversations. J Oncol Pract. 2017;13(10):e844–50. https://doi.org/10.1200/jop.2016.018796.
64. Daubman BR, Bernacki R, Stoltenberg M, Wilson E, Jacobsen J. Best practices for teaching clinicians to use a serious illness conversation guide. Palliat Med Rep. 2020;1(1):135–42. https://doi.org/10.1089/pmr.2020.0066.
65. Janet LA, Bethany-Rose D, Molly C. Comprehensive guide to supportive and palliative care for patients with cancer. 4th ed. Johns Hopkins University Press; 2022.
66. Kruser JM, Nabozny MJ, Steffens NM, et al. "Best case/worst case": qualitative evaluation of a novel communication tool for difficult in-the-moment surgical decisions. J Am Geriatr Soc. 2015;63(9):1805–11. https://doi.org/10.1111/jgs.13615.
67. Madariaga A, Lau J, Ghoshal A, et al. MASCC multidisciplinary evidence-based recommendations for the management of malignant bowel obstruction in advanced cancer. Support Care Cancer. 2022;30(6):4711–28. https://doi.org/10.1007/s00520-022-06889-8.

68. Krouse RS. Invasive treatment options for malignant bowel obstruction #119. J Palliat Med. 2009;12(12):1152–3. https://doi.org/10.1089/jpm.2009.9922.
69. von Gunten CF, Muir JC. Medical management of bowel obstructions, 2nd edition #45. J Palliat Med. 2009;12(12):1151–2. https://doi.org/10.1089/jpm.2009.9923.
70. Banting SP, Waters PS, Peacock O, et al. Management of primary and metastatic malignant small bowel obstruction, operate or palliate. A systematic review. ANZ J Surg. 2021;91(3):282–90. https://doi.org/10.1111/ans.16188.
71. Rath KS, Loseth D, Muscarella P, et al. Outcomes following percutaneous upper gastrointestinal decompressive tube placement for malignant bowel obstruction in ovarian cancer. Gynecol Oncol. 2013;129(1):103–6. https://doi.org/10.1016/j.ygyno.2013.01.021.
72. LeBlanc K, Arnold RM. Palliative treatment of malignant ascites #177. J Palliat Med. 2010;13(8):1028–9. https://doi.org/10.1089/jpm.2010.9799.
73. Narayanan G, Pezeshkmehr A, Venkat S, Guerrero G, Barbery K. Safety and efficacy of the PleurX catheter for the treatment of malignant ascites. J Palliat Med. 2014;17(8):906–12. https://doi.org/10.1089/jpm.2013.0427.
74. Randle RW, Swett KR, Swords DS, et al. Efficacy of cytoreductive surgery with hyperthermic intraperitoneal chemotherapy in the management of malignant ascites. Ann Surg Oncol. 2014;21(5):1474–9. https://doi.org/10.1245/s10434-013-3224-y.
75. Karnes B. Gone from my sight: the dying experience. Rev. ed. Barbara Karnes Books; 2009.
76. Weissman D. Determining prognosis in advanced cancer #13a. J Palliat Med. 2003;6(3):433–4. https://doi.org/10.1089/109662103322144763.
77. Marrelli TM. In: Marrelli TM, editor. Hospice & palliative care handbook: quality, compliance, and reimbursement. 3rd ed. Sigma Theta Tau International; 2018.
78. Gazelle G. Understanding hospice–an underutilized option for life's final chapter. N Engl J Med. 2007;357(4):321–4. https://doi.org/10.1056/NEJMp078067.
79. Organization NHaPC. Hospice Care Overview for Professionals. www.nhpco.org/hospice-care-overview/
80. Raijmakers NJH, van Zuylen L, Costantini M, et al. Artificial nutrition and hydration in the last week of life in cancer patients. A systematic literature review of practices and effects. Ann Oncol. 2011;22(7):1478–86. https://doi.org/10.1093/annonc/mdq620.
81. Blundon EG, Gallagher RE, Ward LM. Electrophysiological evidence of preserved hearing at the end of life. Sci Rep. 2020;10(1):10336. https://doi.org/10.1038/s41598-020-67234-9.

Peritoneal Surface Malignancies

Jackson Baril and Trang Nguyen

Introduction

- Majority of PSM are metastatic with most common primaries being ovarian, gastric, and colon cancer. Less common but more often surgically treated are appendiceal primaries.
- Only 3% are of primary peritoneal origin (mesothelioma).
- Pseudomyxoma peritonei (PMP) was originally a clinical description of mucinous ascites, now with WHO pathology classification.
- Surgical treatment typically involves cytoreductive surgery (CRS) +/- intraperitoneal chemotherapy.
- Hyperthermic intraperitoneal chemotherapy (HIPEC) first developed by Dr. Spratt in 1980 treating a patient with heated intraperitoneal chemotherapy for pseudomyxoma peritonei [1] and early work on peritoneal metastases for gastric cancer in Japan by Dr. Koga in the 1980s [2, 3].
- Peritoneum—mesothelial cells overlying a network of lymphatics and blood vessels.
  - Thin basal lamina acts as a filter for proteins and cells and allows for transport of fluid. This allows for peritoneal dialysis [4].
  - Malignant cells should not pass this basement membrane, thus making peritoneal carcinomatosis a locoregional spread of disease.
  - The flow of peritoneal fluid is based on primary site of origin, negative pressure from respirations, and gravity-dependent area.

J. Baril
Department of Surgery, Indiana University School of Medicine, Indianapolis, IN, USA
e-mail: jbaril@iu.edu

T. Nguyen (✉)
School of Medicine Department of Surgery, Washington University in St. Louis, Saint Louis, MO, USA

- Primary sites of absorption and peritoneal tumors are the greater and lesser omentum, under the diaphragm and areas of fluid stagnation such as the pericolic gutters [5]. Macroscopic tumor is often adhered to greater and lesser omentum and under the diaphragm.
- Small bowel is somewhat protected by peristaltic movement reducing the seeding of cancerous cells.

Diagnosis and Workup

- Symptoms may include abdominal pain, abdominal distention, and early satiety or be found incidentally on imaging or during surgery.
- Obtaining tissue diagnosis:
  - Percutaneous biopsy if possible (omental, peritoneal) of metastatic deposits
    - Mucinous ascites often difficult to sample and associated with false negatives and low cellularity
    - Tumor genomic profiling can be helpful in unknown primaries and for potential targeted therapies
  - EGD/colonoscopy—to evaluate for primary site; colonoscopy to also rule out synchronous tumors
  - Diagnostic laparoscopy may be needed for biopsy (consider appendectomy, bilateral salpingo-oophorectomy) and to evaluate extent of disease
  - Consider secondary review on pathology, especially for rare cancers
  - Various classification systems exist for peritoneal disease/pseudomyxoma peritonei (Table 15.1)
- Imaging—CT chest to rule out extraabdominal disease and CT or MRI abdomen and pelvis
  - Mucin and miliary disease are often not FDG avid during PET.
  - Imaging can underestimate extent of peritoneal disease:
    - CT imaging has a sensitivity and specificity of 83% and 86%, respectively, for detecting peritoneal metastases; however, the performance is worse for smaller tumors and CT underpredicts the extent of disease or peritoneal carcinomatosis index (PCI) score [6, 7]. It is easier to obtain than MRI.

Table 15.1 Classification systems for peritoneal disease/pseudomyxoma peritonei

		Low-grade mucinous carcinoma peritonei	High-grade mucinous carcinoma peritonei	
2016 PSOGI [6]	Acellular mucin without epithelial cells	Low-grade mucinous carcinoma peritonei	High-grade mucinous carcinoma peritonei	High-grade mucinous carcinoma peritonei with signet ring cells
2019 WHO [7]	pM1a	pM1b, grade 1	pM1b, grade 2	pM1b, mucinous tumor deposits with signet ring cells
9th version AJCC [8]	M1a	M1b, well differentiated (grade 1)	M1b, moderately differentiated (grade 2)	M1b, poorly differentiated (grade 3)

- Contrast-enhanced MRI is superior for detecting smaller tumors <1 cm with sensitivity 85–90% but limited by a lack of access and standardized protocols [7].
- Labs—Tumor markers are nonspecific but can follow trends (CEA, CA19-9, CA125), nutrition assessment, CBC, and CMP.
- Extent and severity of peritoneal disease
  - Peritoneal cancer index (PCI) is calculated as a sum of the lesion sizes (score 0–3: 0 is no disease, 1 point is <2 cm, 2 points is 2–5 cm, 3 points is >5 cm of disease) seen in each of the 13 defined abdominopelvic regions (numbered 0 through 12) as noted in Fig. 15.1 for a maximum score of 39 [8].
  - Estimated PCI by imaging may miss smaller radiographically occult lesions.
  - Peritoneal surface disease severity score (PSDSS) incorporates both PCI and tumor histology (Table 15.2).
    - Score 2–3 is stage I, score 4–7 stage II, score 8–10 stage III, and score >10 stage IV.
    - PSDSS correlates with resectability with stages III and IV having little chance of resectability [10].

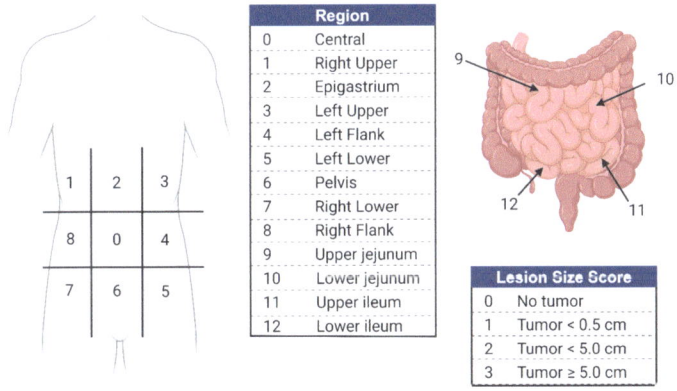

Fig. 15.1 Peritoneal cancer index. (Image created with Biorender)

Table 15.2 Peritoneal surface disease severity score (PSDSS) for colon [9]

Clinical disease	PCI	Histology
No symptoms = 0 points	PCI <10 = 1 point	Well-moderately differentiated and N0 = 0 points
Mild symptoms = 1 point	PCI 10–20 = 3 points	Moderately differentiated/N1 or N2 = 3 points
Severe symptoms = 6 points	PCI >20 = 7 points	Poor differentiated, any signet ring cancer = 9 points

Treatment

- It depends on primary tumor type and functional status to tolerate chemotherapy or surgery.
- At this time, radiation plays no role outside of clinical trials in peritoneal disease.

Survival data can be difficult to interpret due to varying descriptions of pathology.

- NCCN guidelines are limited. Consensus groups offer some guidelines—Peritoneal Surface Oncology Group International (PSOGI) and the Yale Peritoneal Surface Malignancy Consortium formerly Chicago Consensus.
  - *Appendiceal neoplasms and tumors*
    - Low-grade and high-grade appendiceal mucinous neoplasms do not respond to systemic therapy, and therefore CRS/HIPEC is considered upfront if there is disseminated peritoneal disease:
      - For positive margins on appendectomy without peritoneal dissemination, resection of the appendiceal cuff or partial cecectomy is recommended over resection requiring anastomosis.
      - LAMN and HAMN have similar survival rates of 100% at three years, 86% at five years, and 45% at ten years [11], but HAMNs believed to have a slightly higher recurrence risk.
    - Goblet cell carcinoma (formerly goblet cell carcinoid)—chemotherapy upfront considered for high grade (Tang classification group B or C with group B having signet ring cell morphology and C having additional features of poorly differentiated adenocarcinoma) or when incomplete CRS predicted (Table 15.3) [12, 13]
    - Adenocarcinoma—consider neoadjuvant chemotherapy if incomplete cytoreduction predicted or higher-grade (moderately or poorly differentiated) peritoneal disease [13]. Goal is improvement or stable disease with progression being a poor prognostic factor (Table 15.4).
    - Right colectomy is indicated for goblet cell carcinoma and appendiceal adenocarcinoma confined to the appendix. Observation without right colectomy can be considered for well-differentiated mucinous adenocarcinoma [13].
    - Survival for low- and high-grade adenocarcinomas after CRS/HIPEC is 80–90% [15].
  - *Colorectal/small bowel primaries*—chemotherapy and CRS +/- HIPEC in select cases.

Table 15.3 Disease-specific survival of goblet cell carcinoma

Tang subtype	Five years	Five years
A	100%	85%
B	85%	36%
C	17%	0%

Table 15.4 Outcomes of mucinous appendiceal adenocarcinoma by grade [14]

Grade	Five-year OS	Five-year DFS
Well differentiated	94%	66%
Moderately differentiated	71%	21%
Poorly differentiated	30%	0%

- Considerations include progression-free interval, BRAF wild-type, low PCI, peritoneal metastasis-only disease, response to systemic therapy, and MSI (immunotherapy considered for MSI high).
- Typically 3–6 months of neoadjuvant chemotherapy prior to consideration of CRS +/- HIPEC.
- Verwaal 2003—Randomized controlled trial of CRS+HIPEC vs chemotherapy alone (5-FU) for colorectal cancer with peritoneal carcinomatosis showed benefit with CRS+HIPEC (22.3 vs 12.6 months, p = 0.032) [16].
  – 105 patients, not modern chemo regiment
- PRODIGE 7—No survival benefit for CRS and HIPEC (30-min oxaliplatin) over CRS alone (41.7 vs 41.2 months, p = 0.99)
  – Subset analysis showed survival advantage for PCI 11-15 with CRS-HIPEC, but study was not powered for this subset analysis [17].
– *Primary peritoneal tumors*
  - Peritoneal mesothelioma [18]
    – CRS/HIPEC upfront for epithelioid histology, low Ki-67%
    – Systemic therapy upfront for high-risk biphasic/sarcomatoid histology, high tumor burden, and Ki-67 >10%
    – Assess for BAP1 mutation (related cancers—uveal melanoma, clear cell and renal cell carcinoma)
  - Well-differentiated papillary mesothelial tumor—can observe if asymptomatic, otherwise consider repeat biopsy and CRS+/-HIPEC.
  - There are no randomized controlled trials in mesothelioma.
  - Median survival for epithelial subtype is 79 months; biphasic/sarcomatoid is 10 months (p = 0.001) in patients who received CRS/HIPEC [19]
  - All subtypes, three-year OS 50–65% [20–22].
– See corresponding chapters for other primary tumor types.
- Consider palliative interventions and surgery if unable to undergo curative intent treatment. This can include limited debulking, perfusion alone for mucinous tumors, intestinal bypass, and draining gastrostomy.

Surgical Treatment

- Selection Criteria for Surgery
  – Histologies with regional rather than systemic spread
    - Region being peritoneal cavity (no extraabdominal metastasis)
  – Good tumor behavior—Progression-free or recurrence-free survival >2 years and response to chemotherapy

- Considered when it is the only treatment option (low-grade appendiceal neoplasms)—not sensitive to chemotherapy
 - Favorable peritoneal carcinomatosis index (PCI) or extent of metastases:
   - For colorectal cancer, more favorable outcomes with CRS and intraoperative intraperitoneal chemo if PCI <20 or lymph node negative and in the original Verwaal study if five or less of seven regions (pelvis and sigmoid; right lower abdomen; small bowel and mesentery; omentum and transverse colon; subhepatic space and stomach; right subphrenic space; and left subphrenic space) were involved [16, 23].
 - Ability to achieve complete cytoreduction (e.g., cannot cover entire small bowel or require portal resection)
 - Malignant small bowel obstruction is typically a relative contraindication as a sign of aggressive biology. An exception would be a small bowel primary (typically treated like colorectal) that is causing an obstruction.
- Preoperative considerations: nutrition optimization, prehabilitation, splenectomy vaccination, ostomy nursing, and fertility counseling
- Cytoreductive surgery +/− HIPEC indicated for primary malignancies of the appendix and peritoneum. Selectively indicated for colorectal cancers, ovarian cancer, neuroendocrine tumors, sarcomatosis, and gastric cancers
- Cytoreductive surgery
  - Goal is to remove all macroscopic diseases of cancer via visceral resection and peritonectomies
  - CCR (completeness of cytoreduction) [8]
    - CC-0 = no visible tumor
    - CC-1 = largest remaining tumor implants <0.25 cm in diameter
    - CC-2 = largest remaining tumor implants 0.25–2.5 cm in diameter
    - CC-3 = largest remaining tumor implants >2.5 cm in diameter
      - CC-2 and CC-3 are considered debulking surgeries instead of cytoreduction.
  - Consider diagnostic laparoscopy to evaluate tumor burden and disease along major vessels and screen for extensive serosal involvement.
  - Stepwise CRS depending on extent of disease can include resection of lesser and greater omentum, splenectomy, left upper quadrant peritonectomy, right upper quadrant peritonectomy, lesser omentectomy-cholecystectomy with stripping of the omental bursa, pelvic peritonectomy with or without sleeve resection of sigmoid colon, hysterectomy with bilateral salpingo-oophorectomy, and bowel resections [24].
- HIPEC
  - Closed abdomen technique: after CRS, inflow and outflow catheters are placed in the abdomen along with temperature probes. Outflow catheters are placed in dependent areas in the pelvis and under right diaphragm. The skin is closed in a water-tight fashion and heated chemotherapy solution is administered. Generally the heat exchanger is set at 44–46 °C such that the perfusate is maintained at 41–43 °C for 30–90 min of therapy. External manual agitation is performed to promote distribution of the chemotherapy [25].

- Open abdomen technique: catheters are placed in the abdomen through the midline incision or separate lateral incisions to tunnel subcutaneously and enter the abdomen at the midline facial incision. Skin edges are lifted using a self-retaining retractor with elevation creating an open reservoir in the abdominal cavity. A plastic sheet covers the midline incision to prevent spillage, through which the surgeon may manually stir the chemotherapy perfusate. A smoke evacuator is placed under the sheet to prevent vapors and small droplets from dissipating [11].
- General safety components: correct instrument counts prior to initiating HIPEC; proper PPE including double gloves, eye protection, impervious gowns, and shoe covers; and absorbent towels for possible spills
- No difference in postoperative morbidity or mortality between the open and closed techniques [11]
- Chemotherapeutic agents:
  - Mitomycin C and oxaliplatin commonly used for appendiceal and colorectal primaries with no difference in outcomes in randomized controlled trial (This is the only randomized controlled trial in appendiceal cancers.) [15]
  - Platinum compounds: cisplatin, carboplatin, and oxaliplatin
    - Cisplatin nephrotoxicity limits the dose. Doses under 240 mg may reduce risk of renal injury, as well as IV sodium thiosulfate prior to cisplatin use [12, 13].
  - Alkylating agents: mitomycin C and melphalan
  - Antimicrobials: docetaxel and paclitaxel
  - Antimetabolites: 5-FU and gemcitabine
  - Topoisomerase inhibitors: doxorubicin, mitoxantrone, irinotecan, and topotecan
  - Penetration depth 1–3 mm depending on agent

Commonly used HIPEC agents by primary disease [13, 18, 26–28]

Appendiceal tumors	Mitomycin C, oxaliplatin, and mitomycin C + doxorubicin
Colorectal cancer	Mitomycin C (favored over oxaliplatin after PRODIGE 7)
Mesothelioma	Cisplatin +/− doxorubicin, mitomycin C, and carboplatin

- PIPAC (pressurized intraperitoneal aerosol chemotherapy)
  - Currently used in a clinical trial setting. PIPAC therapy increases the depth of chemotherapy penetration. Oxaliplatin, cisplatin, and doxorubicin are commonly used chemotherapy [29].
- NIPEC (normothermic intraperitoneal chemotherapy), EPIC (early postoperative intraperitoneal chemotherapy)
  - Used in select centers, typically as part of a clinical trial. Utilizes cell cycle-dependent chemotherapy such as paclitaxel and 5-FU [30]
- Prevention of complications
  - Hold antiangiogenic agents such as bevacizumab for five weeks prior to CRS-HIPEC (strong recommendation, low evidence) [15].
  - Hold systemic chemotherapy four weeks prior to surgery.

- ERAS components recommended [15]: epidural neuraxial analgesia or blocks, multimodal pain regimen, early oral intake, glucose and nutrition monitoring, removal of urinary catheter by post op day #3, and perioperative venous thromboembolism prophylaxis
- Surgical Complications
  - Overall morbidity 33% and mortality 2.9% [31]
  - Bowel obstruction: Rates range from 20% to 37% [14]
  - Perforations/leak:
     (i) Anastomosis before or after HIPEC not shown to affect leak rates [16]
     (ii) Leak rates similar with and without HIPEC [32]
  - Ileus
  - Infection
  - Neutropenia: risk factors—neoadjuvant chemotherapy, female, and mitomycin C dose/BSA (body surface area). Mitomycin C has more of a WBC decrease than oxaliplatin typically between POD 5 and 10 [15, 33].
  - Long term—hernia and GI dysfunction.
  - Readmission 11% [31].

Follow-Up

- Imaging every 3–6 months for adenocarcinomas and peritoneal mesothelioma and every 6–12 months for appendiceal mucinous neoplasm for 5–10 years with tumor markers such as CEA and others that were abnormal at diagnosis [13, 18].
- Adjuvant FOLFOX can be considered for stage III appendiceal adenocarcinoma [13].
- Utility of prophylactic HIPEC colorectal cancers at high risk for peritoneal metastases is debatable
  - COLOPEC trial—No difference in a five-year overall survival between adjuvant chemotherapy and oxaliplatin HIPEC for patients with high-risk colorectal cancer (perforated or T4N0-2M0) [34].
  - PROPHYLOCHIP-PRODIGE 15—No difference in a three-year overall survival with second look laparoscopy and oxaliplatin HIPEC after adjuvant systemic chemotherapy for perforated or metastatic colon cancers [35]
  - HIPECT4—Addition of mitomycin C HIPEC to cytoreductive surgery for T4 colon cancer showed improved locoregional control but no disease free or overall survival difference at three years without increased morbidity [36].

References

1. Spratt JS, Adcock RA, Muskovin M, Sherrill W, McKeown J. Clinical delivery system for intraperitoneal hyperthermic chemotherapy. Cancer Res. 1980;40(2):256–60.
2. Koga S, Shimizu N, Maeta M, Hamazoe R, Izumi A. Application of heat combined with antineoplastic agent administration in the treatment of cancer (with special reference to malignancy of the digestive system). Gan To Kagaku Ryoho. 1983;10(2 Pt 2):358–65.

3. Yonemura Y, Sako S, Wakama S, Ishibashi H, Mizumoto A, Takao N, et al. History of peritoneal surface malignancy treatment in Japan. Indian J Surg Oncol. 2019;10(Suppl 1):3–11.
4. van Baal JO, Van de Vijver KK, Nieuwland R, van Noorden CJ, van Driel WJ, Sturk A, et al. The histophysiology and pathophysiology of the peritoneum. Tissue Cell. 2017;49(1):95–105.
5. Waniewski J. Peritoneal fluid transport: mechanisms, pathways, methods of assessment. Arch Med Res. 2013;44(8):576–83.
6. Carr NJ, Cecil TD, Mohamed F, Sobin LH, Sugarbaker PH, González-Moreno S, Taflampas P, Chapman S, Moran BJ, Peritoneal Surface Oncology Group International. A consensus for classification and pathologic reporting of pseudomyxoma peritonei and associated appendiceal neoplasia: the results of the peritoneal surface oncology group international (PSOGI) modified delphi process. Am J Surg Pathol. 2016;40(1):14–26.
7. Misdraji J, Carr N, Pai R. Appendiceal serrated lesions and polyps. Appendiceal mucinous neoplasm. WHO classification of tumours of digestive system 2019:141–6.
8. Overman MJ, Kakar S, Carr NJ, et al. AJCC cancer staging system: appendix: AJCC cancer staging system. Version 9. American Joint Committee on Cancer, American College of Surgeons; 2023.
9. Laghi A, Bellini D, Rengo M, Accarpio F, Caruso D, Biacchi D, et al. Diagnostic performance of computed tomography and magnetic resonance imaging for detecting peritoneal metastases: systematic review and meta-analysis. Radiol Med. 2017;122(1):1–15.
10. Low RN, Barone RM. Imaging for peritoneal metastases. Surg Oncol Clin N Am. 2018;27(3):425–42.
11. Misdraji J, Yantiss RK, Graeme-Cook FM, Balis UJ, Young RH. Appendiceal mucinous neoplasms: a clinicopathologic analysis of 107 cases. Am J Surg Pathol. 2003;27(8):1089–103.
12. Tang LH, Shia J, Soslow RA, Dhall D, Wong WD, O'Reilly E, Qin J, Paty P, Weiser MR, Guillem J, et al. Pathologic classification and clinical behavior of the spectrum of goblet cell carcinoid tumors of the appendix. Am J Surg Pathol. 2008;32:1429–43.
13. Chicago Consensus Working Group. The Chicago consensus on peritoneal surface malignancies: management of appendiceal neoplasms. Ann Surg Oncol. 2020;27(6):1753–60.
14. Grotz TE, Royal RE, Mansfield PF, Overman MJ, Mann GN, Robinson KA, Beaty KA, Rafeeq S, Matamoros A, Taggart MW, Fournier KF. Stratification of outcomes for mucinous appendiceal adenocarcinoma with peritoneal metastasis by histological grade. World J Gastrointest Oncol. 2017;9(9):354–62.
15. Levine EA, Votanopoulos KI, Shen P, Russell G, Fenstermaker J, Mansfield P, Bartlett D, Stewart JH. A multicenter randomized trial to evaluate hematologic toxicities after hyperthermic intraperitoneal chemotherapy with oxaliplatin or mitomycin in patients with appendiceal tumors. J Am Coll Surg. 2018;226(4):434–43.
16. Verwaal VJ, van Ruth S, de Bree E, van Sloothen GW, van Tinteren H, Boot H, Zoetmulder FA. Randomized trial of cytoreduction and hyperthermic intraperitoneal chemotherapy versus systemic chemotherapy and palliative surgery in patients with peritoneal carcinomatosis of colorectal cancer. J Clin Oncol. 2003;21(20):3737–43.
17. Quénet F, Elias D, Roca L, Goéré D, Ghouti L, Pocard M, et al. Cytoreductive surgery plus hyperthermic intraperitoneal chemotherapy versus cytoreductive surgery alone for colorectal peritoneal metastases (PRODIGE 7): a multicentre, randomised, open-label, phase 3 trial. Lancet Oncol. 2021;22(2):256–66.
18. Chicago Consensus Working Group. The Chicago consensus on peritoneal surface malignancies: management of peritoneal Mesothelioma. Ann Surg Oncol. 2020;27(6):1774–9.
19. Yan TD, Deraco M, Elias D, Glehen O, Levine EA, Moran BJ, Morris DL, Chua TC, Piso P, Sugarbaker PH, Peritoneal Surface Oncology Group. A novel tumor-node-metastasis (TNM) staging system of diffuse malignant peritoneal mesothelioma using outcome analysis of a multi-institutional database*. Cancer. 2011;117(9):1855–63.

20. Yan TD, Deraco M, Baratti D, Kusamura S, Elias D, Glehen O, Gilly FN, Levine EA, Shen P, Mohamed F, Moran BJ, Morris DL, Chua TC, Piso P, Sugarbaker PH. Cytoreductive surgery and hyperthermic intraperitoneal chemotherapy for malignant peritoneal mesothelioma: multi-institutional experience. J Clin Oncol. 2009;27(36):6237–42.
21. Deraco M, Casali P, Inglese MG, Baratti D, Pennacchioli E, Bertulli R, Kusamura S. Peritoneal mesothelioma treated by induction chemotherapy, cytoreductive surgery, and intraperitoneal hyperthermic perfusion. J Surg Oncol. 2003;83(3):147–53.
22. Deraco M, Nonaka D, Baratti D, Casali P, Rosai J, Younan R, Salvatore A, Cabras Ad AD, Kusamura S. Prognostic analysis of clinicopathologic factors in 49 patients with diffuse malignant peritoneal mesothelioma treated with cytoreductive surgery and intraperitoneal hyperthermic perfusion. Ann Surg Oncol. 2006;13(2):229–37.
23. da Silva RG, Sugarbaker PH. Analysis of prognostic factors in seventy patients having a complete cytoreduction plus perioperative intraperitoneal chemotherapy for carcinomatosis from colorectal cancer. J Am Coll Surg. 2006;203(6):878–86.
24. Pelz JO, Stojadinovic A, Nissan A, Hohenberger W, Esquivel J. Evaluation of a peritoneal surface disease severity score in patients with colon cancer with peritoneal carcinomatosis. J Surg Oncol. 2009;99(1):9–15.
25. Yoon W, Alame A, Berri R. Peritoneal surface disease severity score as a predictor of resectability in the treatment of peritoneal surface malignancies. Am J Surg. 2014;207(3):403–7; discussion 6–7.
26. Turaga K, Levine E, Barone R, Sticca R, Petrelli N, Lambert L, Nash G, Morse M, Adbel-Misih R, Alexander HR, Attiyeh F, Bartlett D, Bastidas A, Blazer T, Chu Q, Chung K, Dominguez-Parra L, Espat NJ, Foster J, Fournier K, Garcia R, Goodman M, Hanna N, Harrison L, Hoefer R, Holtzman M, Kane J, Labow D, Li B, Lowy A, Mansfield P, Ong E, Pameijer C, Pingpank J, Quinones M, Royal R, Salti G, Sardi A, Shen P, Skitzki J, Spellman J, Stewart J, Esquivel J. Consensus guidelines from The American Society of Peritoneal Surface Malignancies on standardizing the delivery of hyperthermic intraperitoneal chemotherapy (HIPEC) in colorectal cancer patients in the United States. Ann Surg Oncol. 2014;21(5):1501–5.
27. Kepenekian V, Sgarbura O, Marchal F, et al. 2022 PSOGI consensus on HIPEC regimens for peritoneal malignancies: diffuse malignant peritoneal mesothelioma. Ann Surg Oncol. 2023;30:7803–13.
28. Hübner M, van Der Speeten K, Govaerts K, de Hingh I, Villeneuve L, Kusamura S, Glehen O. 2022 peritoneal surface oncology group international consensus on HIPEC regimens for peritoneal malignancies: colorectal cancer. Ann Surg Oncol. 2024;31(1):567–76.
29. Mortensen MB, Casella F, Düzgün Ö, Glehen O, Hewett P, Hübner M, Jørgensen MS, Königsrainer A, Marin M, Pocard M, Rezniczek G, So J, Fristrup CW. Second annual report from the ISSPP PIPAC database. Pleura Peritoneum. 2023;8(4):141–6.
30. Goodman MD, McPartland S, Detelich D, Saif MW. Chemotherapy for intraperitoneal use: a review of hyperthermic intraperitoneal chemotherapy and early post-operative intraperitoneal chemotherapy. J Gastrointest Oncol. 2016;7(1):45–57. https://doi.org/10.3978/j.issn.2078-6891.2015.111. PMID: 26941983; PMCID: PMC4754301.
31. Jafari MD, Halabi WJ, Stamos MJ, Nguyen VQ, Carmichael JC, Mills SD, Pigazzi A. Surgical outcomes of hyperthermic intraperitoneal chemotherapy: analysis of the American college of surgeons national surgical quality improvement program. JAMA Surg. 2014;149(2):170–5.
32. Chouliaras K, Levine EA, Fino N, Shen P, Votanopoulos KI. Prognostic factors and significance of gastrointestinal leak after cytoreductive surgery (CRS) with heated intraperitoneal chemotherapy (HIPEC). Ann Surg Oncol. 2017;24(4):890–7.
33. Lambert LA, Armstrong TS, Lee JJ, Liu S, Katz MH, Eng C, Wolff RA, Tortorice ML, Tansey P, Gonzalez-Moreno S, Lambert DH, Mansfield PF. Incidence, risk factors, and impact of severe neutropenia after hyperthermic intraperitoneal mitomycin C. Ann Surg Oncol. 2009;16(8):2181–7.

34. Zwanenburg ES, El Klaver C, Wisselink DD, Punt CJA, Snaebjornsson P, Crezee J, Aalbers AGJ, Brandt-Kerkhof ARM, Bremers AJA, Burger PJWA, Fabry HFJ, Ferenschild FTJ, Festen S, van Grevenstein WMU, Hemmer PHJ, de Hingh IHJT, Kok NFM, Kusters M, Musters GD, Schoonderwoerd L, Tuynman JB, van de Ven AWH, van Westreenen HL, Wiezer MJ, Zimmerman DDE, van Zweeden A, Dijkgraaf MGW, Tanis PJ, COLOPEC Collaborators Group; COLOOPEC Collaborators Group. Adjuvant hyperthermic intraperitoneal chemotherapy in patients with locally advanced colon cancer (COLOPEC): 5-year results of a randomized multicenter trial. J Clin Oncol. 2024;42(2):140–5.
35. Goéré D, Glehen O, Quenet F, Guilloit JM, Bereder JM, Lorimier G, Thibaudeau E, Ghouti L, Pinto A, Tuech JJ, Kianmanesh R, Carretier M, Marchal F, Arvieux C, Brigand C, Meeus P, Rat P, Durand-Fontanier S, Mariani P, Lakkis Z, Loi V, Pirro N, Sabbagh C, Texier M, Elias D, BIG-RENAPE group. Second-look surgery plus hyperthermic intraperitoneal chemotherapy versus surveillance in patients at high risk of developing colorectal peritoneal metastases (PROPHYLOCHIP-PRODIGE 15): a randomised, phase 3 study. Lancet Oncol. 2020;21(9):1147–54.
36. Arjona-Sánchez A, Barrios P, Boldo-Roda E, Camps B, Carrasco-Campos J, Concepción Martín V, García-Fadrique A, Gutiérrez-Calvo A, Morales R, Ortega-Pérez G, Pérez-Viejo E, Prada-Villaverde A, Torres-Melero J, Vicente E, Villarejo-Campos P, Sánchez-Hidalgo JM, Casado-Adam A, García-Martin R, Medina M, Caro T, Villar C, Aranda E, Cano-Osuna MT, Díaz-López C, Torres-Tordera E, Briceño-Delgado FJ, Rufián-Peña S. HIPECT4: multicentre, randomized clinical trial to evaluate safety and efficacy of Hyperthermic intra-peritoneal chemotherapy (HIPEC) with Mitomycin C used during surgery for treatment of locally advanced colorectal carcinoma. BMC Cancer. 2018;18(1):183.

Soft Tissue Sarcomas

16

Cameron Keramati and Anthony Scholer

Introduction

- Represent a rare and diverse group of malignancies, accounting for approximately 1% of all cancer diagnoses [1].
  - SEER database 2018
    - Incidence is 3.46 per 100,000 or roughly 56,529 new cases between 2014-2018.
    - Mortality is 5,000–6,000.
- National Cancer Institute and American Cancer Society, five-year relative survival for STS [2]
  - Overall 65%
  - Localized 81%
  - Locally advanced 58%
  - Metastatic 17%
- Arises from various connective tissues, including tendons, muscles, adipose tissue, and vascular/neural structures in the extremities and retroperitoneum
- Primary location(s) [3, 4]
  - 50–60% extremities
  - 15–20% retroperitoneum
- Over 60 subtypes, with a range of clinical behaviors (highly aggressive to indolent).
  - Classification is based on anatomical location, histological features, and, in some cases, specific genetic translocation profiles (Table 16.1).

C. Keramati
Department of Surgery, University of Texas Southwestern Medical Center, Dallas, TX, USA
e-mail: Cameron.keramati@utsouthwestern.edu

A. Scholer (✉)
Department of Surgery, Division of Surgical Oncology, Jersey Shore University Medical Center Hackensack Meridian, Neptune, NJ, USA
e-mail: Anthony.Scholer@hmhn.org

Table 16.1 Characteristics of sarcoma subtypes

Sarcoma subtype	Most common location	Chromosomal abnormality	Genes	Recurrence (%) and site	Metastatic site	Risk of lymph node metastasis[a]	Five-year survival rate
Well-differentiated and atypical liposarcoma [5]	Extremity	t(12;16)(q13;p11)	FUS-DDIT3	50% local	Minimal risk	No	80%
Myxoid/round cell LPS [3, 6, 7]		t(12;16)(q13;p11) t(12;22)(q13;q12)	FUS-DDIT3 EWSR1-CHOP	20–50% local and distant	Spine Soft tissue abdomen and pelvis	No	55–80%
Dedifferentiated liposarcoma [8]	Retroperitoneum	Amplification of 12q13-15	MDM2 and CDK4	80% Local and distant	Lung and liver	No	50%
Leiomyosarcoma [9]	RP > Extremity	13q Deletion	RB1	40% Distant > local	Lung and liver Abdomen and pelvis	No	60%
Desmoid tumor [10]	Trunk			50% Local	Minimal risk	No	95%
Angiosarcoma [11]	Primary (tissue) Scalp/face and extremity Secondary (skin) Breast	Secondary Amplification of MYC and FLT4 (VEGFR3) [12, 13]		20–40% Local and distant Regional	Lung and liver Abdomen and pelvis Central nervous system	Yes	50%
Dermatofibrosarcoma protuberans [8, 14–24]	Skin and subcutaneous tissue	t(17;22)(q22;q13)	COL1A1-PDGFB	1–20% local	Minimal risk	No	95%

Fibrosarcoma [25]	Extremities and head/neck	t(12;15)(p13;q25) (infantile variant)	ETV6-NTRK3 (infantile variant)	55% local and distant	Lung	No	80%
Malignant nerve sheath tumors [26]	Extremities and head/neck			40–65% local and distant	Lung	No	65%
Undifferentiated pleomorphic sarcoma [27]	Soft tissues			30% Local and distant regional	Lung	No	75%
Synovial sarcoma [28, 29].	Extremity	t(X;18)(p11;q11)	SYT-SSX1 or SYT-SSX2	Local and distant regional	Lung and liver	Yes	65%
Rhabdomyosarcoma [30]	Head/neck and extremity	Various (t(2;13), t(1;13), etc.)	PAX3-FOXO1 or PAX7-FOXO1	25–30% Local and distant	Lungs and liver Bone Brain	Yes	55%
Ewing's sarcoma [31]	Bone and extremity	t(11;22)(q24;q12)	EWSR1-FLI1	50% Local and distant	Lung Bone	No	65%
Myxofibrosarcoma [32]	Extremity			Local	Lung Pleura Adrenal	No	70%
Epithelioid sarcoma [33, 34]	Extremity	t(11;22)(p13;q12)	EWSR1-ATF1	45% Local and distant Regional	Lungs Abdomen and pelvis	Yes	60%

(continued)

Table 16.1 (continued)

Sarcoma subtype	Most common location	Chromosomal abnormality	Genes	Recurrence (%) and site	Metastatic site	Risk of lymph node metastasis[a]	Five-year survival rate
Clear cell sarcoma [35–37]	Extremity	t(11;22)(p13;q12)	EWSR1-ATF1	84% Local and distant regional	Lung	Yes	60%
Alveolar soft part sarcoma	Extremity	t(X;17)(p11;q25)	ASPSCR1-TFE3	Local and distant	Lung Central nervous system		60% for adults

[a]STS subtypes with a higher likelihood for lymph node involvement should undergo consideration for sentinel lymph node biopsy

- The most common subtypes
  - Liposarcoma (LPS), leiomyosarcoma (LMS), synovial sarcoma, epithelioid sarcoma, undifferentiated Pleomorphic sarcoma (UPS), malignant peripheral nerve sheath tumors (MPNST), and rhabdomyosarcoma (RMS).
- This chapter will focus on STS aligned with the typical clinical focus of a complex general surgical oncologist, excluding non-STS neoplasms (such as osteosarcoma and chondrosarcoma).
  - Gastrointestinal stromal tumors (GIST) have a dedicated chapter within this textbook.

Classification and Characteristics of Subtypes

- The 2020 World Health Organization (WHO) Classification of Soft Tissue and Bone Sarcomas
  - Categorized by histopathologic type and tumor biology
  - Subtype categories
    - Adipocytic, fibroblastic, myofibroblastic, vascular, pericytic (perivascular), smooth muscle, skeletal muscle, chondro-osseous, peripheral nerve sheath, and tumors of uncertain differentiation [3].
- Risk Factors
  - Generally, STS occurs in individuals without known risk factors.
  - Incidence is relatively equal in men versus women, except for certain subtypes.
  - Prior radiation therapy is associated with a delayed risk of less than 1% (with an onset of approximately seven years) of developing angiosarcoma and undifferentiated pleomorphic sarcoma.
  - Lymphedema (especially when associated with radiation exposure) has up to a 0.05% risk of developing lymphangiosarcoma (Stewart-Treves syndrome).
  - Other risk factors:
    - Arsenic, thorotrast, arsenic (angiosarcoma), immunosuppression (HIV, HHV-8, and immunosuppressive agents), herbicides (phenoxyacetic acid), and wood preservatives (chlorophenol).
  - 3% of cases are associated with underlying genetic syndromes (Table 16.2).
    - Cases that arise in association with genetic syndromes tend to be younger at onset (median age of 37 vs. 53 compared to sporadic cases) [38–49].

Table 16.2 Genetic syndromes associated with sarcomas

Syndrome	Mutation	Inheritance pattern	Sarcoma type
Carney-Stratakis	SDH	Autosomal dominant	GIST
Hereditary retinoblastoma	RB1	Autosomal dominant	Increased risk overall, but particularly LMS
Neurofibromatosis (NF)-1 and NF-2	NF1/NF2	Autosomal dominant	MPNSTs
Li-Fraumeni syndrome	TP53	Autosomal dominant	Pediatric rhabdomyosarcoma and adult undifferentiated pleomorphic sarcoma
Familial adenomatous polyposis (FAP)	APC	Autosomal dominant	Intraabdominal desmoid tumors

GIST Gastrointestinal stromal tumor, *LMS* leiomyosarcoma, and *PMNST* malignant peripheral nerve sheath tumor

Liposarcoma [50–52]

- Common subtype in the USA.
- Most common subtype globally.
- Frequently found in the extremities, trunk, and retroperitoneum.
- Originates from lipoblasts.
- WHO subclasses LPS based on histological features.
  - Well-differentiated (WD)/dedifferentiated (DD), round cell/myxoid, and undifferentiated pleomorphic sarcoma
  - LPS found in the extremities is more likely to be of the myxoid or WD LPS.
  - LPS located in the retroperitoneum is more often categorized as a DD-LPS.
  - WD LPS
    - Can be further categorized into the following.
      - Lipoma-like subtype shares similarities with lipomas, typically contains a significant number of lipoblasts.
      - Sclerosing subtype is characterized by an abundance of fibrosis, whereas the inflammatory subtype exhibits prominent B-cell infiltration.
      - Inflammatory subtype exhibits prominent B-cell infiltration.
  - Myxoid LPS
    - Characterized on histology by abundance of curved "chicken-wire" capillaries, bland nuclei, and a dearth of cellularity.
  - Round Cell LPS
    - Can be thought of as a high-grade version of Myxoid LPS
    - Similar histological characteristics with abundant "chicken-wire" capillaries, but with the addition of thick sheets of round cells [53]
  - Undifferentiated Pleomorphic Sarcoma
    - Previously known as malignant fibrous histiocytoma (MFH)
      - Modern classification schema has reclassified many of the tumors that were formally belonged in this group.

- Histologically defined by presence of at least 65% pleomorphic cells within the sample, along with intervening areas showing typical liposarcoma differentiation [53].
  - Atypical Lipomatous Tumors (ALT)
    - Formally categorized as a WD LPS subtype, now a distinct diagnosis
    - Two subtypes:
      - Atypical lipomatous spindle cell tumors
      - Atypical pleomorphic lipomatous tumors
    - These tumors display alarming histological characteristics but often have indolent clinical courses with metastasis and recurrence being rare.
    - Often lack driver mutations found in other LPSs [3]

Leiomyosarcoma (LMS)

- One of the most common subtypes
- Most common subtype found within the abdomen
  - Also found in the retroperitoneum and uterus and arising from large blood vessels (vena cava)
- Originates from smooth muscle and mesenchymal cells
- Risk Factors
  - Men are more at risk to develop cutaneous LMS.
  - Women are more at risk of developing LMS of the retroperitoneum, vena cava, and aorta [54].
- Histopathology
  - Characterized by intersecting, sharply marginated fascicles of spindle cells with elongated, hyperchromatic nuclei and abundant eosinophilic cytoplasm.
  - Spindle-cell variants are most common; however, nonspindle-cell variants exist.
  - Can be difficult to differentiate between LMS and benign leiomyoma.
  - The presence of abrupt necrosis heavily suggests LMS [55, 56].

Synovial Sarcoma [28]

- Represents 10% of all STS
- Highest prevalence in individuals <30 years of age
- Characteristic translocation, t(X;18)(p11;q11)
- Histopathology
  - Monophasic pattern: spindle cell or epithelial morphology.
  - Biphasic pattern: both fibroblast-like spindle-shaped cells and epithelial cells.
  - Cytokeratin (CK)7 and cytokeratin (CK)19 are highly specific markers of synovial sarcoma [57].

Angiosarcoma

- Constitutes <1% of all STS
- Endothelial origin
- Significantly aggressive
- Subtypes [12, 13, 58]
    - Categorized by the location in which the tumor develops.
        - Primary—tissue parenchyma
            - Higher risk of early metastasis
        - Secondary—skin overlying the tissue
            - Defined by its risk factors
            - Higher risk of local recurrence
            - Displays unique genetic alterations, such as the amplification of MYC and FLT4 (VEGFR3)
- Risk factors [11]
    - Primary angiosarcoma
        - Environmental exposures (arsenic, polyvinyl chloride, and thorotrast, a radiopaque contrast agent not used in the USA since the 1950s)
        - Women aged 30–50
    - Secondary angiosarcoma
        - Radiation therapy (commonly in the context of chest wall radiation for breast cancer)
        - Chronic lymphedema (Stewart-Treves syndrome)
- Histopathology [59]
    - In early stages, challenging to differentiate from benign endothelial tissue due to the lack of capsule
    - In late stages, challenging to differentiate from melanoma
    - Immunohistochemical staining
        - Markers of vascular endothelial origin
            - Vascular endothelial growth factor (VEGF) and Von Willebrand Factor (VWF)
        - For poorly differentiated
            - Ulex europaeus agglutinin 1 and CD31 may help identify endothelial origin

Fibrosarcoma

- Rare
  - Historically more common, many now reclassified due to new classification schema and improved diagnostic capabilities
- Two distinct disease entities
  - Congenital infantile fibrosarcoma and adult-type sarcoma
    - Adult type has a much worse prognosis.
- Risk factors [60]
  - Prior trauma, radiation, and chemotherapy
- Histopathology [25]
  - Spindle-cell "herringbone" pattern
  - Immunohistochemical staining.
    - Vimentin, a marker of mesenchymal origin.
    - Actin and desmin may indicate a degree of myofibroblastic differentiation.

Myxofibrosarcoma

- Estimated to be 5% of all STS.
- High local recurrence rate.
- Risk Factors
  - Male sex and elderly (6th–8th decades)
- Histopathology
  - "Curvilinear" capillaries (vs. the "chicken-wire" capillaries found in myxoid LPS)
- Unlike myxoid LPS, myxofibrosarcoma does not display consistent genetic alterations [61].

Malignant Peripheral Nerve Sheath Tumors (MPNSTs)

- Originates from nerve sheath differentiation
- Can occur spontaneously or arise from existing neurofibromas
- Risk Factors
  - 50% of cases linked to neurofibromatosis
  - Approximately 10% of all patients with neurofibromatosis will develop an MPNST
    - These patients should undergo yearly neurological and ophthalmological examination.
- Histopathology [62]
  - Spindle cells arranged in a palisade or rosette-like pattern
  - Immunohistochemical staining
    - S100 protein

Dermatofibrosarcoma Protuberans (DFSP)

- Slow growing.
- 1–5% of all STS cases
- Typically presents as a firm truncal plaque in young adults
- Can present with rapid growth during pregnancy
  - The behavior of these tumors after pregnancy is not well defined, although recurrence and metastasis has been reported.
  - Can be treated during or after pregnancy.
  - The influence of oral contraceptives on DFSP behavior is under investigation [63].
- Histopathology:
  - COL1A1-PDGF-beta fusion gene is diagnostic for DFSP.
  - Displays features of fibroblastic, muscular, and neurological differentiation.
  - DFSP lesions exhibit cells that are arranged in a storiform pattern.
  - The presence fibrosarcomatous changes with atypical cytological features within the tumor margins indicates a more aggressive form of DFSP and a poorer prognosis.
- In the absence of these features, a 10-year survival rates exceed 99% [64].

Desmoid Tumor

- Also known as aggressive fibromatosis (AF)
- Locally invasive tumors with high recurrence rates
- Low rates of metastasis
- High association with familial adenomatous polyposis (FAP)
  - All patients with desmoid tumors should be evaluated for germline APC mutations.

- Associated with pregnancy
  - Postpartum cases have improved outcomes.
- Histopathology
  - Most sporadic common mutation: CTNNB1
  - Resemble the proliferative stage of wound healing with a rich vascular network, abundant collagenous stroma, and an abundance of myofibroblasts.
  - May resemble fibrosarcoma, myxofibrosarcoma, or myxoid liposarcoma but without significant cellular atypia.
  - Immunohistochemical staining [65, 66]:
    - Nuclear β-catenin, vimentin, PDGF-beta, androgen receptor, and estrogen receptor beta

Rhabdomyosarcoma (RMS) [67, 68]

- Most common STS in children and adolescents
- Four main subtypes that commonly occur within specific age ranges:
  - Botryoid sarcoma
    - Most favorable prognosis
    - Infants and young children
    - Originates specifically within hollow organs, such as the bladder or vagina.
  - Embryonal rhabdomyosarcoma
    - Worse prognosis than botryoid sarcoma
    - Children in early childhood and adolescence
  - Alveolar rhabdomyosarcoma
    - Worse prognosis than embryonal rhabdomyosarcoma
    - Adolescents
    - Identified by specific chromosomal translocations: PAX3-FOXO1 or PAX7-FOXO1
  - Pleomorphic rhabdomyosarcoma
    - Affects adults
    - Worst prognosis of the RMS subtypes
- Histopathology
  - Poorly circumscribed, highly infiltrative
  - Characteristic pattern of cells with eccentric eosinophilic cytoplasm filled with granules and thick and thin filaments, reflecting their rhabdomyoblastic origin

Clinical Evaluation

- The National Comprehensive Cancer Network (NCCN) guidelines categorize the management of STS according to their location.
  - Extremity, trunk, or head/neck (referred to as extremity unless specified)
  - Retroperitoneal or intraabdominal (RP unless specified)

- Specific subtypes such as desmoid tumors, RMS, and DFS [4, 69]
- Evaluation should focus on the following:
  - Identify the primary tumor location.
  - Signs or symptoms of local-regional or distant metastasis.
  - Explore presence of subtype-specific risk factors.
  - Discuss any possible genetic predisposition within the family.

Extremity and Trunk STS

- Most common location (63%) of all STS [50, 51]
  - Upper thigh (44%)
  - Other sites include the following:
    - Lower extremity (27%)
    - Upper extremity (12%)
    - Shoulder/axilla (11%)
    - Trunk (10%)
    - Forearm (6%)
- Most common subtypes [50, 51]
  - Undifferentiated pleomorphic sarcoma (24%)
  - LPS (21%)
  - Synovial sarcoma and myxofibrosarcoma (each 10%)
  - LMS (8%)
- Presentation and evaluation
  - Painless mass of the extremity (most likely proximal thigh) [50, 51]
    - Differential diagnosis
      - Exclude traumatic injury
      - Benign etiologies
        - Cysts, leiomyomas, schwannomas, neurofibromas, ganglions, nodular fasciitis, sebaceous cysts, hypertrophic scarring, hematomas, lipomas, myositis ossificans, myxomas, infections, and hemangiomas
      - Malignancy causes
        - Lymphoma, skin cancers, and metastatic diseases
        - Increased risk of malignancy if [70]
          - Larger than 4 cm
          - Increase in size
          - Located deep to the fascia
          - Painful
          - Recurrence after previous excision
  - Comprehensive physical exam of the mass, focusing on the following:
    - Size and immobility.
    - Consider complexity of wound closure and potential for reconstruction.
    - Potential neurovascular involvement.
    - Lymph node evaluation.

Retroperitoneum and Intraabdominal STS

- RP and intraabdominal sarcomas make up 15% of STS compared to visceral STS (22%) [50, 51].
- LPS and LMS are the most common.
- Presentation
  - Vague abdominal pain, palpable mass (average size at presentation 15 cm), compressive symptoms secondary to mass effect (early satiety and obstruction), or an incidental mass found on imaging.
- Broad differential, with specific history taking aimed at cancers of the following:
  - Adrenal gland, kidney, pancreas, duodenum, metastatic urologic and gynecological malignancies, extrarenal paragangliomas, lymphomas, schwannomas, and germ cell tumors
- Exam should include a thorough abdominal, regional lymph node, and testicular (in young men) examination.

Diagnosis

Extremity and Trunk STS

- Preferred imaging modality:
  - Magnetic resonance imaging (MRI) with gadolinium contrast
    - Some evolving roles for CT and ultrasound
    - WD-LPS has high signal intensity during the T1 phase with lower intensity in the T2 phase compared to Myxoid STS (high T2 intensity).
    - Non-WD-LPS have varying intensities.
    - High-grade STS is T1 isointense to muscle, T2 (fat-suppressed) hyperintense, and contrast enhancement in the delay phase.
  - Poor prognostic signs
    - Satellite lesions
    - Enhancement or nodularity which suggests a high-grade tumor component within the STS
  - WD-LPS with classic MRI findings do not require tissue diagnosis to initiate treatment.
- Biopsy recommendations for tissue diagnosis
  - Core needle biopsy no smaller than an 18 gauge.
  - Aimed at nodular or enhancing lesions.
  - It is imperative to carefully plan the biopsy track.
    - The biopsy track should be aimed in such a way that a subsequent resection would encompass the track.
      - This is to not seed the surrounding tissues.
  - Up to 15% of biopsies do not yield a definitive diagnosis.
    - An incisional biopsy is appropriate if it would alter treatment.

- Performed along the axis of the extremity so that it can be incorporated into the definitive surgical resection with minimal dissection.
    - For superficial lesions <3 cm, excisional biopsy can be an appropriate choice.
- Pathological testing
    - Hemotoxin and eosin.
    - Immunohistochemistry
    - Identification of chromosomal abnormalities with fluorescence in situ hybridization (FISH)

Retroperitoneum and Intraabdominal STS

- Preferred imaging
    - Cross-sectional contrast computed tomography (CT)
        - To determine location and size relative to surrounding structures
    - PET scans rarely aid diagnosis or change management and are therefore usually not indicated.
        - Some recent use in differentiating WD-LPS from DD-LPS and determining response to neoadjuvant treatment.
- Biopsy
    - Given the risk of undergoing an intraabdominal or RP biopsy due to tumor location and size, biopsy is pursued only when.
        - Suspicion of a dedifferentiated component.
        - Imaging is inconclusive.
        - Tissue diagnosis would alter treatment and the risk of biopsy is acceptable.
        - Adrenal masses should particularly be ruled out to avoid inadvertent biopsy of a hormone secreting adrenal mass or paraganglioma (**Chapter: Adrenal and/or Endocrine Tumors** for adrenal mass workup and biopsy indications).

Subtype Special Considerations

Clinical Evaluation, Diagnosis, and Stage and Grade

- Subtypes that have a propensity for metastasis at specific sites should have contrast imaging of the potential metastatic site at the initial diagnostic workup, during surveillance, and with recurrence regardless of the primary site location [4]:
    - CT or MRI of the abdomen and pelvis
        - Angiosarcoma, leiomyosarcoma, myxoid/round cell sarcoma, and epithelioid sarcoma
    - Chest CT scans

- Intermediate- and high-grade STS and subtypes with a tendency for lung metastasis (Table 16.1).
- Can avoid Chest CT in WD-LPS, ATL, and low-grade desmoid tumors because of their low metastatic potential.
  - Whole-body MRI
    - Myxoid/round cell LPS given propensity for soft tissue metastasis
      - MRI should map outside the CT chest, abdomen, and pelvis
  - MRI of the total spine:
    - Myxoid/round cell LPS because of the likelihood of spinal metastasis
  - MRI of all CNS structures:
    - Angiosarcoma and alveolar soft part sarcoma
  - CT or PET/CT of regional lymph node basins:
    - Angiosarcoma, epithelioid sarcoma, clear cell sarcoma, synovial sarcoma, and RMS, given their high propensity for lymph node metastasis [71].
  - PET/CT can be useful for selecting histologies for neoadjuvant therapy when further assistance is required for determining staging, prognosis, grading, and response to subsequent neoadjuvant therapy [4].

Stage and Grade

- Sarcomas are staged in accordance with the guidelines set forth by the American Joint Committee on Cancer (AJCC) in their Cancer Staging Manual, Eighth Edition, using the Tumor, Node, Metastasis (TNM) system [72] (Tables 16.3, 16.4, 16.5, and 16.6).
- Histologic grade plays a critical role in the staging process of sarcomas.
- The Fédération Nationale des Centres de Lutte Contre le Cancer (FNCLCC) system standardizes the grading of sarcomas by the following:
  - Tumor differentiation, mitotic rate, and necrosis (Table 16.3) [73]
- Within this system, the grading of the following sarcomas is not recommended.
  - Gastrointestinal stromal tumors, malignant peripheral nerve sheath tumors, embryonal and alveolar rhabdomyosarcomas, angiosarcomas (rapid growth and dissemination common), extraskeletal myxoid chondrosarcomas, alveolar soft part sarcomas, clear cell sarcomas, and epithelioid sarcomas.
- Sarculator
  - Online validated nomogram developed to aid in prognostication.
    - https://www.sarculator.com/
  - Resected, primary extremity and trunk [75–77]
    - Age, size, grade, and histology
    - Predicts five- and ten-year OS and distant metastasis-free survival
  - Resected RP STS [78]
    - Age, size, grade, histology, multifocality, and completeness of resection
    - Predicts five-year OS and DFS for high-volume and low-volume sarcoma centers

Table 16.3 FNCLCC histologic grading system [72, 73]

Tumor differentiation score	Definition
1	Resemble normal mesenchymal tissue (low-grade LMS)
2	Histologic subtype is certain (myxoid/round cell LPS)
3	Embryonal and undifferentiated sarcomas, sarcomas of doubtful type, synovial sarcomas, soft tissue osteosarcoma, and Ewing sarcoma/primitive neuroectodermal tumor (PNET) of soft tissue
Subtype-specific tumor differentiation score	**Score**
ALT, WD-LPS, and WD-LMS	1
Myxoid LPS, fibrosarcoma, myxofibrosarcoma, LMS (conventional)	2
LPS (round cell, pleomorphic, DD), undifferentiated pleomorphic sarcoma, poorly differentiated/pleomorphic/epithelioid LMS, synovial sarcoma (biphasic/monophasic or poorly differentiated), RMS (pleomorphic), mesenchymal chondrosarcoma, extraskeletal osteosarcoma, Ewing sarcoma/PNET, malignant rhabdoid tumor, undifferentiated sarcoma, not otherwise specified	3
Mitotic count score[a]	**Definition**
1	0–9 mitoses per 10 HPF
2	10–19 mitoses per 10 HPF
3	≥20 mitoses per 10 HPF
Tumor necrosis score[b]	**Definition**
0	No necrosis
1	<50% tumor necrosis
2	≥50% tumor necrosis
Grade	**Definition**
GX	Grade cannot be assessed
G1	Total differentiation, mitotic count, and necrosis score of 2 or 3
G2	Total differentiation, mitotic count, and necrosis score of 4 or 5
G3	Total differentiation, mitotic count, and necrosis score of 6, 7, or 8

Fédération Nationale des Centres de Lutte Contre le Cancer (FNCLCC)
[a]In the most mitotically active area of the sarcoma, ten successive high-power fields (HPF; one HPF at 400× magnification = 0.1734 mm^2) were assessed using a 40× objective.
[b]Evaluated on gross examination and validated with histologic sections.

Table 16.4 Extremity and Trunk STS AJCC Tumor, Node, Metastasis Staging System [74]

Primary tumor (T)

T category	T criteria
TX	Primary tumor cannot be assessed
T0	No evidence of primary tumor
T1	Tumor 5 cm or less in greatest dimension
T2	Tumor more than 5 cm and less than or equal to 10 cm in greatest dimension
T3	Tumor more than 10 cm and less than or equal to 15 cm in greatest dimension
T4	Tumor more than 15 cm in greatest dimension

Regional lymph nodes (N)

N category	N criteria
NX	Regional lymph nodes cannot be assessed
N0	No regional lymph node metastasis or unknown lymph node status
N1	Regional lymph node metastasis

Distant metastasis (M)

M category	M criteria
MX	Distant metastases cannot be assessed
M0	No distant metastasis
M1	Distant metastasis

Definition of grade (G)

G	G definition
GX	Grade cannot be assessed
G1	Total differentiation, mitotic count, and necrosis score of 2 or 3
G2	Total differentiation, mitotic count, and necrosis score of 4 or 5
G3	Total differentiation, mitotic count, and necrosis score of 6, 7, or 8

Prognostic stage groups

T stage	N stage	M stage	Grade	Stage
T1	N0	M0	G1, GX	IA
T2, T3, T4	N0	M0	G1, GX	IB
T1	N0	M0	G2, G3	II
T2	N0	M0	G2, G3	IIIA
T3, T4	N0	M0	G2, G3	IIIB
Any T	N1	M0	Any G	IV
Any T	Any N	M1	Any G	IV

STS Soft tissue sarcoma, *TNM* tumor, node, metastasis, *AJCC* American Joint Committee on Cancer

Table 16.5 Retroperitoneum STS AJCC Tumor, Node, Metastasis Staging System [74]

Primary tumor (T)	
T category	T criteria
TX	Primary tumor cannot be assessed
T0	No evidence of primary tumor
T1	Tumor 5 cm or less in greatest dimension
T2	Tumor more than 5 cm and less than or equal to 10 cm in greatest dimension
T3	Tumor more than 10 cm and less than or equal to 15 cm in greatest dimension
T4	Tumor more than 15 cm in greatest dimension
Regional lymph nodes (N)	
N category	N criteria
NX	Regional lymph nodes cannot be assessed
N0	No regional lymph node metastasis or unknown lymph node status
N1	Regional lymph node metastasis
Distant metastasis (M)	
M category	M criteria
MX	Distant metastasis cannot be assessed
M0	No distant metastasis
M1	Distant metastasis
Definition of grade (G)	
G	G definition
GX	Grade cannot be assessed
G1	Total differentiation, mitotic count, and necrosis score of 2 or 3
G2	Total differentiation, mitotic count, and necrosis score of 4 or 5
G3	Total differentiation, mitotic count, and necrosis score of 6, 7, or 8

Prognostic stage groups				
T stage	N stage	M stage	Grade	Stage group
T1	N0	M0	G1, GX	IA
T2–T4	N0	M0	G1, GX	IB
T1	N0	M0	G2, G3	II
T2	N0	M0	G2, G3	IIIA
T3-T4	N0	M0	G2, G3	IIIB
Any T	N1	M0	Any G	IIIB
Any T	Any N	M1	Any G	IV

STS Soft tissue sarcoma, *TNM* tumor, node, metastasis, *AJCC* American Joint Committee on Cancer

Table 16.6 Intraabdominal and Intrathoracic Viscera STS AJCC Tumor, Node, Metastasis Staging System [74][a]

Primary tumor (T)
T category	T criteria
TX	Primary tumor cannot be assessed
T1	Organ confined
T2	Tumor extension into tissue beyond organ
T2a	Invades serosa or visceral peritoneum
T2b	Extension beyond serosa (mesentery)
T3	Invades another organ
T4	Multifocal involvement
T4a	Multifocal (two sites)
T4b	Multifocal (three to five sites)
T4c	Multifocal (>5 sites)

Regional lymph nodes (N)
N category	N criteria
NX	Regional lymph nodes cannot be assessed
N0	No lymph node involvement or unknown lymph node status
N1	Lymph node involvement present

Distant metastasis (M)
M category	M criteria
MX	Distant metastasis cannot be assessed
M0	No metastases
M1	Metastases present

STS Soft tissue sarcoma, *TNM* tumor, node, metastasis, *AJCC* American Joint Committee on Cancer

[a]There is no recommended prognostic stage grouping currently

Multidisciplinary Management

Resectable and Locally Advanced Extremity and Trunk STS

- Treatment is multifaceted; however, surgery remains the primary modality.
  - If margins are positive, reresection is strongly advised.
  - Careful consideration of radiation and systemic therapy where appropriate.
- Limb-Sparing Surgery
  - Prior to Rosenburg et al.'s groundbreaking study, STS of the extremity was treated with amputation with local recurrences < 5% (nonamputation approaches had recurrences of 30–50%) [79].
    - However, high rates of distant metastasis remained a significant challenge when undergoing such a morbid operation.
  - This led to a shift toward limb-sparing surgery followed by XRT (Table 16.7).
    - Equivalent five-year disease-free survival (DFS) and overall survival (OS)
    - Less than 5% rate of amputation [80]
    - Over time, as XRT techniques have improved [81–83, 89]
      - Local recurrence rates have dropped to between 10% and 20%.
      - XRT is associated with a 50% relative risk reduction.

Table 16.7 Extremity STS surgery and radiation studies

Study	Design	Results	Interpretation
Surgery Studies			
Rosenberg (1982) [80]	LSS + adjuvant XRT (6000–7000 Gy) vs. amputation Low- and high-grade extremity STS	Similar five-year DFS (71% vs. 78%, $p = 0.75$) and OS (83% vs. 88%, $p = 0.99$) but LSS had an increased LR (15% vs. 0%, $p = 0.06$) however < 5% needed an amputation.	LSS + adjuvant XRT becomes the new standard of care.
Adjuvant Brachytherapy Studies			
Pisters (1996) [81]	LSS +/− adjuvant BRT Low- and high-grade extremity and trunk STS	Improved five-year local control with BRT (overall, 82% vs. 69%, $p = 0.04$ and high grade, 89% vs. 66%, $p = 0.0025$) but not for low grade. BRT did not improve. Five-year DSS or the risk of distant metastasis.	Local control is achieved in high-grade STS with little effect on preventing systemic disease or survival.
Adjuvant radiation studies			
Yang (1985) [82]	LSS +/- adjuvant XRT Low- and high-grade extremity STS Only high-grade STS received concurrent chemotherapy (doxorubicin + cyclophosphamide)	Overall, 5-year LR decreased with XRT, 13% vs. 26% with no difference in 5-year OS 66% vs. 57%. Low-grade five-year LR decreased with XRT (7% vs. 21%, $p = 0.016$) with no difference in five-year OS (78% vs. 71%). High-grade five-year LR decreased with XRT (20% vs. 33%, $p = 0.0028$) with no difference in five-year OS (58% vs. 46%). XRT LR (17.9-years 1.4% vs. 25%, $p = 0.0001$).	The benefit of XRT for high grade is because they have a greater risk of LR (vs. low grade) despite toxicity profile.
Beane (2010) [83]	Long-term follow-up	XRT trend toward more wound complications (17% vs. 12.5%) and edema (25% vs. 12%) with worse functional outcomes (15% vs. 12%)	XRT reduced LR <10% (vs. 30–50% history control) with nonsignificant rate of complications.
Pisters (2007) [84]	LSS for T1 ($n = 88$) Adjuvant XRT for R1+	R0 five-year and ten-year LR 7.9% and 10.6%, respectively R1 + XRT (14/88) with 6 LR of which 2 required amputation	XRT can be omitted in T1 tumors. Achieving a negative margin is essential to improving LR in this subset of patients

(continued)

Table 16.7 (continued)

Study	Design	Results	Interpretation
Neoadjuvant vs. adjuvant radiation studies			
O'Sullivan (2002) [85]	Neoadjuvant (50 Gy) vs. adjuvant (66 Gy) XRT	No difference in LR, OSS, and DSS Neoadjuvant had increased acute wound complications (35% vs. 17%, p=0.01).	Adjuvant XRT had worse long-term functional outcomes while neoadjuvant XRT had more initial wound complications
Davis (2005) [86]		Adjuvant XRT had increased grade or higher fibrosis (48.2% vs. 31.5%, $p = 0.07$) with trend toward increased edema and joint stiffness which correlated with significant worse functional outcomes ($p < 0.01$).	
Chemoradiation studies			
Kraybill (2006) [87]	Neoadjuvant chemoradiation Three cycles pre- and postop (mesna, doxorubicin, ifosfamide, and dacarbazine)	High toxicity (5% grade 5 and 83% grade 4) with 59% completing treatment Three-year LR 17.6% (5 amputations) with 56.6% disease-free survival (DFS), 64.5% distant disease-free survival (DFS) 64.5%, and 75.1% overall survival (OS)	Feasibility and efficacy of chemoradiation however the benefit must be weighed against the toxicity profile
RTOG 9514 (2010) [88]		97% grade 3 toxicity at 5 years with 28% distant metastasis (7.7-year follow-up) with lung being most common site	

LSS Limb-sparing surgery, *XRT* radiation, *BRT* brachytherapy, *DFS* disease-free survival, *LR* local recurrence, *OS* overall survival, *DSS* disease-specific survival, *DFS* distant disease-free survival

- XRT
  - General indications
    - Intermediate- and high-grade tumors, where the most significant clinical benefit is anticipated.
    - Tumors are proximate to critical structures and pose a risk for suboptimal margins [4].
  - Tumor stage and grade considerations
    - Low-grade tumors <5 cm, such as T1G1 (stage IA), surgery without radiation may be appropriate.
    - Larger low-grade stage IB (T2–T4G1) tumors typically undergo surgery alone, provided that a satisfactory margin of at least 1 cm is achievable.
      - Local recurrence rates of 7.9% and 10.6% at five and ten years, respectively, with specific histologic subtypes considered [4, 81, 85, 90–94].

- Small high-grade stage II (T1G2-3) and large high-grade stage IIIA/IIIB (T2-T4, G2-3) extremity STS are generally considered for XRT.
    - Due to higher rates of local recurrence (16.7% at ten years) for high-grade neoplasms [81].
- Timing of XRT (neoadjuvant vs. adjuvant)
    - Multidisciplinary discussions are warranted.
    - No significant differences in OS, LR, or progression-free survival (PFS) (Table 16.7).
    - Consider patient factors, tumor characteristics, and toxicity profile (*radiation therapy*) [85, 95].
    - Neoadjuvant XRT may improve the likelihood of a negative surgical margin.
        - Delivering radiation to an intact mass may facilitate more precise radiation planning but must be balanced against the increased risk of acute wound complications [85, 96].
            - For example, in individuals who are at risk for poor wound healing (smokers, peripheral arterial disease, poorly controlled diabetes), favoring an adjuvant approach could be preferred despite a higher risk of limb dysfunction.
        - Conversely, in young healthy patients, neoadjuvant therapy can be considered because of the lower risk of long-term limb dysfunction.
- Systemic Therapy
    - Integration of chemotherapy into the treatment regimen for stage II and III sarcomas remains a contentious issue due to the disparate evidence found in the literature.
        - In a subset of patients with stage III extremity STS exhibiting adverse prognostic indicators, the addition of chemotherapy, whether in a neoadjuvant or adjuvant setting, has been suggested to confer benefits.
            - This is evidenced by a limited number of clinical trials (Tables 16.7, 16.11, and 16.12).
    - Timing of systemic therapy (neoadjuvant vs. adjuvant)
        - Optimal timing of systemic therapy and its concomitant use with radiotherapy (chemoradiation) in the treatment of extremity soft tissue sarcomas remains a subject of debate [87, 88].
        - Neoadjuvant chemoradiation is considered for stage II and III extremity STS due to an association with improved DFS, OS, and local control [108, 109] (Table 16.7).
            - However, data supporting this approach is not uniform and remains a point of clinical investigation.
- In summary
    - Stage I are treated with wide local excision with adequate margin.
        - Reresection is preferred for postoperative positive margin if there is an acceptable cosmetic and functional outcome.
    - Resectable and locally advanced stage II and III extremity STS are most commonly treated via surgical excision complemented by neoadjuvant

radiotherapy, preferably over adjuvant radiotherapy, particularly when there is a concern for potential positive surgical margins [85, 96, 108, 110].

Resectable and Locally Advanced RP and Intraabdominal STS

- Surgery remains the backbone of treatment with the goal of a macroscopically negative resection (R0/R1).
    - To achieve this, en bloc resection of organs or other vital structures is indicated when tumor invasion is present (*surgical technique, intraoperative decision-making, and outcomes*).
- Unfortunately, many patients with RP sarcoma eventually develop unresectable local disease.
    - As such, treatment is focused on reducing LR.
- XRT
    - Complex decision with multidisciplinary review [111].
    - Historically, conflicting retrospective and small single institution studies (Table 16.8)

Table 16.8 Retroperitoneal STS surgery and radiation studies

Study	Design	Results	Interpretation
Surgery studies			
Bonvalot (2009) [112]	Retrospective multiinstitutional Simple vs. macroscopic en bloc vs. compartmental resection	Compartmental resection was associated with improved three-year LR HR 3.86 ($p = 0.01$) but no difference in five-year OS compared to macroscopic resection HR 1.37 (0.06). Number of resected organs did not differ between macroscopic and compartmental resections and was not associated with improved three-year LR.	Suggests the need for a prospective study before making definitive conclusions. Does not factor in chemotherapy or radiation bias.
Gronchi (2009) [113]	Retrospective single institution Compartmental vs. macroscopic en block resection (>/= 2 visceral resections)	Ten-year OS 36%, LR 47%, and distant metastasis 20%. Prior 2001, 20% multivisceral resections compared to 50% after 2001 (18% simple resection) Compartmental improved five-year LR (48% vs. 28%, $p = 0.01$) and distant metastases 22% vs. 13% ($p = 0.01$).	2001 the institution changed to a compartment resection policy Extrapolation of this data should be done with caution. Had short-term follow-up for the surgery group after 2001. Does not factor in chemotherapy or radiation bias.

(continued)

Table 16.8 (continued)

Study	Design	Results	Interpretation
Gronchi (2012) [114]	Retrospective Reassessment of initial single institution study	Compartmental had an improved five-year OS 66.5% vs. 44.8% ($p = 0.009$) and five-year LR 27.8% vs. 49.3% ($p < 0.0001$) compared to macroscopic resection but a decreased five-year distant metastasis 24.5% vs. 12.1%	Long-term follow-up to initial study. Worse distant metastasis suggest more aggressive surgery may not influence outcomes past five years especially for certain subtypes.
Radiation studies			
Nussbaum (2016) [115]	Retrospective Neoadjuvant XRT vs. surgery and surgery vs. adjuvant XRT	Neoadjuvant improved median OS 110 months (110 months, 95% CI 75-not estimable vs. 66 months 95% CI 0.59–0.82; HR 0.70, $p < 0.0001$) Adjuvant improved mOS (89 months, 95% CI 79–100 vs. 64 months 95% CI 0.71–0.85; HR 0.78, $p < 0.0001$)	The addition of XRT can improve OS.
EORTC-62092 STRASS (2020) [116]	Phase III neoadjuvant XRT (50.4 Gy, 28 fractions) vs. surgery	No difference in median AFRS (4.5 XRT vs. five-year surgery, $p = 0.095$) Posthoc analysis showed the potential for improved local control with XRT for WD LPS and grade 1–2 DD LPS.	The addition of neoadjuvant XTR does not improve local control except for certain LPS subtypes.
Callegaro (2023) [117]	Pooled data from the STREXIT (propensity matched) and STRASS trials	Neoadjuvant XRT was associated with improved AFRS (HR 0.61; 95% CI, 0.42–0.82) and AFRI in WD LPS and grade 1–2 DD LPS	XRT had a similar effect on AFRS in both studies.

XRT Radiation, *DFS* disease-free survival, *LR* local recurrence, *OS* overall survival, *DSS* disease-specific survival, *DFS* distant disease-free survival, *AFRS* abdominal recurrence-free survival, *AFRI* abdominal recurrence-free interval, *LPS* liposarcoma, *WD* well-differentiated, *DD* dedifferentiated

- STRASS (Surgery with or without Radiation Therapy in Untreated Nonmetastatic Retroperitoneal Sarcoma) Trial
    - No difference in abdominal recurrence-free survival (ARFS) between neoadjuvant XRT and curative surgery alone [116].
    - This controversial result was further analyzed in a follow-up study which suggested in posthoc analysis that LPS specifically may benefit from neoadjuvant XRT, warranting further study [117].
- When XRT is administered, it is generally recommended in the neoadjuvant setting.
    - As the mass effect of the tumor can displace nearby bowel
        - Theoretically decreases the risk of seeding nearby structures at the time of the operation (*radiation therapy*).

- Systemic Therapy
  - Benefits of chemotherapy for high-grade RP STS are being investigated (STRASS2).
  - Current recommendations are based on data from extremity STS clinical trials (Table 16.12) (*systemic therapy*) [101, 118, 119].

Metastatic Extremity and RP STS [4, 120]

- 30% have synchronous or metachronous metastatic disease (8% extremity and 10% RP) [121, 122]
  - Most frequent sites
    - Liver and lung
      - Lung slightly more common in metastatic extremity
      - Liver slightly more common in metastatic RP
  - Tumor grade, size, and incomplete resection increase likelihood of metastasis
  - Tumor subtype can also influence metastatic potential (Table 16.1)
    - Tumor subtypes with the greatest metastatic potential
      - LMS, epithelioid sarcoma, clear cell sarcoma, angiosarcoma, RMS, synovial sarcoma, fibrosarcoma, PMNST, DD-LPS, alveolar soft part sarcoma, myxoid/round cell LPS, undifferentiated pleomorphic sarcoma, and myxofibrosarcoma
  - Stage IV disease (any T, N1, M0, any G, or any T, any N, M1, any G)
    - Generally poor prognosis (17% five-year relative survival)
      - Due to the limited clinical benefits of most modern therapies [2–4] (Table 16.12)
- Systemic Therapy
  - Largely doxorubicin-based regimens either alone or in combination
    - Commonly combined with ifosfamide depending on patient functional status and toxicity tolerance
  - Next-generation sequencing can be used to identify targetable mutations.
- All patients with metastatic STS should be considered for enrollment into clinical trials.
  - Due to poor outcomes of current first-line therapy
- Surgical Resection
  - Synchronous metastasis
    - Resection of primary is considered when anatomically feasible with minimal morbidity AND if the site of metastatic disease can also be adequately controlled with surgery, local therapy, or systemic therapy.
      - Metastasectomy is controversial, but several prognostic factors can help aid in identifying patients who would benefit (*surgical technique, intraoperative decision-making, and outcomes, metastasectomy*) [123–126].
  - Consider palliative resection after other treatment modalities fail to control symptomatology.

Unresectable Extremity and RP STS [4, 75, 111, 120]

- Tumors may be deemed unresectable if:
  - Involvement of vital structures.
  - Those whose surgery would cause unacceptable morbidity.
  - Those that are unfit for surgery due to frailty and comorbidities (*surgical technique, intraoperative decision-making, and outcomes*)
- Biopsy is recommended prior to initiating treatment.
- Treatment
  - Typically consists of any of the following in isolation or in combination with another modality:
    - XRT
    - Systemic therapy (chemotherapy, targeted therapy, or immunotherapy)
    - Regional therapy
      - Isolated limb infusion reserved for select extremity STS patients
  - Conversion to resectability is low with treatment and the intent of therapy is palliative.
- Surgical Resection
  - Palliative surgery can be considered for patients who remain symptomatic after other therapies.
    - Includes amputation in extremity STS
- Observation can be considered in patients who are asymptomatic.

Recurrent Extremity and RP STS [75, 111]

- 20–50% develop recurrence after treatment (including local and metachronous metastasis).
  - Five-year DSS 20–70%, largely dependent on STS subtype [121, 127]
  - Recurrence rate dependent on location, grade, subtype, and surgical margin [128–130]
- Extremity STS is less likely to develop local recurrence compared to RP sarcoma.
  - Extremity (15–30%) vs. RP (30–70%)
    - This is largely due to extremity accessibility and amenability to surgery as well as advances in limb-sparing surgery with XRT.
      - Results in a greater R0 rate (Table 16.7)
    - R0 surgical margins for RP sarcoma are less likely due to invasion into RP fat and nearby structures (*surgical technique, intraoperative decision-making, and outcomes*).
- Subtypes with higher recurrence rates
  - DD-LPS (20–30%)
  - High-grade STS (30–50% vs. 20–25% in low grade) [131]
    - High-grade tends to be more infiltrative with poorly defined margins.
- Evaluation of Recurrent Extremity STS

- Clinical evaluation, diagnosis, stage, and grade of LR should mirror the initial management of extremity STS (*clinical evaluation and diagnosis, extremity and trunk*, and *stage and grade*).
- Multimodality treatment (*multidisciplinary management, extremity and trunk STS*) should be offered when indicated.
  - Surgery can be offered to resectable recurrent tumors when good functional and cosmetic outcomes are anticipated.
    - Palliative resections when other treatment modalities fail to control symptomatology.
  - XRT and Systemic Therapy
    - Indications for systemic therapy and XRT remain the same as a primary occurrence.
      - If a patient has previously received XRT, should be reevaluated by a radiation oncologist.
    - Patients with nonoperable recurrence can be offered palliative XRT/chemotherapy.
- Evaluation of Recurrent Intrabdominal and RP Sarcoma
  - Like the management of extremity STS local recurrence, RP and intraabdominal STS LR follow the initial primary tumor management (*Clinical Evaluation and Diagnosis, RP and Intraabdominal STS* and *Stage and Grade* and *Multidisciplinary Management, RP and Intraabdominal STS*).
    - Surgery is indicated for tumors that can be resected with a negative margin and acceptable morbidity.
      - Palliative surgery when other treatment modalities fail to control symptomatology.
    - XRT and Systemic Therapy:
      - Multidisciplinary discussion for indications and sequence of treatment.
      - Indications for systemic therapy and XRT remain the like primary occurrence.
        - If a patient has previously received XRT, should be reevaluated by a radiation oncologist.
        - XRT can be offered with a preference for neoadjuvant XRT.
      - Patients who are not candidates for surgery can under palliative local or systemic therapy as indicated (*Multidisciplinary Management, Unresectable and Metastatic Extremity and RP STS*).

Surgical Technique, Intraoperative Decision-Making, and Outcomes

- Goals of surgery
  - Obtain an R0/R1 margin:
    - Negative margin is highly prognostic for LR.
    - STS in difficult anatomic locations (RP and head/neck) have higher LR.
      - Likely due to difficulty in obtaining negative margin [132, 133].

- Avoid pseudocapsule or intratumoral violation.
- Achieve functional outcome.

Extremity and Trunk STS

- Limb-salvage surgery
  - Standard of care
    - Amputation reserved for salvage therapy
  - Preoperative planning to determine the extent of resection
    - Based on tumor subtype, grade, and depth
  - Margin width
    - 1–2 cm margin of normal tissue is acceptable.
      - Decreases rate of R1
    - Narrower margin is acceptable when.
      - Need to preserve functional outcome.
        - STS are more likely to push neurovascular and osseous structures rather than invade or encase.
          - Adventitia (vascular structures), nerve sheath, perineurium (bone), and/or fascia (muscle) is used as a barrier when possible [134–136].
        - Deep tumors are more likely to involve critical structures.
  - Intraoperative decisions
    - Involvement of neurovascular structures
      - With exception of malignancy arising from the nerve sheath (MPNST), extremity STS rarely invades neural tissue.
        - Major nerves can safely be left intact with the nerve sheath utilized as the margin [137, 138].
      - If the presence of a major nerve or artery impedes surgical margin:
        - Attempt to open the neurovascular bundle and lift the nerve or artery away from the tumor (neurolysis or arteriolysis) [138, 139].
        - If this does not facilitate a proper surgical margin
          - Resection of major neurovascular structures is indicated, with subsequent vascular reconstruction to improve limb function.
      - Unlike nerves and arteries, major veins can often be resected with minimal morbidity.
    - Involvement of osseous structures
      - Given the absence of frank bone invasion.
      - Deploying the use of periosteal stripping can facilitate a surgical margin in tumors that abut bone.
        - Complications of periosteal stripping
          - Increased risk of radiation dose-dependent fractures.
          - Increased rate of nonunion.
          - The femur is especially susceptible to these complications [138, 140].

- Surgical clips can be placed in the operative bed to aid planning of XRT, especially when there is suspicion of a positive surgical margin.
- Use of surgical drains:
  - Drains may be left within the operative bed to decrease fluid retention.
  - Insert drains through skin near the edge of the wound so that the site can be incorporated into XRT field or reexcised as needed.
- If margins are positive
  - Reresection is indicated.
    - T1G1 (stage IA) and T2–T4G1 (stage IB) [4, 81, 85, 90–94]
    - Improved LR at 5, 10, and 15 years with reresection compared to those who did not undergo surgery (5%, 85%, and 82% vs. 78%, 73%, and 73%, respectively, $p = 0.03$) [4, 81, 85, 90–94].
  - Proceed with XRT (reresection not indicated)
    - Invasion of blood vessel, bone, and nerve
    - Nonacceptable functional outcome or morbidity

Regional Node Evaluation in Extremity and Trunk STS

- <5% of STS spreads to regional lymph nodes [141]
  - Exception is lymphotropic STS (15% of all STS)
    - 20–40% involvement of lymph nodes [29, 142, 143]
    - Synovial cell sarcoma, clear cell sarcoma, angiosarcoma, RMS, and epithelioid sarcoma (SCARE) [144].
      - Synovial cell sarcoma and clear cell sarcoma have demonstrated up to 40% regional lymph node metastasis [28, 34, 36, 37, 144].
- Lack of evidence to support routine intraoperative lymphatic staging.
  - True incidence of occult lymph node metastasis in extremity STS is unknown.
  - Clinical benefit needs to be determined.
    - Sentinel lymph node biopsy (SLBN)
      - With goal of removal of occult lymph node metastasis
  - Dearth of well-designed phase 3 clinical studies
    - 62 patients with lymphotropic sarcoma subtypes who underwent SNLB [144]
    - Eight patients with +SNLB (12.9%)
      - Two with evidence of regional disease upon completion of lymph node dissection (CLND).
        - Both patients went on to develop distant metastatic disease.
    - Three patients with -SNLB went on to develop regional metastatic disease.
- The American College of Surgeons Operative Standards for STS does not recommend routine regional lymph node evaluation due to limited known clinical utility of SNLB [138].
  - However, regional lymphatic staging may be considered in select patients at high risk for lymph node metastasis.

- When to Consider Lymphadenectomy
  - Clinically positive lymph nodes noted on physical exam
  - Suspicious lymph nodes seen on imaging
  - Lymphotropic subtypes
    - May have significantly longer median survival (4.3 months vs. 16.3 months) with lymphadenectomy [143]

RP and Intraabdominal STS

- Preoperative imaging can determine tumor extent and possible invasion of adjacent structures.
  - Unresectable disease
    - Peritoneal carcinomatosis, spinal cord invasion extensive involvement of the superior mesenteric vessels, aorta, and/or porta hepatis.
    - Those that would require and unacceptably morbid operation such as proximity to vertebrae, the lumbar plexus, or other neurovascular structures.
  - Relative contraindications (must weigh the morbidity of the operation)
    - Involvement of the IVC
      - LMS can originate from the IVC and require IVC resection with or without reconstruction.
    - Involvement of iliac vessels
      - These can in some cases be resected with or without subsequent reconstruction.
- Surgical Technique
  - R0/R1 resection associated with a decrease in LR vs. R2 (gross tumor) [112].
    - Depending on subtype and study, LR can be >40% at ten years [145],
  - Resect visible tumor with a margin of normal tissue.
    - RP can be difficult to achieve R0/R1 [138, 146].
      - Large tumor size (15–20 cm)
      - Proximity to critical structures
      - Difficulty differentiating gross tumor from retroperitoneal fat
        - Indistinct borders with low-grade tumors (WD LPS) whereas LMS have more distinct borders.
    - Avoidance of tumor rupture (friable tumors)
      - Rupture and subsequent dissemination are associated with increased LR similar outcomes to R2 [138, 147, 148].
  - Macroscopic complete resection
    - Comparable oncologic outcomes to compartmental resection with less morbidity [112, 127, 138, 145, 146, 148–156] (Table 16.8).
    - En bloc resection of organs involved with gross tumor invasion.
      - Structure is resected because it cannot be removed from the tumor (R2).
      - Direct organ invasion
        - Splenectomy, nephrectomy, distal pancreatectomy, diaphragm resection, and small intestine or colon resections

- Preoperative spleen vaccines and bowel preparation should be administered when indicated should be provided when appropriate.
- Renal involvement
  - Evaluate the functionality of the spared counterpart.
    - For example, renal scintigraphy
  - Consider neoadjuvant vs. adjuvant chemotherapy, as toxicity may be better tolerated with both kidneys intact.
- Pancreatic involvement
  - Pancreaticoduodenectomy can be considered for right-sided disease.
    - Increases the morbidity of the operation.
    - When appropriate, partial resection of the duodenum is preferred.
  - It is recommended to place an intraabdominal drain at the level of the pancreas when pancreatectomy is performed, especially when performing concomitant vascular reconstruction, bowel anastomosis, or diaphragm resection [157].
- Compartmental resection
  - Systematic removal of the tumor en bloc with "normal" appearing adjacent organs and surrounding soft tissue
    - Removal of adjacent organs with no direct tumor invasion
      - Most common organs are surrounding muscle, kidney, or colon.
    - Only perform neurovascular and osseous resections and Whipple with direct tumor invasion
  - Generally, not recommended due to insufficient data (Table 16.8) [112–114]
    - Retrospective studies
    - Limited survival benefit
      - Only with long-term follow-up in WD-LPS
    - No comparison to the morbidity or mortality with macroscopic resection
      - No quality of life or patient-reported outcomes
    - Increased organ resection with either compartmental or macroscopic resection was not associated with improved LR or OS.
      - Suggests routine resection of grossly normal organs may not be the underlying mechanism to prevent LR or increase OS.
- Subtype and genomic profiles may determine the extent of surgical resection [158].
  - Belief that compartmental resection improves LR because it removes microscopic tumor that would have been left behind with a macroscopic resection.
    - Residual tumor (microscopic invasion) can be seen after reexcision with macroscopic en bloc resection.
  - Importance of microscopic invasion needs to be elucidated.
    - Certain subtypes are at greater risk for microscopic invasion.
      - WD-LPS > LMS

- Subtypes may determine the extent of surgery needed.
  - Low-grade tumors (WD-LPS) increased LR.
    - May benefit from compartmental resection given indistinct borders and possible survival benefit.
  - High-grade tumors (LMS) increased distant recurrence.
    - May benefit from macroscopic complete resection given oncologic outcomes would be less likely effected by a LR.
- However, residual tumor after complete resection has been shown to be associated with OS and distant metastasis but not LR.
- Removing residual tumor with compartmental resection may not improve OS given the propensity for high distant metastasis.

Metastasectomy

- Patients whose primary disease is controlled, have favorable prognostic factors, are fit for surgery, have limited metastatic disease, and have improved survival with metastasectomy (Table 16.9).

Table 16.9 Metastasectomy in STS studies

Study	Design	Results	Interpretation
Pulmonary metastasectomy			
Canter (2007) [159]	Retrospective (extremity) Neoadjuvant chemotherapy vs. pulmonary metastasectomy	No difference in median DSS (24 vs. 33 months, $p = 0.19$) and PFS (10 vs. 11 months, $p = 0.063$, neoadjuvant and surgery, respectively)	Lack of benefit of neoadjuvant chemotherapy
Blackmon (2009) [160]	Retrospective Pulmonary metastasectomy vs. extrapulmonary resection (synchronous and metachronous)	No difference in median survival (pulmonary resection 35.5 vs. extrapulmonary resection 37.8 months, $p = 0.96$) however worse median survival in patients who were not offered resection (13.5 months, $p < 0.001$)	Extrapulmonary metastases should not be a contraindication for resection when complete resection is possible
Predina (2011) [161]	Retrospective Pulmonary metastasectomy	5-year OS 52% and DFS 10% with <2 cm and <2 pulmonary metastases associated with better survival.	Improved OS compared to historic controls (10–40%)
Treasure (2012) [162]	Systematic review (no clinical trials) Pulmonary metastasectomy	Metastasectomy median five-year survival 34% STS and 25% for bone sarcoma Median five-year survival for patients with any site of metastatic disease 15% STS and 25% bone sarcoma	Improved survival in patients who undergo pulmonary metastasectomy compared to other metastatic sites of disease

(continued)

Table 16.9 (continued)

Study	Design	Results	Interpretation
Chudgar (2017) [163]	Retrospective Pulmonary metastasectomy	Median OS, 33.2 months (95% CI, 29.9–37.1) Improved prognosis with LMS, primary $\le$ 10 cm, time to recurrence, solitary lung metastasis, and minimally invasive resection	Help define which patients might benefit most from pulmonary metastasectomy
Hepatic metastasectomy			
DeMatteo (2001) [164]	Retrospective Surgery vs. control	Improved five-year survival with hepatic resection (30% vs. 4%) with median survival of 39 months A two-year recurrence interval associated with better prognosis	Hepatic resection improved survival.
Adam (2006) [79]	Multivariate analysis Hepatic metastasis resection Noncolorectal and neuroendocrine cancers (n = 205; 13.5% GIST and sarcoma)	Median five-year survival GIST 70% Other types 58% Adenocarcinoma 36% Sarcoma 31% Melanoma 21% Squamous cell carcinoma 19%	Sarcoma patients benefit from hepatectomy compared to other cancers.
Groeschl (2012) [165]	Retrospective Hepatic metastasis resection Noncolorectal and neuroendocrine cancers (n = 98; 23% sarcoma)	Overall, five-year survival 31% with median OS 49 months with no difference among cancer types 66% recurred after resection with lymphovascular invasion and metastases $\ge$5 cm associated with a poor prognosis	Hepatic resection has acceptable morbidity and mortality however most patients recur.
Brudvik (2015) [166]	Retrospective Hepatic metastasis resection	Five-year overall survival. GIST: 55.3% LMS: 48.4% Sarcoma: 44.9% Imatinib improved five-year RFS GIST (47.1% vs. 9.5%, p = 0.013). Lung recurrence most common in LMS (36%, p < 0.0001)	GIST and LMS appear to have better outcomes with hepatic resection.

STS Soft tissue sarcoma, *DFS* disease-free survival, *OS* overall survival, *DSS* disease-specific survival, *LMS* leiomyosarcoma, *GIST* gastrointestinal stromal tumor, *LPS* liposarcoma, *WD* well differentiated, *DD* dedifferentiated

- Tumor biology plays a vital role in selecting appropriate patients.
  - Surrogates of tumor biology
    - Longer time from recurrence
    - Good response to systemic therapy
  - Prognostic factors
    - Low-grade tumors

- Number of tumors (<3)
- Size (<2 cm)
- Location
- Hepatectomy has slightly improved outcomes over pulmonary metastasectomy.
  - Median disease-free survival (38–43-month hepatectomy vs. 12–26-month pulmonary resection).
  - Five-year OS (27–32% hepatectomy vs. 14–38% pulmonary resection).
  - Five-year relapse-free survival (20% hepatectomy vs. 7–35% pulmonary resection).
- Nonsurgical candidates may be offered ablative therapies (lung and liver) and additional arterial-based liver-directed therapies.

Management of Peritoneal Sarcomatosis

- Sarcomatosis is a very poor prognostic indicator.
- Palliative systemic therapy is recommended in most cases.
- Cytoreductive surgery with heated hyperthermic intraperitoneal chemotherapy is indicated in select patient populations with a low peritoneal carcinomatosis index.
  - Uterine leiomyosarcoma
  - Pediatric desmoplastic small round cell tumors

Postoperative Care and Complications

- For all extremity and RP STS:
  - Assess neurological and vascular function.
  - Early drain removal when appropriate.
  - Aspiration for symptomatic fluid collection.
  - Adequate pain control.
  - Wound care, especially if adjuvant XRT is planned.
  - Physical therapy for patients with neurovascular defects.

Radiation Therapy

- External beam radiation using intensity-modulated radiotherapy (IMRT) is the standard of care (Table 16.10).
  - Intraoperative XRT can be used at the time of surgery when R0 resection is not feasible or if a positive margin is suspected.
- Neoadjuvant vs. Adjuvant XRT (Table 16.11)
  - NCCN guidelines discourages the use of adjuvant XRT in RP STS.
    - With a suspected positive margin in RP sarcoma, regardless of reresection, patients should be closely followed for recurrence.
      - If patient recurs, at that time, they can be offered neoadjuvant XRT [4].

Table 16.10 Radiation modalities for soft tissue sarcomas

	Modality	Dose
Retroperitoneal STS		
Neoadjuvant	IMRT	50–50.4 Gy or 1.8–2.0 Gy per fraction
Intraoperative	IORT	Microscopic disease (10–12.5 Gy)
		Macroscopic disease (15 Gy)
Extremity/trunk STS		
Neoadjuvant		50–50.4 Gy or 1.8–2.0 Gy per fraction
Adjuvant	IMRT	50–50.4 Gy or 1.8–2.0 Gy per fraction
		Boost for + margin (10–20 Gy)

STS Soft tissue sarcoma, *IMRT* intensity modulated radiotherapy, *IORT* intraoperative radiotherapy, *Gy* Gray

Table 16.11 Comparison of neoadjuvant and adjuvant radiation

	Neoadjuvant XRT	Adjuvant XRT
Dose	Lower (50 Gy)	Higher (66 Gy)
Target volume	Small	Large
Toxicity		
Wound complication, overall	35%	17%
Wound complication, upper extremity	6%	0%
Wound complication, lower extremity	35%	25%
Grade 2+ dermatitis	36%	68%
Fibrosis, edema, and stiff joints	Less	Higher
Function	Better	Worse

XRT Radiation

Systemic Therapy

- Doxorubicin continues to be the first-line systemic agent for STS despite its toxicity.
- Difficulty in selecting additional lines of systemic therapy (second or higher) due to poor quality data.
- Next-generation sequencing is recommended in all patients.
  - Targeted therapy can have rapid tumor response in select circumstances.
- Tyrosine kinase inhibitors (TKIs) have prolonged survival in STS.
  - Combination with chemotherapy may provide a much-needed breakthrough.
- Immunotherapy's benefit is limited to certain subtypes.
- Sarculator (*stage and grade*)
  - Online validated nomogram developed to aid in prognostication.
    - https://www.sarculator.com/
    - Predicts survival in resected, primary extremity and trunk STS [75–77]
    - Predicts survival in resected, RP STS in high- and low-volume centers [78]
  - Recent studies have demonstrated chemotherapy response (neoadjuvant and perioperative) [167, 168].

Chemotherapy

- Lack of consensus regarding when to incorporate chemotherapy into the multimodality treatment of STS owing to its limited benefit.
- The absolute clinical benefit from chemotherapy has been studied (Tables 16.7, 16.8, 16.9, and 16.12).
  - Prognostic factors for patient selection
  - Timing (neoadjuvant vs. adjuvant)
  - Benefit of its combination with XRT (chemoradiation)
  - Largely reserved for high-grade, unresectable disease, and stage IV [169, 170] (*multidisciplinary management, unresectable, and metastatic STS*).
    - Can improve survival in high-grade STS.
- Doxorubicin remains the first-line chemotherapy drug.
- The selection of second line or higher therapeutic agents remains a challenge.
  - Several nonanthracycline or anthracycline (nondoxorubicin) clinical trials have been conducted in the hope of improving upon the survival seen with doxorubicin while decreasing its associated toxicity.
    - No agent is superior to doxorubicin's efficacy and safety profile even though they may have good efficacy in certain subtypes.
      - Including but not limited to taxanes, trabectedin, cisplatin, vinca alkaloid agents, etoposide, dacarbazine, pemetrexed, gemcitabine, eribulin, and methotrexate
      - Various response rates, safety, and efficacy
- Extremity and Trunk STS
  - Most clinical trials have failed to show substantial benefit with adjuvant chemotherapy in resectable extremity STS.
    - Due to the design, dosage, stratification, and lack of knowledge regarding STS subtype tumor biology

Table 16.12 STS Systemic Therapy Metanalysis and Clinical Trials

Study	Design	Results
Adjuvant, locally advanced, and metastatic chemotherapy		
Sarcoma Metanalysis Collaboration (1997) [97]	Metanalysis (14 clinical trials) Adjuvant doxorubicin-based chemotherapy	Doxorubicin improved OS, LR, and distant recurrence with 4–10% absolute 10-year benefit.
Sarcoma Metanalysis Collaboration-Update (2008) [98]	Metanalysis (18 trials) Adjuvant doxorubicin-based chemotherapy	Doxorubicin improves OS. OR 0.84 (95% CI, 0.68–1.03; $p = 0.09$). The addition of ifosfamide to doxorubicin improves OS OR 0.56 (95% CI, 0.36–0.85; $p = 0.01$).
EORTC 62931 (2012) [99]	Multicenter phase III Grade II-III STS Any site No metastasis Adjuvant doxorubicin + ifosfamide vs. surgery	No difference in five-year OS (66.5% vs. 67.8%, $p = 0.72$) adjuvant and surgery, respectively) or relapse-free survival.

(continued)

Table 16.12 (continued)

Study	Design	Results
EORTC 62012 (2014) [100]	Multicenter phase III High-grade locally advanced, unresectable, or metastatic Doxorubicin vs. doxorubicin + ifosfamide	No difference in median OS (12.8 vs. 14.3 months, $p = 0.076$ doxorubicin vs. doxorubicin + ifosfamide, respectively) Doxorubicin + ifosfamide had improved median PFS (7.4 vs. 4.6 months, $p = 0.003$) with a better overall response (26% vs. 14%, $p < 0.0006$).
La Cense (2014) [101]	Pooled analysis (phase III clinical trials, n = 2) Adjuvant doxorubicin + ifosfamide vs. surgery	No difference in OS Adjuvant chemotherapy associated with better RFS HR 0.7, 95% CI 0.6–0.9; $p = 0.01$.
GeDDIS (2017) [102]	Phase III Locally advanced and metastatic Gemcitabine + docetaxel vs. doxorubicin	No difference in median PFS (23.3 vs. 23.7 months, $p = 0.06$ for doxorubicin and gemcitabine + docetaxel, respectively)
Neoadjuvant chemotherapy		
Gortzak (2001) [103]	Phase II Neoadjuvant doxorubicin + ifosfamide) vs. surgery High-risk extremity	No difference in five-year OS (64% vs. 65%, p = 0.2204) or DFS (56% vs. 52%, $p = 0.3548$) for neoadjuvant and surgery, respectively.
Grobmyer (2004) [104]	Retrospective Neoadjuvant doxorubicin + ifosfamide vs. surgery High grade, deep, > 5 cm Extremity sarcoma	Neoadjuvant doxorubicin + ifosfamide was associated with improved DSS but not metastasis-free survival.
ISG-STS 0101 (2016) [105]	Phase III Neoadjuvant vs. perioperative epirubicin +ifosfamide High-risk	No difference in ten-year OS (64% vs. 59%, HR 95% CI 0.68–1.23) neoadjuvant and perioperative, respectively Better response rates in UPS than LMS.
Targeted therapy		
PALETTE (2012) [106]	Phase III Pazopanib vs. control 143 placebo) Nonadipocytic Metastatic Progressed on chemotherapy	Pazopanib improved median PFS (4.6 vs. 1.6 months, $p < 0.01$) with no difference in OS (12.5 vs. 10.7 months, $p = 0.25$).
Immunotherapy		
SARC028 (2017) [107]	Two-cohort, single-arm, open-label study Pembrolizumab Metastatic or unresectable STS with ≥3 previous lines of systemic therapy At least one measurable lesion and one lesion accessible for biopsy	Overall objective response (7/40) with responses in 4/10 UPS 2/10 LPS 1/10 Synovial 0/10 LMS 1/22 Osteosarcoma 1/5 Chondrosarcoma 0/10 Ewing

LMS Leiomyosarcoma, *UPS* undifferentiated pleomorphic sarcoma, *RFS* recurrence-free survival, *DFS* disease-free survival, *OS* overall survival, *DSS* disease-specific survival, *LMS* leiomyosarcoma

- Sarcoma Metanalysis Collaboration pooled data from these trials (1997–2008)
  - Improvement in local recurrence and distant recurrence with the combination of doxorubicin and ifosfamide [97, 98]
  - However, higher toxicity and minimal clinical improvement compared to single-agent doxorubicin
    - Many patients do not complete therapy due to toxicity (Table 16.12).
- In 2012, EORTC 62931 showed no difference in survival or recurrence between surgery and adjuvant ifosfamide to doxorubicin.
  - Suggests there is minimal clinical benefit of adjuvant multiagent adjuvant chemotherapy.
  - Must weigh the toxicity of multiagent therapy compared to single-agent doxorubicin.
- Conflicting data exists supporting the use of chemoradiation for locally advanced resectable extremity STS (*Multidisciplinary Management of STS, Resectable and Locally Advanced Extremity STS*).
- RP STS
  - Data supporting the use of chemotherapy is largely extrapolated from extremity STS (Table 16.12).
  - One meta-analysis found that when used selectively in patients with FNCLCC grades of 3.
    - Adjuvant chemotherapy had improved five-year OS and five-year metastasis-free survival [118].
  - In another study, which included pooled data from two prior studies.
    - R1 treated with cyclophosphamide, vincristine, doxorubicin, and dacarbazine
    - Improved OS and RFS with significant short-term toxicity [101]
  - The largest retrospective study investigating the use of chemotherapy in RP sarcoma
    - Patients either underwent surgery or surgery with adjuvant or neoadjuvant chemotherapy
      - Decrease in OS in patients receiving chemotherapy [119]
  - NCCN guidelines [4]
    - Does not recommend routine use of chemotherapy in R1 and R2 resections
      - Limited data, marginal benefit, and toxicity
    - Consideration in cases where there is a high likelihood for recurrence based on pathological findings.
  - STRASS2 Trial is currently enrolling patients to further investigate the role of chemotherapy in RP sarcoma [4, 171].

Targeted Therapy and Immunotherapy (Table 16.12)

- All patients should undergo next-generation sequencing and receive appropriate therapy if a targetable mutation is identified.
  - Enrollment into clinical trials is recommended for those that do not tolerate treatment due to toxicity.

- Targeted therapy has been utilized over the past decade in STS.
  - For example, pazopanib has improved survival.
    - Antivascular endothelial factor receptor multitarget tyrosine kinase inhibitors (TKIs)
  - Combination with chemotherapy was a breakthrough.
    - Phase II: Doxorubicin + olaratumab (platelet-derived growth factor α (anti-PDGFα) antibody) vs. doxorubicin
      - Dual-agent therapy improved survival (26.5 months vs. 14.7 months, respectively).
      - 18% objective response rate.
    - Differences in efficacy when tailoring a chemotherapy agent and different targeted agents.
      - Selection of a particular combination should consider the STS subtype to attempt to improve efficacy.
        - Limited data to support the selection of a certain chemotherapy agent to be combined with a particular targeted therapy.
- Immunotherapy has not been as successful in treating STS when compared to lung cancer or melanoma.
  - Further investigation to delineate appropriate indications is ongoing [107].
    - Programmed cell death protein 1 inhibitors have some clinic benefit in certain STS subtypes [107, 172, 173].

Neoadjuvant and Adjuvant Regimens [4]

- Regimens are for general STS (*STS Subtype Regimens below*)
- First line
  - Doxorubicin, ifosfamide, and mesna (AIM, preferred neoadjuvant and adjuvant regimen) [100] (Table 16.12).
    - Synovial sarcoma is more sensitive to this combination.
- Second line
  - Double agent (doxorubicin and dacarbazine)
    - LMS or if ifosfamide cannot be used.
  - Single agent (doxorubicin)
  - Gemcitabine and docetaxel
- Useful in certain situations
  - Trabectedin (myxoid liposarcoma)

Unresectable and Metastatic Regimens [4]

- Regimens are for general STS (*Systemic Therapy*, *STS Subtype Regimens* for subtype recommendations)
- First-line preferred regimens
  - Anthracycline-based regimens (doxorubicin, epirubicin) or in combination with dacarbazine or ifosfamide/mesna
    - Double agent (doxorubicin and dacarbazine)

- If +*NTRK* gene fusion (any subtype)
  - Larotrectinib or entrectinib
- Other recommended regimens.
  - Gemcitabine-based regimens (alone or with docetaxel, vinorelbine, or dacarbazine)
- Useful situations
  - Pazopanib
    - Contraindication to IV systemic therapy or anthracycline toxicity
  - Trabectedin and doxorubicin (LMS)
  - If + *RET* gene fusion, Selpercatinib
- Subsequent lines of therapy
  - Preferred regimens
    - Recommended for palliative therapy only.
      - Pazopanib (nonadipocyte sarcomas)
      - Eribulin (especially LPS)
      - Trabectedin (especially LPS and LMS)
  - Useful in certain circumstances
    - Pembrolizumab or nivolumab +/- ipilimumab
      - Myxofibrosarcoma, UPS, DD-LPS, cutaneous angiosarcoma, undifferentiated sarcoma
      - Regardless of subtype if tumor mutational burden high (>/= 10 mutations/mega base)
    - Pembrolizumab
      - MSI-H or dMMR regardless of subtype

STS Subtype Regimens [4] (Table 16.12)

- There is conflicting data regarding the sensitivity of STS subtypes to a given therapeutic agent.
- No agent has convincing data to support its superiority over doxorubicin.
  - However, NCCN guidelines suggest the use of nondoxorubicin agents in certain clinical situations for different subtypes.
- Considered to be the more favorable chemosensitive STS.
  - Synovial sarcoma, RMS, and myxofibrosarcoma [28]
- Desmoid
  - Sorafenib (preferred)
  - Methotrexate with vinorelbine or vinblastine
  - Imatinib
  - Doxorubicin regimens
  - Pazopanib
- Angiosarcoma
  - Paclitaxel (preferred) followed by anthracycline or gemcitabine-based regimens
  - TKIs

- Pembrolizumab
  - Cutaneous angiosarcoma
- DFSP with fibrosarcomatous transformation
  - Imatinib (preferred)
  - Anthracycline or gemcitabine-based regimens
  - Pazopanib
    - Contraindication to systemic therapy or anthracycline toxicity
- Epithelioid sarcoma
  - Tazemetostat single-agent therapy
    - Metastatic or locally advanced epithelioid sarcoma (nonsurgical candidates)
- Malignant perivascular epithelioid cell tumor (PEComa)
  - Sirolimus-albumin bound
    - Locally advanced unresectable or metastatic disease
- Solitary fibrous tumor
  - Preferred regimens
    - Bevacizumab and temozolomide
    - Sunitinib or sorafenib
    - Pazopanib
- RP WD and DD-LPS
  - Palbociclib
    - Unresectable

Follow-Up and Surveillance [4]

- Surveillance based on stage
- Extremity stages IA and IB
  - History and physical q3–6 months for 2–3 years.
  - Then, annually for ten years.
  - Imaging:
    - If physical exam is unchanged, can forgo routine imaging at the time of physical exam.
    - Chest CT and primary site imaging is based on sarcoma subtype (local, regional, distant) (*Subtype Special Considerations*, *Clinical Evaluation, Diagnosis, and Stage and Grade*).
- Extremity stage II–III and RP stage I–III STS
  - History and physical q3–6 months for 2–3 years
  - Then q6 months for two years.
  - Then annually for ten years
  - Imaging:
    - Based on subtype STS risk of local-regional recurrence and distant metastasis.
- Extremity and RP stage IV STS
  - History and physical q2–6 months for 2–3 years

- Then q6 months for two years
- Then annually if there is no evidence of disease
- Imaging:
  - CT of the chest and other known metastatic sites with imaging of the primary site based on subtype local regional risk

Subtypes with Special Considerations

Multidisciplinary Management

Dermatofibrosarcoma Protuberans
- Excellent overall survival
- Poor prognostic factors
  - Head/neck DFSP, high mitotic rate, fibrosarcomatous transformation, male sex, and African American patients
  - Fibrosarcomatous transformation = high-grade tumor
    - Increased risk of metastasis and LR
    - Recommend multidisciplinary management and treatment like other high-grade STS
- Treatment:
  - Mohs Excision and Peripheral and Deep Margin Assessment (PDEMA)
    - Preferred over wide resection
    - Provides better evaluation of histologic margins (crucial in DFSP)
    - Several studies have indicated significantly lower recurrence rates and improved cosmesis with Mohs vs. wide resection
      - 1–3% vs. 20%, respectively [8, 14–20, 22–24]
  - Wide resection
    - Can be performed when PDEMA and Mohs are not available or the primary tumor is in a less cosmetically sensitive area.
    - Must meticulously evaluate margin.
- Follow-up
  - High LR rates.
  - NCCN guidelines
    - Physical exam q6–12 months with focus on primary disease site
    - Rebiopsy any suspicious regions [69]
- Recurrent DFSP
  - Recurrent disease can be treated with reexcision and adjuvant XRT.
- Locally advanced or unresectable DFSP
  - Consider neoadjuvant imatinib [69]

Desmoid
- Benign, yet locally aggressive tumors with no metastatic potential
- High recurrence rate despite wide margins (Table 16.13)
- Treatment

Table 16.13 Desmoid tumor surgery and targeted therapy studies

Study	Design	Results	Interpretation
Penel (2017) [174]	Prospective Wait and see vs. surgery Favorable locations (abdominal wall, intraabdominal, breast, digestive viscera, and lower limb) Nonfavorable locations	No difference in two-year event-free survival (EFS) (53% vs. 58%, $p = 0.42$). Improved two-year EFS with favorable locations (66% vs. 41% $p = 0.0001$). Favorable locations two-year EFS was similar for wait and see and surgery (70% vs. 63%; $p = 0.41$) Whereas unfavorable locations, had improved 2-year EFS with Wait & see (52% vs. 25%; $p = 0.001$).	Location is prognostic. Validation of these findings is needed.
Janssen (2017) [175]	Cochrane meta-analysis Surgery (R1 vs. R0) Adjuvant XRT	R1 associated with increased LR (RR 1.78, 95% CI 1.40–2.26) and can benefit from adjuvant XRT (RR 1.54, 1.05–2.27)	Local recurrence is more likely in desmoid tumors after R1 therefore benefit from adjuvant XRT.
Targeted therapy			
Grounder (2018) [176]	Phase III Sorafenib vs. control	Sorafenib improved two-year PFS (81% vs. 36%, $p < 0.001$).	Sorafenib prolongs PFS in desmoid tumors.
Grounder (2023) [177]	Phase III Nirogacestat vs. control Desmoids with progression	Improved PFS (HR 0.28) and response rate (41% vs. 8%) Decreased two-year event-free (76% vs. 44%)	Nirogacestat improved outcomes and quality of life in the setting of low toxicity profile

- Shift toward a period of observation
- Patients with symptomatic tumors or tumors with continued growth in areas where resection would cause large surgical defects and/or morbidity should be offered surgery
- Spontaneous regression possible
  - Systemic therapy can reduce LR [178].
- Multidisciplinary discussion imperative to delineate which patients would benefit from observation, surgery, or systemic therapy.
- Systemic Therapy
  - Nirogacestat was recently approved by FDA (150 mg PO, BID).
    - A gamma secretase inhibitor
    - Phase III trial demonstrated.
      - Improved PFS, response rates (40%), and patient-reported outcomes (less symptoms and improved quality of life) compared to placebo [177].
      - Side effects

- Ovarian dysfunction in women of child-bearing potential (75% low-grade fatigue, nausea, and diarrhea
    - Ovarian dysfunction resolved in 74% of affected patients
- Desmoid tumors involving small intestine:
    - R1 resection appropriate to limit potential of small bowel devascularization [138]

Atypical Lipomatous Tumor
- Typically well-circumscribed, low-grade tumors with a capsule, facilitating resection
- In cases of neurovascular invasion, preservation of these structures is paramount
- If pathologic margins are positive:
    - Observation vs. reresection is recommended.
    - If dedifferentiation is observed, recommend reresection with negative margins [138].

Liposarcoma (LPS)
- Surgery for RP liposarcoma (LPS) involves removing the tumor en bloc with the fascia of the psoas muscle and surrounding adipose tissue to decrease marginal involvement and improve surveillance [138].

Leiomyosarcoma (LMS)
- RP leiomyosarcoma (LMS) of the IVC require resection of the IVC due to their high metastatic potential.
- When invasion into adjacent organs is present, visceral resection is required.

Malignant Peripheral Nerve Sheet Tumor (MPNST)
- Malignant peripheral nerve sheath tumors (MPNST) of the RP require surgical resection of the nerve of origin.
- Like LMS, may also require multiorgan resection of the invaded structures.

Solitary Fibrous Tumor
- Solitary fibrous tumors have a low risk of a local recurrence therefore a marginal resection rather than radical resection is preferred [25, 75, 82, 145].

Myxofibrosarcoma
- Extremity myxofibrosarcoma is highly infiltrative with fibrous septae.
    - Often septae extend beyond surgical field.
- Difficult-to-obtain R0/R1 resection [32].
- High risk of LR.
- Imaging
    - Recommend MRI, which may assist preoperative planning if fibrous septae are identified.

Angiosarcoma
- Goal of R0 resection
- Primary breast angiosarcoma
  - Wide local excision preferred
  - Mastectomy reserved for tumors where R0 cannot be obtained with wide local excision
- Secondary breast angiosarcoma
  - Mastectomy is required due to more aggressive tumor biology [179].
  - Removal of irradiated skin is important to improve local control.
- Low rate of regional lymph node metastasis
  - Lymphadenectomy reserved for clinically suspicious nodes

References

1. Siegel RL, Miller KD, Jemal A. Cancer statistics, 2018. CA Cancer J Clin. 2018;68(1):7–30.
2. Cancer.Net. Sarcomas, Soft Tissue: Statistics. 2023 March 2023 [cited 2023 December 30]; Available from: https://www.cancer.net/cancer-types/sarcomas-soft-tissue/statistics#:~:text=The%205%2Dyear%20relative%20survival%20rate%20for%20people%20with%20locally,for%20sarcoma%20every%205%20years.
3. Sbaraglia M, Bellan E, Dei Tos AP. The 2020 WHO classification of soft tissue tumours: news and perspectives. Pathologica. 2021;113(2):70–84.
4. Network, N.C.C. NCCN clinical practice guidelines in oncology: soft tissue sarcoma. April 25, 2023 December 1, 2023]; Available from: https://www.nccn.org/professionals/physician_gls/pdf/sarcoma.pdf.
5. Singer S, et al. Prognostic factors predictive of survival for truncal and retroperitoneal soft-tissue sarcoma. Ann Surg. 1995;221(2):185–95.
6. Lansu J, et al. Time trends and prognostic factors for overall survival in Myxoid Liposarcomas: a population-based study. Sarcoma. 2020;2020:2437850.
7. Amer KM, et al. Epidemiology and survival of liposarcoma and its subtypes: a dual database analysis. J Clin Orthop Trauma. 2020;11(Suppl 4):S479–84.
8. Alvarenga JC, et al. Limitations of surgery in the treatment of retroperitoneal sarcoma. Br J Surg. 1991;78(8):912–6.
9. Gladdy RA, et al. Predictors of survival and recurrence in primary leiomyosarcoma. Ann Surg Oncol. 2013;20(6):1851–7.
10. Peng PD, et al. Management and recurrence patterns of desmoids tumors: a multi-institutional analysis of 211 patients. Ann Surg Oncol. 2012;19(13):4036–42.
11. Young RJ, et al. Angiosarcoma. Lancet Oncol. 2010;11(10):983–91.
12. Guo T, et al. Consistent MYC and FLT4 gene amplification in radiation-induced angiosarcoma but not in other radiation-associated atypical vascular lesions. Genes Chromosomes Cancer. 2011;50(1):25–33.
13. Manner J, et al. MYC high level gene amplification is a distinctive feature of angiosarcomas after irradiation or chronic lymphedema. Am J Pathol. 2010;176(1):34–9.
14. Chen Y, Jiang G. Association between surgical excision margins and outcomes in patients with dermatofibrosarcoma protuberans: a meta-analysis. Dermatol Ther. 2021;34(4):e14954.
15. DuBay D, et al. Low recurrence rate after surgery for dermatofibrosarcoma protuberans: a multidisciplinary approach from a single institution. Cancer. 2004;100(5):1008–16.
16. Foroozan M, et al. Efficacy of Mohs micrographic surgery for the treatment of dermatofibrosarcoma protuberans: systematic review. Arch Dermatol. 2012;148(9):1055–63.
17. Gloster HM Jr, Harris KR, Roenigk RK. A comparison between Mohs micrographic surgery and wide surgical excision for the treatment of dermatofibrosarcoma protuberans. J Am Acad Dermatol. 1996;35(1):82–7.

18. Meguerditchian AN, et al. Wide excision or Mohs micrographic surgery for the treatment of primary dermatofibrosarcoma protuberans. Am J Clin Oncol. 2010;33(3):300–3.
19. Bogucki B, Neuhaus I, Hurst EA. Dermatofibrosarcoma protuberans: a review of the literature. Dermatol Surg. 2012;38(4):537–51.
20. Durack A, et al. A 10-year review of surgical management of dermatofibrosarcoma protuberans. Br J Dermatol. 2021;184(4):731–9.
21. Lowe GC, et al. A comparison of Mohs micrographic surgery and wide local excision for treatment of dermatofibrosarcoma protuberans with long-term follow-up: the Mayo clinic experience. Dermatol Surg. 2017;43(1):98–106.
22. Malan M, Xuejingzi W, Quan SJ. The efficacy of Mohs micrographic surgery over the traditional wide local excision surgery in the cure of dermatofibrosarcoma protuberans. Pan Afr Med J. 2019;33:297.
23. Paradisi A, et al. Dermatofibrosarcoma protuberans: wide local excision vs. Mohs micrographic surgery. Cancer Treat Rev. 2008;34(8):728–36.
24. Veronese F, et al. Wide local excision vs. Mohs Tubingen technique in the treatment of dermatofibrosarcoma protuberans: a two-centre retrospective study and literature review. J Eur Acad Dermatol Venereol. 2017;31(12):2069–76.
25. Bahrami A, Folpe AL. Adult-type fibrosarcoma: a reevaluation of 163 putative cases diagnosed at a single institution over a 48-year period. Am J Surg Pathol. 2010;34(10):1504–13.
26. James AW, et al. Malignant Peripheral Nerve Sheath Tumor. Surg Oncol Clin N Am. 2016;25(4):789–802.
27. Peiper M, et al. Malignant fibrous histiocytoma of the extremities and trunk: an institutional review. Surgery. 2004;135(1):59–66.
28. Blay JY, et al. Synovial sarcoma: characteristics, challenges, and evolving therapeutic strategies. ESMO Open. 2023;8(5):101618.
29. Mazeron JJ, Suit HD. Lymph nodes as sites of metastases from sarcomas of soft tissue. Cancer. 1987;60(8):1800–8.
30. Heske CM, Mascarenhas L. Relapsed Rhabdomyosarcoma. J Clin Med. 2021;10:4.
31. Bacci G, et al. Therapy and survival after recurrence of Ewing's tumors: the Rizzoli experience in 195 patients treated with adjuvant and neoadjuvant chemotherapy from 1979 to 1997. Ann Oncol. 2003;14(11):1654–9.
32. Roland CL, et al. Myxofibrosarcoma. Surg Oncol Clin N Am. 2016;25(4):775–88.
33. Zhang S, et al. Epithelioid sarcoma: a single-institutional retrospective cohort study of 36 cases. J Orthop Surg (Hong Kong). 2021;29(3):23094990211029349.
34. Armah HB, Parwani AV. Epithelioid sarcoma. Arch Pathol Lab Med. 2009;133(5):814–9.
35. Mavrogenis A, et al. Clinicopathological features, diagnosis and treatment of clear cell sarcoma/melanoma of soft parts. Hippokratia. 2013;17(4):298–302.
36. Deenik W, et al. Clear cell sarcoma (malignant melanoma) of soft parts: a clinicopathologic study of 30 cases. Cancer. 1999;86(6):969–75.
37. Finley JW, et al. Clear cell sarcoma: the Roswell Park experience. J Surg Oncol. 2001;77(1):16–20.
38. Kleinerman RA, Schonfeld SJ, Tucker MA. Sarcomas in hereditary retinoblastoma. Clin Sarcoma Res. 2012;2(1):15.
39. Nieuwenhuis MH, et al. Family history, surgery, and APC mutation are risk factors for desmoid tumors in familial adenomatous polyposis: an international cohort study. Dis Colon Rectum. 2011;54(10):1229–34.
40. Korf BR. Neurofibromatosis. Handb Clin Neurol. 2013;111:333–40.
41. Kleihues P, et al. Tumors associated with p53 germline mutations: a synopsis of 91 families. Am J Pathol. 1997;150(1):1–13.
42. Galiatsatos P, Foulkes WD. Familial adenomatous polyposis. Am J Gastroenterol. 2006;101(2):385–98.
43. Kleinerman RA, et al. Risk of soft tissue sarcomas by individual subtype in survivors of hereditary retinoblastoma. J Natl Cancer Inst. 2007;99(1):24–31.

44. Penel N, et al. Frequency of certain established risk factors in soft tissue sarcomas in adults: a prospective descriptive study of 658 cases. Sarcoma. 2008;2008:459386.
45. Gill AJ, et al. Immunohistochemistry for SDHB divides gastrointestinal stromal tumors (GISTs) into 2 distinct types. Am J Surg Pathol. 2010;34(5):636–44.
46. Carney JA, Stratakis CA. Familial paraganglioma and gastric stromal sarcoma: a new syndrome distinct from the Carney triad. Am J Med Genet. 2002;108(2):132–9.
47. Gaal J, et al. SDHB immunohistochemistry: a useful tool in the diagnosis of Carney-Stratakis and Carney triad gastrointestinal stromal tumors. Mod Pathol. 2011;24(1):147–51.
48. Li FP, et al. A cancer family syndrome in twenty-four kindreds. Cancer Res. 1988;48(18):5358–62.
49. Pasini B, et al. Clinical and molecular genetics of patients with the Carney-Stratakis syndrome and germline mutations of the genes coding for the succinate dehydrogenase subunits SDHB, SDHC, and SDHD. Eur J Hum Genet. 2008;16(1):79–88.
50. Brennan MF, et al. Lessons learned from the study of 10,000 patients with soft tissue sarcoma. Ann Surg. 2014;260(3):416–21; discussion 421-2.
51. Brennan MF, Singer S. Five decades of sarcoma care at Memorial Sloan Kettering Cancer Center. J Surg Oncol. 2022;126(5):896–901.
52. Crago AM, Brennan MF. Principles in management of soft tissue sarcoma. Adv Surg. 2015;49(1):107–22.
53. Zafar R., Wheeler Y. Liposarcoma, in *StatPearls*. 2023: Treasure Island (FL).
54. George S, et al. Soft tissue and uterine leiomyosarcoma. J Clin Oncol. 2018;36(2):144–50.
55. Ip PP, Cheung AN. Pathology of uterine leiomyosarcomas and smooth muscle tumours of uncertain malignant potential. Best Pract Res Clin Obstet Gynaecol. 2011;25(6):691–704.
56. Serrano C, George S. Leiomyosarcoma. Hematol Oncol Clin North Am. 2013;27(5):957–74.
57. Eilber FC, et al. Chemotherapy is associated with improved survival in adult patients with primary extremity synovial sarcoma. Ann Surg. 2007;246(1):105–13.
58. Hillenbrand T, et al. Primary and secondary angiosarcomas: a comparative single-center analysis. Clin Sarcoma Res. 2015;5:14.
59. Ohsawa M, et al. Use of immunohistochemical procedures in diagnosing angiosarcoma. Evaluation of 98 cases. Cancer. 1995;75(12):2867–74.
60. Augsburger D, et al. Current diagnostics and treatment of fibrosarcoma -perspectives for future therapeutic targets and strategies. Oncotarget. 2017;8(61):104638–53.
61. Mentzel T, et al. Myxofibrosarcoma. Clinicopathologic analysis of 75 cases with emphasis on the low-grade variant. Am J Surg Pathol. 1996;20(4):391–405.
62. Knight SWE, et al. Malignant peripheral nerve sheath tumors-a comprehensive review of pathophysiology, diagnosis, and multidisciplinary management. Children (Basel). 2022;9(1)
63. Kibbi N, et al. Dermatofibrosarcoma protuberans in pregnancy: a case series and review of the literature. Int J Dermatol. 2021;60(9):1114–9.
64. Brooks J, Ramsey ML. Dermatofibrosarcoma Protuberans: *StatPearls [Internet]*. Treasure Island: StatPearls Publishing; 2023.
65. Kotiligam D, et al. Desmoid tumor: a disease opportune for molecular insights. Histol Histopathol. 2008;23(1):117–26.
66. Couto Netto SD, et al. Sporadic abdominal wall desmoid type fibromatosis: treatment paradigm after thirty two years. BMC Surg. 2018;18(1):37.
67. Weiss AR, Harrison DJ. Soft Tissue Sarcomas in Adolescents and Young Adults – PubMed. J Clin Oncol. 2024;42(6)
68. Martin-Giacalone BA, et al. Pediatric Rhabdomyosarcoma: Epidemiology and Genetic Susceptibility – PubMed. J Clin Med. 2021;10(9)
69. Network, N.C.C. NCCN clinical practice guidelines in oncology: dermatofibrosarcoma protuberans. November 9, 2023 December 1, 2023; Available from: https://www.nccn.org/guidelines/guidelines-detail?category=1&id=1430.
70. George A, Grimer R. Early symptoms of bone and soft tissue sarcomas: could they be diagnosed earlier? Ann R Coll Surg Engl. 2012;94(4):261–6.

71. Basile G, et al. Curability of patients with lymph node metastases from extremity soft-tissue sarcoma. Cancer. 2020;126(23):5098–108.
72. Amin MB, Edge SB, Greene FL, Byrd DR, editors. AJCC, American Joint Committee on Cancer Cancer Staging Manual. 8th ed. Springer; 2017.
73. Coindre JM, et al. Grading of soft tissue sarcomas: guidelines for study and diagnosis from the French Federation of Cancer Centers Sarcoma Group (FNLCC). Ann Pathol. 2018;38(1):37–48.
74. AJCC. Soft tissue sarcoma. In: Amin MB, Edge SB, Greene FL, Byrd DR, editors. AJCC Cancer Staging Manual. Springer; 2017. p. 507–22, 531–538.
75. Tseng WW, et al. Management of locally recurrent retroperitoneal sarcoma in the adult: an updated consensus approach from the transatlantic Australasian retroperitoneal sarcoma working group. Ann Surg Oncol. 2022;29(12):7335–48.
76. Voss RK, et al. Sarculator is a good model to predict survival in resected extremity and trunk sarcomas in US patients. Ann Surg Oncol. 2022;29:4376.
77. Callegaro D, et al. Development and external validation of two nomograms to predict overall survival and occurrence of distant metastases in adults after surgical resection of localised soft-tissue sarcomas of the extremities: a retrospective analysis. Lancet Oncol. 2016;17(5):671–80.
78. Callegaro D, et al. New sarculator prognostic nomograms for patients with primary retroperitoneal sarcoma: case volume does matter. Ann Surg. 2023;279:857.
79. Adam R, et al. Hepatic resection for noncolorectal nonendocrine liver metastases: analysis of 1,452 patients and development of a prognostic model. Ann Surg. 2006;244(4):524–35.
80. Rosenberg SA, et al. The treatment of soft-tissue sarcomas of the extremities: prospective randomized evaluations of (1) limb-sparing surgery plus radiation therapy compared with amputation and (2) the role of adjuvant chemotherapy. Ann Surg. 1982;196(3):305–15.
81. Pisters PW, et al. Long-term results of a prospective randomized trial of adjuvant brachytherapy in soft tissue sarcoma. J Clin Oncol. 1996;14(3):859–68.
82. Yang JC, et al. Randomized prospective study of the benefit of adjuvant radiation therapy in the treatment of soft tissue sarcomas of the extremity. J Clin Oncol. 1998;16(1):197–203.
83. Beane JD, et al. Efficacy of adjuvant radiation therapy in the treatment of soft tissue sarcoma of the extremity: 20-year follow-up of a randomized prospective trial. Ann Surg Oncol. 2014;21(8):2484–9.
84. Pisters PW, et al. Long-term results of prospective trial of surgery alone with selective use of radiation for patients with T1 extremity and trunk soft tissue sarcomas. Ann Surg. 2007;246(4):675–81; discussion 681-2.
85. O'Sullivan B, et al. Preoperative versus postoperative radiotherapy in soft-tissue sarcoma of the limbs: a randomised trial. Lancet. 2002;359(9325):2235–41.
86. Davis AM, et al. Late radiation morbidity following randomization to preoperative versus postoperative radiotherapy in extremity soft tissue sarcoma. Radiother Oncol. 2005;75(1):48–53.
87. Kraybill WG, et al. Phase II study of neoadjuvant chemotherapy and radiation therapy in the management of high-risk, high-grade, soft tissue sarcomas of the extremities and body wall: Radiation Therapy Oncology Group Trial 9514. J Clin Oncol. 2006;24(4):619–25.
88. Kraybill WG, et al. Long-term results of a phase 2 study of neoadjuvant chemotherapy and radiotherapy in the management of high-risk, high-grade, soft tissue sarcomas of the extremities and body wall: Radiation Therapy Oncology Group Trial 9514. Cancer. 2010;116(19):4613–21.
89. Roland CL, van Houdt W, Gronchi A. The landmark series: multimodality treatment of extremity sarcoma. Ann Surg Oncol. 2020;27(10):3672–82.
90. Fiore M, et al. Adequate local control in high-risk soft tissue sarcoma of the extremity treated with surgery alone at a reference centre: should radiotherapy still be a standard? Ann Surg Oncol. 2018;25(6):1536–43.
91. Gundle KR, et al. Analysis of margin classification systems for assessing the risk of local recurrence after soft tissue sarcoma resection. J Clin Oncol. 2018;36(7):704–9.

92. Blay JY, et al. Surgery in reference centers improves survival of sarcoma patients: a nationwide study. Ann Oncol. 2019;30(7):1143–53.
93. McKee MD, et al. The prognostic significance of margin width for extremity and trunk sarcoma. J Surg Oncol. 2004;85(2):68–76.
94. Fleming JB, et al. Long-term outcome of patients with American Joint Committee on Cancer stage IIB extremity soft tissue sarcomas. J Clin Oncol. 1999;17(9):2772–80.
95. Salerno KE, et al. Radiation therapy for treatment of soft tissue sarcoma in adults: executive summary of an ASTRO clinical practice guideline. Pract Radiat Oncol. 2021;11(5):339–51.
96. Davis AM, et al. Function and health status outcomes in a randomized trial comparing preoperative and postoperative radiotherapy in extremity soft tissue sarcoma. J Clin Oncol. 2002;20(22):4472–7.
97. Adjuvant chemotherapy for localised resectable soft-tissue sarcoma of adults: meta-analysis of individual data. Sarcoma Meta-analysis Collaboration. Lancet. 1997;350(9092):1647–54.
98. Pervaiz N, et al. A systematic meta-analysis of randomized controlled trials of adjuvant chemotherapy for localized resectable soft-tissue sarcoma. Cancer. 2008;113(3):573–81.
99. Woll PJ, et al. Adjuvant chemotherapy with doxorubicin, ifosfamide, and lenograstim for resected soft-tissue sarcoma (EORTC 62931): a multicentre randomised controlled trial. Lancet Oncol. 2012;13(10):1045–54.
100. Judson I, et al. Doxorubicin alone versus intensified doxorubicin plus ifosfamide for first-line treatment of advanced or metastatic soft-tissue sarcoma: a randomised controlled phase 3 trial. Lancet Oncol. 2014;15(4):415–23.
101. Le Cesne A, et al. Doxorubicin-based adjuvant chemotherapy in soft tissue sarcoma: pooled analysis of two STBSG-EORTC phase III clinical trials. Ann Oncol. 2014;25(12):2425–32.
102. Seddon B, et al. Gemcitabine and docetaxel versus doxorubicin as first-line treatment in previously untreated advanced unresectable or metastatic soft-tissue sarcomas (GeDDiS): a randomised controlled phase 3 trial. Lancet Oncol. 2017;18(10):1397–410.
103. Gortzak E, et al. A randomised phase II study on neo-adjuvant chemotherapy for 'high-risk' adult soft-tissue sarcoma. Eur J Cancer. 2001;37(9):1096–103.
104. Grobmyer SR, et al. Neo-adjuvant chemotherapy for primary high-grade extremity soft tissue sarcoma. Ann Oncol. 2004;15(11):1667–72.
105. Gronchi A, et al. Short, full-dose adjuvant chemotherapy (CT) in high-risk adult soft tissue sarcomas (STS): long-term follow-up of a randomized clinical trial from the Italian Sarcoma Group and the Spanish Sarcoma Group. Ann Oncol. 2016;27(12):2283–8.
106. van der Graaf WT, et al. Pazopanib for metastatic soft-tissue sarcoma (PALETTE): a randomised, double-blind, placebo-controlled phase 3 trial. Lancet. 2012;379(9829):1879–86.
107. Tawbi HA, et al. Pembrolizumab in advanced soft-tissue sarcoma and bone sarcoma (SARC028): a multicentre, two-cohort, single-arm, open-label, phase 2 trial. Lancet Oncol. 2017;18(11):1493–501.
108. Sampath S, et al. Preoperative versus postoperative radiotherapy in soft-tissue sarcoma: multi-institutional analysis of 821 patients. Int J Radiat Oncol Biol Phys. 2011;81(2):498–505.
109. Al-Absi E, et al. A systematic review and meta-analysis of oncologic outcomes of pre- versus postoperative radiation in localized resectable soft-tissue sarcoma. Ann Surg Oncol. 2010;17(5):1367–74.
110. Kachare SD, et al. Radiotherapy associated with improved survival for high-grade sarcoma of the extremity. J Surg Oncol. 2015;112(4):338–43.
111. Callegaro D, et al. Retroperitoneal sarcoma: the Transatlantic Australasian Retroperitoneal Sarcoma Working Group Program. Curr Opin Oncol. 2021;33(4):301–8.
112. Bonvalot S, et al. Primary retroperitoneal sarcomas: a multivariate analysis of surgical factors associated with local control. J Clin Oncol. 2009;27(1):31–7.
113. Gronchi A, et al. Aggressive surgical policies in a retrospectively reviewed single-institution case series of retroperitoneal soft tissue sarcoma patients. J Clin Oncol. 2009;27(1):24–30.

114. Gronchi A, et al. Frontline extended surgery is associated with improved survival in retroperitoneal low- to intermediate-grade soft tissue sarcomas. Ann Oncol. 2012;23(4)
115. Nussbaum DP, et al. Preoperative or postoperative radiotherapy versus surgery alone for retroperitoneal sarcoma: a case-control, propensity score-matched analysis of a nationwide clinical oncology database. Lancet Oncol. 2016;17(7):966–75.
116. Bonvalot S, et al. Preoperative radiotherapy plus surgery versus surgery alone for patients with primary retroperitoneal sarcoma (EORTC-62092: STRASS): a multicentre, open-label, randomised, phase 3 trial. Lancet Oncol. 2020;21(10):1366–77.
117. Callegaro D, et al. Preoperative radiotherapy in patients with primary retroperitoneal sarcoma: EORTC-62092 Trial (STRASS) versus off-trial (STREXIT) results. Ann Surg. 2023;278(1):127–34.
118. Italiano A, et al. Effect of adjuvant chemotherapy on survival in FNCLCC grade 3 soft tissue sarcomas: a multivariate analysis of the French Sarcoma Group Database. Ann Oncol. 2010;21(12):2436–41.
119. Miura JT, et al. Impact of chemotherapy on survival in surgically resected retroperitoneal sarcoma. Eur J Surg Oncol. 2015;41(10):1386–92.
120. Trans-Atlantic Retroperitoneal Sarcoma Working Group. Electronic address, a.m.b.b.c. Management of metastatic retroperitoneal sarcoma: a consensus approach from the Trans-Atlantic Retroperitoneal Sarcoma Working Group (TARPSWG). Ann Oncol. 2018;29(4):857–71.
121. Italiano A, et al. Trends in survival for patients with metastatic soft-tissue sarcoma. Cancer. 2011;117(5):1049–54.
122. Li RH, et al. A nomogram to predict metastasis of soft tissue sarcoma of the extremities. Medicine (Baltimore). 2020;99(21):e20165.
123. Chudgar NP, et al. Is repeat pulmonary metastasectomy indicated for soft tissue sarcoma? Ann Thorac Surg. 2017;104(6):1837–45.
124. Okiror L, et al. Survival following pulmonary metastasectomy for sarcoma. Thorac Cardiovasc Surg. 2016;64(2):146–9.
125. Ferguson PC, et al. Soft tissue sarcoma presenting with metastatic disease: outcome with primary surgical resection. Cancer. 2011;117(2):372–9.
126. Kane JM, et al. The treatment and outcome of patients with soft tissue sarcomas and synchronous metastases. Sarcoma. 2002;6(2):69–73.
127. Li B, Luo CH, Zheng W. Risk factors for recurrence and survival in patients with primary retroperitoneal tumors. J BUON. 2013;18(3):782–7.
128. Lahat G, et al. Angiosarcoma: clinical and molecular insights. Ann Surg. 2010;251(6):1098–106.
129. Gronchi A, et al. Extremity soft tissue sarcoma: adding to the prognostic meaning of local failure. Ann Surg Oncol. 2007;14(5):1583–90.
130. Lewis JJ, et al. Association of local recurrence with subsequent survival in extremity soft tissue sarcoma. J Clin Oncol. 1997;15(2):646–52.
131. Coindre JM. Grading of soft tissue sarcomas: review and update. Arch Pathol Lab Med. 2006;130(10):1448–53.
132. Kirane A, Crago AM. The importance of surgical margins in retroperitoneal sarcoma. J Surg Oncol. 2016;113(3):270–6.
133. O'Donnell PW, et al. The effect of the setting of a positive surgical margin in soft tissue sarcoma. Cancer. 2014;120(18):2866–75.
134. Eilber FR, Eckardt J. Surgical management of soft tissue sarcomas. Semin Oncol. 1997;24(5):526–33.
135. Geer RJ, et al. Management of small soft-tissue sarcoma of the extremity in adults. Arch Surg. 1992;127(11):1285–9.
136. Karakousis CP, et al. Limb salvage in soft tissue sarcomas with selective combination of modalities. Eur J Surg Oncol. 1991;17(1):71–80.
137. Fujiwara T, et al. The role of surgical margin quality in myxofibrosarcoma and undifferentiated pleomorphic sarcoma. Eur J Surg Oncol. 2021;47(7):1756–62.

138. Surgeons, A.C.o. Operative standards for cancer surgery: soft tissue sarcoma, vol. III. American College of Surgeons.
139. Ghert MA, et al. The surgical and functional outcome of limb-salvage surgery with vascular reconstruction for soft tissue sarcoma of the extremity. Ann Surg Oncol. 2005;12(12):1102–10.
140. Pak D, et al. Dose–effect relationships for femoral fractures after multimodality limb-sparing therapy of soft-tissue sarcomas of the proximal lower extremity. Int J Radiat Oncol Biol Phys. 2012;83(4):1257–63.
141. Jacobs AJ, Morris CD, Levin AS. Synovial sarcoma is not associated with a higher risk of lymph node metastasis compared with other soft tissue sarcomas. Clin Orthop Relat Res. 2018;476(3):589–98.
142. Ecker BL, et al. Implications of lymph node evaluation in the management of resectable soft tissue sarcoma. Ann Surg Oncol. 2017;24(2):425–33.
143. Fong Y, et al. Lymph node metastasis from soft tissue sarcoma in adults. Analysis of data from a prospective database of 1772 sarcoma patients. Ann Surg. 1993;217(1):72–7.
144. Andreou D, et al. Sentinel node biopsy in soft tissue sarcoma subtypes with a high propensity for regional lymphatic spread–results of a large prospective trial. Ann Oncol. 2013;24(5):1400–5.
145. Tan MC, et al. Histology-based classification predicts pattern of recurrence and improves risk stratification in primary retroperitoneal sarcoma. Ann Surg. 2016;263(3):593–600.
146. Snow HA, et al. Treatment of patients with primary retroperitoneal sarcoma: predictors of outcome from an Australian specialist sarcoma centre. ANZ J Surg. 2018;88(11):1151–7.
147. Toulmonde M, et al. Retroperitoneal sarcomas: patterns of care at diagnosis, prognostic factors and focus on main histological subtypes: a multicenter analysis of the French Sarcoma Group. Ann Oncol. 2014;25(3):735–42.
148. Neuhaus SJ, et al. Surgical management of primary and recurrent retroperitoneal liposarcoma. Br J Surg. 2005;92(2):246–52.
149. Ikoma N, et al. Concomitant organ resection does not improve outcomes in primary retroperitoneal well-differentiated liposarcoma: a retrospective cohort study at a major sarcoma center. J Surg Oncol. 2018;117(6):1188–94.
150. Ito H, et al. Leiomyosarcoma of the inferior vena cava: survival after aggressive management. Ann Surg Oncol. 2007;14(12):3534–41.
151. Keung EZ, et al. Predictors of outcomes in patients with primary retroperitoneal dedifferentiated liposarcoma undergoing surgery. J Am Coll Surg. 2014;218(2):206–17.
152. Molina G, et al. Preoperative radiation therapy combined with radical surgical resection is associated with a lower rate of local recurrence when treating unifocal, primary retroperitoneal liposarcoma. J Surg Oncol. 2016;114(7):814–20.
153. Pacelli F, et al. Retroperitoneal soft tissue sarcoma: prognostic factors and therapeutic approaches. Tumori. 2008;94(4):497–504.
154. Rossi CR, et al. Patient outcome after complete surgery for retroperitoneal sarcoma. Anticancer Res. 2013;33(9):4081–7.
155. Smith HG, et al. Outcome following resection of retroperitoneal sarcoma. Br J Surg. 2015;102(13):1698–709.
156. Zhao X, et al. Prognostic factors predicting the postoperative survival period following treatment for primary retroperitoneal liposarcoma. Chin Med J (Engl). 2015;128(1):85–90.
157. Conlon KC, et al. Prospective randomized clinical trial of the value of intraperitoneal drainage after pancreatic resection. Ann Surg. 2001;234(4):487–93; discussion 493-4.
158. Delisle M, et al. Landmark series: a review of landmark studies in the treatment of primary localized retroperitoneal sarcoma. Ann Surg Oncol. 2022;29(12):7297–311.
159. Canter RJ, et al. Perioperative chemotherapy in patients undergoing pulmonary resection for metastatic soft-tissue sarcoma of the extremity: a retrospective analysis. Cancer. 2007;110(9):2050–60.
160. Blackmon SH, et al. Resection of pulmonary and extrapulmonary sarcomatous metastases is associated with long-term survival. Ann Thorac Surg. 2009;88(3):877–84; discussion 884-5.

161. Predina JD, et al. Improved survival after pulmonary metastasectomy for soft tissue sarcoma. J Thorac Oncol. 2011;6(5):913–9.
162. Treasure T, et al. Pulmonary metastasectomy for sarcoma: a systematic review of reported outcomes in the context of Thames Cancer Registry data. BMJ Open. 2012;2(5)
163. Chudgar NP, et al. Pulmonary metastasectomy with therapeutic intent for soft-tissue sarcoma. J Thorac Cardiovasc Surg. 2017;154(1):319–330 e1.
164. DeMatteo RP, et al. Results of hepatic resection for sarcoma metastatic to liver. Ann Surg. 2001;234(4):540–7; discussion 547-8.
165. Groeschl RT, et al. Hepatectomy for noncolorectal non-neuroendocrine metastatic cancer: a multi-institutional analysis. J Am Coll Surg. 2012;214(5):769–77.
166. Brudvik KW, et al. Survival after resection of gastrointestinal stromal tumor and sarcoma liver metastases in 146 patients. J Gastrointest Surg. 2015;19(8):1476–83.
167. Pasquali S, et al. High-risk soft tissue sarcomas treated with perioperative chemotherapy: Improving prognostic classification in a randomised clinical trial – PubMed. Eur J Cancer (Oxford, UK: 1990). 2018;93
168. Pasquali S, et al. Neoadjuvant chemotherapy in high-risk soft tissue sarcomas: a Sarculator-based risk stratification analysis of the ISG-STS 1001 randomized trial – PubMed. Cancer. 2022;128(1)
169. Savina M, et al. Patterns of care and outcomes of patients with METAstatic soft tissue SARComa in a real-life setting: the METASARC observational study. BMC Med. 2017;15(1):78.
170. Kepka L, et al. Results of radiation therapy for unresected soft-tissue sarcomas. Int J Radiat Oncol Biol Phys. 2005;63(3):852–9.
171. Lambdin J, et al. A randomized phase III study of neoadjuvant chemotherapy followed by surgery versus surgery alone for patients with high-risk retroperitoneal sarcoma (STRASS2). Ann Surg Oncol. 2023;30(8):4573–5.
172. Burgess MA, et al. Clinical activity of pembrolizumab (P) in undifferentiated pleomorphic sarcoma (UPS) and dedifferentiated/pleomorphic liposarcoma (LPS): final results of SARC028 expansion cohorts. Journal of Clinical Oncology. 2019;37(15_suppl)
173. D'Angelo SP, et al. Nivolumab with or without ipilimumab treatment for metastatic sarcoma (Alliance A091401): two open-label, non-comparative, randomised, phase 2 trials. Lancet Oncol. 2018;19(3):416–26.
174. Penel N, et al. Surgical versus non-surgical approach in primary desmoid-type fibromatosis patients: a nationwide prospective cohort from the French Sarcoma Group. Eur J Cancer. 2017;83:125–31.
175. Janssen ML, et al. Meta-analysis of the influence of surgical margin and adjuvant radiotherapy on local recurrence after resection of sporadic desmoid-type fibromatosis. Br J Surg. 2017;104(4):347–57.
176. Gounder MM, et al. Sorafenib for advanced and refractory desmoid tumors. N Engl J Med. 2018;379(25):2417–28.
177. Gounder M, et al. Nirogacestat, a gamma-secretase inhibitor for desmoid tumors. N Engl J Med. 2023;388(10):898–912.
178. Fiore M, et al. Desmoid-type fibromatosis: a front-line conservative approach to select patients for surgical treatment. Ann Surg Oncol. 2009;16(9):2587–93.
179. Li GZ, et al. Cutaneous radiation-associated breast angiosarcoma: radicality of surgery impacts survival. Ann Surg. 2017;265(4):814–20.

Small Intestine Cancers

Mary Read and Laura M. Enomoto

Introduction

- An uncommon location for tumors, <5% of all tumors in the GI tract [1].
- Subtypes: adenocarcinoma, neuroendocrine, and lymphoma.
- Most common imaging modality is CT.
- Treatment is highly variable based on tumor subtype.
- Can be associated with several different familial syndromes.

Adenocarcinoma

- *Background*
  - Average age at diagnosis between the fifth and sixth decades of life
  - Risk factors
    - Small bowel Crohn's disease [2]
    - Celiac disease [3]
    - Familial syndromes
      - Familial adenomatous polyposis (FAP)
      - Hereditary nonpolyposis colorectal cancer (HNPCC)
      - Peutz-Jeugers syndrome
- *Diagnosis*
  - Abdominal pain is the most common symptom followed by nausea, vomiting, obstruction, and anemia/bleeding.
  - Imaging with contrasted CT, best by CT enteroclysis [4].

M. Read · L. M. Enomoto (✉)
Graduate School of Medicine, University Surgical Oncology, University of Tennessee, Knoxville, TN, USA
e-mail: lenomoto@utmck.edu

© The Author(s), under exclusive license to Springer Nature Switzerland AG 2025
C. Schmidt, M. G. Kledzik (eds.), *Complex General Surgical Oncology*,
https://doi.org/10.1007/978-3-031-88954-7_17

- Diagnosis can also be obtained by endoscopic ultrasound (EUS) if duodenal.
- Laboratory evaluation includes a complete blood count, chemistry profile, CA 19-9, and CEA.
- Consider studies for celiac disease.
- Mismatch repair testing.
- PET/CT is not indicated.
• Evaluation and Clinic Stage
  - Pathology
    • Well, moderately, or poorly differentiated
    • Signet ring subtype portends worst prognosis [5]
  - Staging
    • AJC TNM Staging; AJCC 8th edition

Stage	Stage grouping	Stage description
0	Tis N0 M0	The cancer is only in the epithelium (the top layer of cells of the mucosa). It has not grown into the deeper tissue layers (Tis). It has not spread to nearby lymph nodes (N0) or distant parts of the body (M0).
I	T1 or T2 N0 M0	The cancer has grown into deeper layers (the lamina propria or the submucosa) (T1) OR it has grown through the submucosa into the muscularis propria (T2). The cancer has not spread to nearby lymph nodes (N0) or to distant parts of the body (M0).
IIA	T3 N0 M0	The cancer has grown through the muscularis propria and into the subserosa. It has not started to grow into any nearby organs or structures (T3). The cancer has not spread to nearby lymph nodes (N0) or to distant parts of the body (M0).
IIA	T3 N0 M0	The cancer has grown through the muscularis propria and into the subserosa. It has not started to grow into any nearby organs or structures (T3). The cancer has not spread to nearby lymph nodes (N0) or to distant parts of the body (M0).
IIIA	Any T N1 M0	The cancer might have grown into any layers of the wall of the small intestine (Any T). It has spread to one or two nearby lymph nodes (N1) but not to distant parts of the body (M0).
IIIB	Any T N2 M0	The cancer might have grown into any layers of the wall of the small intestine (Any T). It has spread to three or more nearby lymph nodes (N2) but not to distant parts of the body (M0).
IV	Any T Any N M1	The cancer might have grown into any layers of the wall of the small intestine (any T). It might or might not have spread to nearby lymph nodes (any N). It has spread to distant lymph nodes or organs such as the liver or the peritoneum (the inner lining of the abdomen) (M1).

• Choice of Therapy
  - Resectable
    • Upfront surgery confers a survival benefit when resectable.
    • Segmental resection with 5–10 cm margins with en bloc removal of regional lymph nodes.

- If duodenal, Whipple may be indicated.
    - Minimally invasive techniques are frequently utilized such as laparoscopic or robotic approaches.
    - If the tumor is in the terminal ileum, then right hemicolectomy likely indicated.
  - Locally unresectable
    - Palliative bypass
    - Stenting (if obstructed)
  - Metastatic or locally advanced disease
    - No large clinical trials to dictate therapy
    - Chemotherapy regimens for metastatic disease
      - Capecitabine + oxaliplatin
      - FOLFOX
      - 5-Flourouracil + leucovorin
- *Surveillance*
  - Follow-up every 3–6 months for 2 years and then every 6 months for a total of 5 years.
  - Laboratory evaluation with CEA and CA 19-9 every 3–6 months for 2 years and then every 6 months for a total of 5 years
  - CT chest, abdomen, and pelvis every 6–12 months for 2 years and then every 12 months for 3–5 years.

Neuroendocrine

- *Background*
  - Most common location for neuroendocrine tumors is the small bowel.
  - Most commonly diagnosed in the sixth decade of life.
  - More common in Caucasians.
  - Most common location is the terminal ileum.
  - Risk factors
    - Familial syndromes
      - Multiple endocrine neoplasias (MEN) 1 and 2
      - Von Hippel-Lindau
      - Neurofibromatosis type 1 (NF1)
      - Tuberous sclerosis
    - More common in Caucasians
    - Occur more frequently in women than men
- *Diagnosis*
  - Need to determine whether the tumor is functional (hormone producing) or nonfunctional
  - Symptoms
    - Hormonal: serotonin, dopamine, histamine, and tachykinins
      - Flushing
      - Secretory diarrhea
      - Bronchospasm

- Right heart failure
- Edema
  - Obstruction
  - Bleeding
- Labs
  - Urinary 5-HIAA, indicates tumor function
  - Serotonin
  - Chromogranin A
    - Also elevated in postmenopausal women, renal or hepatic disease, and PPI use
  - Pancreastatin
    - Provides information on disease progression and tumor burden within the liver
- Imaging
  - Multiple modalities
    - CT is best for identifying metastasis.
    - CT enteroclysis.
    - MRI and best for identifying local tumor invasion.
    - Both double balloon endoscopy and capsule endoscopy have poor detection rates.
    - Somatostatin receptor scintigraphy
      - SSTR2 receptor is most commonly expressed and utilized for scintigraphy.
    - SRS improved by addition of PET utilizing ^{68}Ga-DOTATOC, ^{68}Ga-DOTANOC, and ^{68}Ga-DOTATATE
  - ECHO to evaluate for disease on the tricuspid and pulmonary valves.
- Tumors can be discovered incidentally on imaging obtained for another reason
  - Primary tumor visualized
  - Ill-defined mesenteric mass with a spiculated/stellate pattern indicating metastatic spread
- Biopsy
  - EUS-FNA is an option for proximal lesions.
  - Colonoscopy.
  - Percutaneous biopsy.
  - Diagnostic laparoscopy with surgical resection for both tissue diagnosis and definitive surgical therapy.
- *Evaluation and Clinic Stage*
  - 2019 WHO Classification and Grading Criteria

Terminology	Differentiation	Grade	Mitotic rate (mitoses/2 mm^2)	Ki-67 index (%)
NET and G1	Well differentiated	Low	< 2	< 3
NET and G2	Well differentiated	Intermediate	2–20	3–20
NET and G3	Well differentiated	High	> 20	> 20

(continued)

Terminology	Differentiation	Grade	Mitotic rate (mitoses/2 mm²)	Ki-67 index (%)
Neuroendocrine carcinoma (NEC) and small cell type (SCNEC)	Poorly differentiated	High	> 20	> 20
NEC and large cell type (LCNEC)	Poorly differentiated	High	> 20	>20
Mixed neuroendocrine nonneuroendocrine neoplasm	Well or poorly differentiated	Variable	Variable	Variable

- TNM Staging, AJCC 8th edition
  - Tis: Carcinoma in situ or dysplasia (size <0.5 mm). Confined to mucosa.
  - T1: Tumor invades mucosa or submucosa. Size ≤1 cm.
  - T2: Tumor invades muscularis propria. Size >1 cm.
  - T3: Tumor invades subserosa without penetrating serosa (jejunal/ileal tumors) or invades pancreas or retroperitoneum (duodenal tumors) or invades into nonperitonealized tissues (any small bowel).
  - T4: Tumor invades peritoneum or other organs.
  - N0: No regional lymph node metastasis.
  - N1: Regional lymph node metastasis.
  - M0: No distant metastasis.
  - M1: Distant metastasis.
- Duodenal
  - Stage I: T1 N0 M0
  - Stage II: T2 or T3 N0, and M0
  - Stage III: Any T, N1, M0, or T4 N0 M0
  - Stage IV: Any T, any N, and M1
- Jejunal/ileal
  - Stage I: T1 N0 M0
  - Stage II: T2 or T3 N0 and M0
  - Stage III: Any T, N1 or N2, M0, or T4 N0 M0
  - Stage IV: Any T, any N, and M1
- *Choice of Therapy*
  - Surgical therapy
    - Generally reserved for well-differentiated low- and intermediate-grade tumors; poorly differentiated, high-grade neuroendocrine carcinoma is typically treated with systemic cytotoxic chemotherapy.
    - Goal of surgical therapy is to achieve debulking greater than 70% of disease including resection of metastatic burden.
    - Most common place for unknown primary in setting of metastatic neuroendocrine tumor is the small bowel.
    - Segmental resection of tumor with en bloc lymphadenectomy of regional lymph nodes (at least 12).
    - Cholecystectomy should be considered at the time of resection due to the high rates of cholecystitis (cholestasis) with adjuvant somatostatin receptor therapy.

- Locoregional disease
  - Duodenal NET
    - Endoscopic resection
    - Local excision via transduodenal approach with regional lymphadenectomy
    - Whipple procedure
  - Jejunal/ileal NET
    - Segmental resection of tumor with en bloc lymphadenectomy of regional lymph nodes (at least 12)
  - Duodenal gastrinoma
    - Occult or unknown primary: observe versus exploratory laparotomy with duodenotomy and intraoperative ultrasound
    - Local resection or enucleation with local lymph node dissection
    - Whipple procedure
- Advanced locoregional disease or resectable metastatic disease
  - Surgical debulking/cytoreductive surgery
  - Goal of debulking >70% of disease
- Unresectable metastatic disease
  - Octreotide or lanreotide
  - Disease progression on octreotide or lanreotide treatment consider
    - Everolimus
    - PRRT with 177Lu-dotatate
    - Liver-directed therapy
    - Radiotherapy for bone metastasis
    - Cytotoxic chemotherapy for high-grade disease
- *Surveillance*
  - No adjuvant treatment in completely resected disease
  - 12-week–12-month postresection: Follow-up, possible biochemical markers, with possible imaging including CT or MRI
  - >1–10 years postresection: follow-up every 1–2 years with possible biochemical markers and possible imaging
  - >10 years: surveillance as clinically indicated

Lymphoma

- *Background*
  - Historically a treatment shift from surgical management to medical.
  - Male predominance, average age at diagnosis in the sixth decade of life.
  - Small bowel lymphoma represents a non-Hodgkin's lymphoma.
  - Risk factors
    - Older age
    - Crohn's disease, active in the small bowel
      - Increased risk associated with thiopurine use
    - Celiac disease associated with T-cell lymphomas

- Immunosuppression, especially organ recipients, and HIV/AIDS
  - *Helicobacter pylori*
- *Diagnosis*
  - Symptoms
    - Abdominal pain
    - Nausea and vomiting
    - Obstructive symptoms
    - Bleeding
    - B symptoms: fevers, night sweats, and weight loss
  - Incidental finding on imaging obtained for another reason
  - Labwork
    - CBC, CMP, LDH, cytology for tumor markers, Beta 2-microglobulin, and hepatitis panel
  - Imaging
    - Most commonly found on CT
    - Best study CT and MR enteroclysis
    - Findings
      - Mesenteric adenopathy
      - Obstruction
      - Intussusception
  - Tissue diagnosis
    - Tissue is imperative for identifying histologic subtype and architecture
    - Options for obtaining tissue
      - EUS
      - Percutaneous biopsy via core needle biopsy to preserve follicle structure
      - Local resection
  - Staging
    - CT chest, abdomen, and pelvis
    - PET dependent on subtype
    - Consider head CT/MRI
  - Pathology
    - DLBCL, follicular, MALT lymphoma, Burkitt lymphoma, and T-cell
    - Tissue sampling is important to identify cell surface proteins, receptors, and genetic abnormalities
- *Evaluation and Clinic Stage*
  - Lugano staging system
    - Stage I: Tumor confined to small bowel: single or multiple primary lesions
    - Stage II: Tumor extending into the abdomen from primary small bowel site
      - II1: Paraintestinal nodal involvement
      - II2: Involving mesenteric, aortic, caval, pelvic, or inguinal nodes
      - E (IIE, II1E, or II2E) with penetration of serosa involving adjacent organs or tissues
    - Stage III: No stage III
    - Stage IV: Disseminated extranodal sites or supradiaphragmatic nodal involvement

- *Therapy*
  - Surgical therapy
    - Relieve obstruction
    - Treat perforation or bleeding
    - Secure a diagnosis
    - Segmental resection with en bloc lymphadenectomy to obtain adequate lymph node sampling
    - Not for curative purpose
  - Medical therapy
    - CHOP (cyclophosphamide, doxorubicin, vincristine, prednisone) and R-CHOP (the addition of anti-CD20 rituximab)
    - R-CHOP is superior to CHOP
      - MabThera International Trial (MInT)
      - Groupe d'Etudes des Lymphomes de l'Adulte trial (GELA)

Summary

Small bowel cancers are a heterogenous group of rare malignancies and are often a diagnostic challenge. Cross-sectional imaging and endoscopy often play a pivotal role in staging and diagnosis. Laboratory studies for tumor markers and differentiating functional versus nonfunctional tumors are critical for workup. Treatment modalities and prognosis vary widely depending on tumor type and extent of disease. It is important for the surgeon to be aware of these uncommon group of tumors including the diagnostic and treatment strategies to allow for the best patient outcomes.

References

1. Overman MJ, Hu CY, Kopetz S, Abbruzzese JL, Wolff RA, Chang GJ. A population-based comparison of adenocarcinoma of the large and small intestine: insights into a rare disease. Ann Surg Oncol. 2012;19(5):1439–45.
2. Elriz K, Carrat F, Carbonnel F, Marthey L, Bouvier AM, Beaugerie L. Incidence, presentation, and prognosis of small bowel adenocarcinoma in patients with small bowel Crohn's disease: a prospective observational study. Inflamm Bowel Dis. 2013;19(9):1823–6.
3. Green PH, Fleischauer AT, Bhagat G, Goyal R, Jabri B, Neugut AI. Risk of malignancy in patients with celiac disease. Am J Med. 2003;115(3):191–5.
4. Pilleul F, Penigaud M, Milot L, Saurin JC, Chayvialle JA, Valette PJ. Possible small-bowel neoplasms: contrast-enhanced and water-enhanced multidetector CT enteroclysis. Radiology. 2006;241(3):796–801.
5. Dabaja BS, Suki D, Pro B, Bonnen M, Ajani J. Adenocarcinoma of the small bowel: presentation, prognostic factors, and outcome of 217 patients. Cancer. 2004;101(3):518–26.

Thyroid and Parathyroid Cancers

18

Melissa LoPinto

Thyroid Cancer

- Introduction [1–4]
    - Common, increasing incidence, female predominance
        - In the United States about 45,000 new cases of thyroid cancer/year
            - 12000 in men and 33000 in women
        - In the United States about 2000 deaths/year from thyroid cancer
    - Most common variants have indolent course and excellent prognosis.
    - Newer pathology classification identifies high-grade and poorly differentiated variants as intermediate prognosis.
    - Follicular cell-derived carcinoma accounts for over 90% of thyroid cancer.
    - Medullary thyroid carcinoma is a parafollicular cell (c-cell)-derived tumor.
        - Occurs as sporadic forms, familial forms, and MEN 2 syndromes
    - Anaplastic thyroid carcinoma is one of the most aggressive and deadly human tumors:
        - By definition is stage IV at diagnosis.
        - Disease-specific mortality is near 100%.
        - Median survival is 5–6 months [2].
    - Surgery is the primary treatment modality for the vast majority of thyroid cancers.

- Diagnosis
    - Thyroid cancer usually presents as a thyroid nodule.
        - May be incidentally discovered on imaging, noted during a physical exam, or patient discovered.

M. LoPinto (✉)
Department of Surgery, West Virginia University, Morgantown, WV, USA
e-mail: melissa.lopinto@hsc.wvu.edu

- Patients are often asymptomatic and euthyroid.
- Symptoms may be from mass effect or direction invasion (e.g., vocal cord paralysis).
  - Symptoms of direction invasion raise concern for poorly differentiated or anaplastic carcinoma.
- History:
  - Assess for symptoms: pressure, mass or mass sensation, dysphagia, hoarseness of voice, and hyperthyroidism/hypothyroidism.
  - Family history: thyroid cancer, benign thyroid disease, and other endocrine tumors
  - Radiation exposure
  - Personal history of thyroid cancers or other malignancies
- Physical exam
  - Nodule may not be palpable.
  - Palpable thyroid nodule is suspicious if hard and fixed.
  - Palpable lateral neck nodes should be evaluated with ultrasound and FNA
- Workup
  - TSH and free T4; consider TPO and TSI as clinically indicated
    - Suppressed TSH suggests hyperthyroidism:
      - Ultrasound may demonstrate diffuse goiter, multinodular goiter, or solitary nodule.
      - Nuclear thyroid uptake scan is useful for surgical planning:
        - Diffuse uptake with elevated TSI (Graves' disease) has two options for definitive management.
          - RAI ablation
          - Total thyroidectomy
            - Thyroidectomy may be preferable for younger patients, those with current tobacco use, and ophthalmopathy.
            - Thyroidectomy is indicated when there are concurrent compressive symptoms.
        - Solidary toxic nodule with negative TSI can be management with lobectomy.
        - Toxic multinodular goiter:
          - If considering RAI, assess nodules as detailed below to rule out malignancy.
          - Total thyroidectomy is the preferred treatment option for concurrent compressive symptoms and mass effect.
    - Preoperative medical management includes antithyroidal medication (methimazole, PTU, SSKI) and betablocker.
    - Risk of perioperative thyroid storm is not well delineated in the literature but reports range from 0% to 14% [5].
  - Preoperative thyroglobulin has little clinical utility.
  - Ultrasound to assess size and features of the nodule [6]:
    - Solid, cystic, and spongiform
    - Well defined vs poorly defined

- Hyper-, hypo-, and isoechoic
- Calcifications and their pattern
- Wider than tall (reassuring) vs taller than wide (suspicious)
- Evaluate for adenopathy in central and lateral neck
- Fine need aspiration biopsy (FNA) as indicated by sonographic findings
  - 2015 ATA Guidelines [1]
    - Pattern of sonographic features conferring increasing risk
      - Benign:
        - Purely cystic
          - ROM 1%
          - Only aspirate if symptomatic
      - Very low suspicion
        - Spongiform
          - ROM <3%
          - FNA ≥2cm: surveillance acceptable

- Low suspicion
  - Solid nodule that is iso- or hyperechoic
  - Partially cystic with solid areas
  - Must lack calcification or extrathyroidal extension
  - Must lack irregularity
  - Must not be taller than wide
    - ROM 5–10%
    - FNA ≥ 1.5cm

- Intermediate suspicion
  - Solid hypoechoic nodule with regular margin
    - ROM 10–20%
    - FNA if ≥ 1cm
- High suspicion
  - Solid hypoechoic nodule with any of the following:
    - Irregular margins
    - Microcalcification
    - Rim calcifications
    - Taller-than-wide shape
    - Evidence of extrathyroidal extension
  - ROM >70–90%
  - FNA ≥ 1cm

  - ACR TI-RADS classification [7]
    - Numerical scoring system based on sonographic features
      - For composition, echogenicity, shape, and margin choose most appropriate description
      - For echogenic foci (calcification), include all that apply.
      - Calculate total to determine TI-RADS (TR) category

- TR categories
  - TR 1: 0 points: no FNA
  - TR 2: 2 points: no FNA
  - TR 3: 3 points, mildly suspicious:
    - FNA if ≥2.5cm
    - Surveillance if ≥1.5cm
  - TR 4: 4–6 points, moderately suspicious:
    - FNA if ≥1.5cm
    - Surveillance if ≥1cm
  - TR 5: 7 or greater points, highly suspicious:
    - FNA if ≥1cm
    - Surveillance if ≥0.5cm

- Bethesda classification for thyroid FNA cytology and clinical management [1, 8]
  - Risk of malignancy (ROM) varies depending on how noninvasive follicular thyroid neoplasm with papillary-like nuclear features (NIFTP) is considered.
    - If NIFTP is considered malignancy, ROM falls toward the higher end of the range.
  - Bethesda I: Insufficient specimen/nondiagnostic
    - ROM 5–10%
    - Plan: repeat FNA
  - Bethesda II: Benign
    - ROM 0–3%
    - Plan: surveillance imaging in 6–12 months
  - Bethesda III: Atypia of uncertain significance/follicular lesion of uncertain significance
    - ROM 6–30%
    - Plan
      - Molecular/gene expression classifier (GEC) testing if available
      - Repeat FNA
      - Repeated Bethesda III and molecular/GEC testing not possible:
        - Surveillance vs diagnostic lobectomy based on risk factors

  - Bethesda IV: follicular neoplasm
    - ROM 10–40%
    - Plan:
      - Molecular/GEC testing if available
      - If molecular testing/GEC is not possible: diagnostic lobectomy

  - Bethesda V: suspicious
    - ROM: 45–75%
    - Plan: resection

  - Bethesda VI: malignant
    - Risk of malignancy: up to 99%
    - Plan: resection

- Role of molecular and gene expression classifier testing
  - Further risk stratify Bethesda III and IV nodules.
  - Identify potential genetic markers of more aggressive behavior.
  - Identify potentially actionable mutation in advanced or unresectable disease.

- Follicular cell-derived thyroid carcinoma
  - Follicular cell-derived carcinoma (nonmedullary thyroid carcinoma) include follicular carcinoma, papillary carcinoma, and variants thereof. Prognosis is generally good to excellent but varies with type and subtype, molecular signature, and histologic features.
  - Accounts for at least 90–95% of thyroid cancer.
  - Low-risk/indolent lesions include (Ras-like lesions):
    - Follicular adenoma (benign)
    - Noninvasive follicular thyroid neoplasm with papillary-like nuclear features (NIFTP) [9]
    - Minimally invasive follicular carcinoma (FTC) or follicular variant papillary thyroid cancer (<4 foci of capsular and/or vascular invasion)

  - Papillary thyroid carcinoma (PTC) histologic subtypes (BRAF-like lesions)
    - Classical
    - Infiltrative follicular variant PTC (BRAF mutations, occasionally NRAS)
    - Subtypes with ATA intermediate prognosis are the following:
      - Columnar cell
      - Tall cell (associated with BRAF V600E and TERT promotor mutations)
      - Hobnail (associated with BRAF V600E, TP53, and TERT promotor mutations)
      - Diffuse sclerosing (associated with lymphocytic thyroiditis)

  - Cribriform morula carcinoma (associated with familial adenomatous polyposis/FAP)
    - Historically classified as a PTC subtype
    - 2022 WHO classification regards separately [10]

  - High-grade differentiated and poorly differentiated subtypes [10]
    - High-grade differentiated thyroid carcinoma
      - May be follicular, papillary, or oncocytic; histologic pattern is similar to well-differentiated tumors but has additional features of the following:
      - Tumor necrosis
      - Elevated mitotic rate
    - Poorly differentiated thyroid carcinoma
      - Solid trabecular or insular growth; "raisin-like" cells or pleomorphic nuclei
      - Tumor necrosis
      - Mitotic count $\geq 5/2mm^2$ fields

  - Familial papillary thyroid carcinoma:
    - Approximately 1–3% of cases may be familial [11], possibly up to 10% [12]

- Unknown genetic signature
- Defined clinically as two or more first-degree relatives with nonmedullary thyroid carcinoma in the absence of other genetic syndromes.
- May be more aggressive than sporadic forms but standard treatment results in similar outcomes, stage for stage.

– Extent of surgery [1]
  - Lobectomy may be adequate treatment for early stage, low- to intermediate-risk tumors
    – Tumor ≤4cm (T1 or T2 tumors)
    – Unilateral involvement
    – Clinically node negative by physical exam and ultrasound
    – No sonographic evidence of extrathyroidal extension or contralateral disease
    – Local recurrence rates may be increased compared with total thyroidectomy
  - Total thyroidectomy is preferred for the following
    – Higher-risk sonographic features including the following:
      - Tumor >4cm
      - Extrathyroidal extension
      - Suspicious lymph nodes
    – Bilateral nodules
    – Familial nonmedullary thyroid cancer
    – History of radiation treatments or exposures
    – Likely need for postoperative RAI ablation
    – Multiple bilateral nodules
    – Patient preference and other patient-specific considerations
  - Role lymph node dissection [1]
    – Prophylactic central neck dissection (levels VI and VII) is controversial:
      - Consider central neck dissection for T3 and T4 tumors
      - Consider central neck dissection if information can help determine the potential benefit radioactive iodine (RAI).
      - Consider if higher-risk mutation is known (e.g., BRAF V600E, and TERT promotor)
    – Therapeutic central neck dissection is performed for clinically positive or biopsy positive central neck nodes.
  - Modified radical neck dissection is performed for biopsy-proven lateral neck metastasis [1, 13]:
    – Compartment-oriented dissection includes levels II, III, IV, and Va.
    – Complete compartment-oriented approach minimizes recurrence to about 5% [13].

– Adjuvant Therapy and Surveillance [1, 14]
  - Radioactive iodine

- Remnant ablation is not routinely recommended; consider patient-specific factors
  - Low-risk patients (tumor <4cm, node-negative disease)
    - RAI not routinely given
    - May consider for aggressive histology
    - May consider based on quality/reliability of follow-up
    - Role in patients with <5 involved nodes with micrometastasis <0.2cm is unclear.
      - These patients may still be low risk in the absence of other increasing risk features.
- Adjuvant therapy: consider for ATA intermediate risk, recommended for ATA high risk
  - Intermediate-risk features
    - Tumor >4cm (pT3)
    - Microscopic extrathyroidal extension
    - Aggressive histology
      - Overall survival improved for diffuse sclerosing variant and tall cell variant with RAI following surgery [15]:
        - Diffuse sclerosing variant patients were 4.9x more likely to die without RAI
        - Tall cell variant patients were 2.1x more likely to die without RAI
    - >5 positive cervical nodes with metastasis no larger than 0.2–3cm
    - Tumor <4cm with BRAF mutation
    - PTC with vascular invasion
    - Data regarding the benefit of RAI in this category is mixed (possible confounding variables, age, sex, and heterogeneous tumor characteristics)
      - Multivariate analysis of SEER data suggests improved overall survival with RAI [16]
        - Overall 29% reduction in risk of death
          - For the subgroup <45 years, risk reduction was 36%.
        - However, absolute risk reduction was 1% for age <45 years and 4% for age >65years [1, 16].
      - Benefit may be greatest for patient with metastasis to the lateral neck nodes (N1b), larger tumors, and larger nodal deposits [17].
      - Advancing age would also favor RAI treatment.
  - High-risk features
    - RAI recommended
    - Gross extrathyroid extension
    - R2 resection
    - Any nodal metastasis >3cm
    - Distant metastases

- Patients >45years, tumor >2cm, positive nodes, and M1 disease experienced overall median survival more than double 7 vs 57 months with RAI [18]
    - TERT promotor mutation
    - Follicular carcinoma with >4 foci of vascular invasion
- TSH suppression goals are based on ATA risk category:
    - High risk: 0.1mU/L
    - Intermediate risk: 0.1–0.5 mU/L
    - Low risk, with RAI and undetectable Tg level: 0.5–2 mU/L
    - Low risk with mildly elevated Tg or no RAI: 0.1–0.5mU/L

- Surveillance
    - Labs: Thyroglobulin, antithyroglobulin antibody, TSH, and initially every 6–12 months, more frequent in higher-risk patients
    - Ultrasound every 6–12 months
    - RAI thyroid uptake scan for suspected persistent or recurrent disease
    - ^{18}FDG-PET to evaluate high-risk patient with Tg>10ng/ml and negative RAI imaging

- Other Adjuvant Therapies
    - Kinase inhibitors
        - Should be considered for RAI refractory disease when metastatic, symptomatic, and/or rapidly progressive [1]
            - Sorafenib [19, 20]
                - Phase 3 DECISION trial, double-blinded RCT
                - FDA-approved metastatic RAI refractory DTC
                - Progression-free survival increased to 10.8 months with sorafenib vs 5.8 months with placebo
                - No difference in overall survival
            - Lenvatinib [20, 21]
                - FDA approved for progressive RAI refractory-differentiated thyroid cancer
                - Phase 3 SELECT trial multicenter RCTs
                - Progression-free survival 18.3 months vs 3.6 with placebo
                - Improved overall survival in the >65-year-old subgroup [22]
            - Cabozantinib [20, 23]
                - Second-line therapy
                - COSMIC-311 trial, phase 3 RCT in patient previously treated with sorafenib and/or lenvatinib
                - Disease stabilization in 43% vs 16% for placebo
                - Survival data limited by small sample size and short follow-up duration
            - Dabrafenib [20]
                - Indicated for metastatic, RAI refractory BRAFV600E positive DTC
                - FDA approved monotherapy

- Phase 2, unblinded comparison of Dabrafenib vs dabrafenib/trametinib concluded no statistically significant benefit over monotherapy [24]:
  - Progression-free survival for monotherapy 10.7 months vs 15.7 for combination therapy
  - Overall survival 37.9 months for monotherapy vs 47.5 combination
- Entrectinib and larotrectinib [20]
  - FDA approved for advanced NKTR fusion-positive tumors
  - Larotrectinib [25]
    - Pooled data from three phase 1 and 2 trials, included 24% anaplastic thyroid cancer patients
    - 24-month progression-free survival 69%
    - 24-month overall survival 76%

- Active surveillance as a management option
  - Data is limited and quality of evidence is generally low [26].
  - May be appropriate for very low-risk cancers in selected circumstances
    - Tumor <1–1.5cm with low-risk histology
    - No clinical or sonographic evidence of extrathyroidal extension or nodal metastasis
    - Older patients
    - Multiple comorbidities/high surgical risk

- Medullary Thyroid Carcinoma (MTC)
  - Preop Workup [3]
    - Presents as a nodule, begin workup as for any thyroid nodule.
    - History to assess risk of familial MTC or MEN2.
    - FNA may reveal MTC; molecular/GEC testing may reveal an MTC signature.
    - Screen for primary hyperparathyroidism and pheochromocytoma.
    - Genetic testing for RET germ-line RET mutations should be considered for any MTC patient.
    - Prophylactic thyroidectomy is recommended before age five years in MEN2A and before age 1 in MEN2B.
    - RET mutations at codons 634 and 918 are subject to early and aggressive cancers and prophylactic node dissection should be discussed.
    - Lymph node dissections for prophylactic thyroidectomy are not recommended.
    - Calcitonin: increasing level corresponds to increasing burden of disease [27, 28]:
      - >20 pg/mL ipsilateral central neck nodes
      - >50 pg/mL ipsilateral lateral neck nodes
      - >200 pg/mL contralateral central neck nodes
      - >500 pg/mL mediastinal nodes
      - >1000 pg/mL bilateral lateral neck nodes

- >10,000 pg/mL surgical cure is unrealistic
- CEA is a marker of nodal metastasis [28].
- Rule out pheochromocytoma preoperatively
  - For concomitant pheochromocytoma, treat the pheochromocytoma first due to perioperative risks.
- R0 Resection offers best chance of cure.

- Surgery [27, 3, 28]:
- Total thyroidectomy with central neck dissection
- Prophylactic ipsilateral lateral neck dissection is controversial but can be considered:
  - If positive central neck nodes
  - If calcitonin>20pg/mL

- Prophylactic contralateral lateral neck dissection may be considered:
  - If clinically positive nodes in the ipsilateral neck
  - If calcitonin >200pg/mL
- Therapeutic modified radical neck dissection for positive nodal disease

- AJCC staging for MTC [3]
  - Stage I: tumor 2cm or less, N0M0
  - Stage II: larger tumors including >4cm but limited to thyroid with minimal to no extrathyroidal extension, N0M0
  - Stage III: any tumor with minimal to no extrathyroidal extension and involved level VI nodes, M0
  - Stage IVa: locally advanced tumor with invasion to surround sutures including trachea, esophagus, recurrent laryngeal nerve, or any size tumor with lateral neck node involvement or level VII node involvement
  - Stage IVb: extensive local disease involving prevertebral fascia, encasing major vessels
  - Stage IVc: distant metastatic disease
- Surveillance [3, 28]
  - Calcitonin and CEA at three months postoperatively
    - Normal CEA and undetectable calcitonin at three months constitute a biochemical cure:
      - Biochemical cure confers 5–10-year recurrence rate of <1–8.5% and survival >97% at five years and >95% at ten years [29]
    - Biochemically incomplete response
      - Detectable calcitonin and/or CEA, no structural lesion
        - 10 year disease-specific survival approaches 100%.
        - 15-year disease-specific survival about 80%.
        - Clinical outcomes are similar to those with biochemical cure.
    - Structurally incomplete response
      - Structural disease present
        - Disease-specific survival: 80% at 5 years, 40% at 10 years, and 25% at 15 years.

- Continue surveillance with calcitonin and CEA q6 monthsx1 year; yearly thereafter.
- If postop calcitonin is elevated but <150pg/mL:
  - Exam, ultrasound, calcitonin, and CEA levels every six months
  - Calcitonin doubling time can predict survival:
    - Doubling time is correlated to rate of structural disease progression.
    - Doubling time <1year: five-year recurrence-free survival 20%
    - Doubling time >1 year: five-year recurrence-free survival 75% [30]
    - Doubling time >2-year disease stability; patients outlived the study period [31]
- If postop calcitonin >150pg/mL
  - Image for metastatic disease: CT chest + contrasted MRI or triple phase liver CT + bone scintigraphy or MRI of pelvis and axial skeleton

- Adjuvant Therapy
  - Since MTC originates from parafollicular c-cells, there is no role for TSH suppression or radioactive iodine ablation
  - Targeted RET and VEGFR
    - Vandetanib
      - FDA approved for symptomatic, progressive, unresectable, and/or metastatic MTC
      - Phase 3 trial ([32]; NCT00410761)
        - Statistically significant improvement in response rate and biochemical control
        - A six-month progression-free survival 83% vs 63% with placebo
        - Predicted progression-free survival 30.5 months vs 19 months for placebo
        - Overall survival data not available
    - Cabozantinib
      - FDA approved for progressive metastatic medullary thyroid carcinoma
      - Phase 3 EXAM trial ([33]; NCT00704730)
        - Increased overall survival by 5.5 months compared to placebo but not statistically significant
        - Larger clinical response for the subgroup with RET M918T mutation
          - Response rate 34% vs 20% in non-RET M918T
          - Increase overall survival 44.3 months vs 18.9 months for placebo
    - Selpercatinib
      - FDA approved for RET mutation metastatic medullar thyroid carcinoma
      - Phase 1–2 clinical trial ([34]; NCT03157128)
        - Patient previously treated with vandetanib and/or cabozantinib had a response rate was 69%, and one-year progression-free survival was 82%.
        - Patients not previously treated had response rate 73% of and one-year progression-free survival of 92%.

- Anaplastic

  – Presents as a rapidly enlarging, sometimes painful neck mass.
  – Age at presentation 60s–early 70s.
  – Other associated symptoms may include airway compromise, vascular compromise, dysphagia, and hoarseness from direct nerve invasion [35].
  – Initial evaluation should be prompt and include the following:
    - Clinical evaluation for impending airway compromise/need for urgent airway protection.
    - Ultrasound, FNA, and FDG PET/CT:
      – Must quickly confirm suspected diagnosis and stage tumor.
    - Larger biopsy, such as a core needle biopsy, may be needed to confirm diagnosis, and provide material for molecular evaluation [2]; can be useful to evaluate for thyroid lymphoma which may have similar presentation.
    - Triple endoscopy to assess invasion into larynx, trachea, and esophagus.
    - Initial workup should include BRAF mutational analysis to determine role of BRAF/MEK inhibitors:
      – Dabrafenib/trametinib is FDA approved for BRAF-mutated anaplastic thyroid carcinoma
        - Overall response rate 69% ([36], NCT02034110)
      – Current phase 2 clinical trial (NCT04675710) assessing effect of dabrafenib/trametinib with pembrolizumab to facilitate R0 resection [37]
    - Data on other potentially actionable targets is insufficient but treatment may be available in clinical trials:
      – ALK fusion (crizotinib)
      – RET fusions
      – PD-L1
      – NTRK (larotrectinib)
  – By definition anaplastic thyroid cancer is stage IV at diagnosis [38, 2]:
    - For tumors confined to thyroid, T1–T3a, and stage IVA, the initial treatment is resection.
    - Tumors with gross extrathyroidal extension and/or lymph node involvement are stage IVB:
      – Some stage IVB tumors may be resectable.
    - Presence of metastatic disease is stage IVC.
    - Surgery for advanced disease may be with therapeutic intent after neoadjuvant therapy or as part of palliative approach.
  – Determining resectability
    - Evaluate cross-sectional imaging and triple endoscopy.
    - Goal is resection of gross cervical and mediastinal disease (R0/R1) with minimal morbidity; vital structures should be preserved.
      – Avoid laryngectomy, esophagostomy, and major vascular resection.
  – Palliative surgery is aimed at preventing airway compromise:
    - Partial thyroidectomy without or without tracheostomy can be considered.
    - Prophylactic tracheostomy:
      – Can be technically difficulty and may delay other adjuvant therapies

- May traverse tumor
- May provide only temporary airway protection
- Radiation
  - Greatest benefit when given at high dose after R0 or R1 resection.
  - High dose >59.4Gy after total thyroidectomy in patients without metastatic disease improved median survival to 16 months and overall survival to 38% at two years [39].
    - Benefit may be limited by treatment toxicity.
    - Likely represents highly selected group of patients.
  - For unresectable or R2 resection [40]
    - 60–75 Gy OS 31% at one year
    - 45–59.9 Gy OS 16% at one year
- Cytotoxic chemotherapy
  - Given in combination with radiation
  - Taxane with or without doxorubicin or platin
    - Paclitaxel produced transient disease regression in 53% of 19 patients [41].
    - Doxorubicin is approved for use in ATC [42].
    - General lack of data to suggest improved survival or quality of life from systemic therapy [2].

- Recent advances in targeted therapy have resulted in improved survival:
  - With aggressive multidisciplinary treatment (BRAF-directed therapy followed by surgery), survival may approach one year [43, 44], but survival at two years is rare [2].

ACR TI-RADS	Points
Composition	
Cystic	0
Spongiform	0
Mixed solid/cystic	1
Solid	2
Echogenicity	
Anechoic	0
Hyperechoic or isoechoic	1
Hypoechoic	2
Very hypoechoic	3
Shape	
Wider-than-tall	0
Taller-than-wide	3
Margin	
Smooth	0
Ill-defined	0
Lobulated or irregular	2
Extrathyroidal extension	3
Echogenic foci	
None	0
Large comet-tail artifact	0
Macrocalcification	1
Peripheral or rim calcification	2
Punctate echogenic foci	3

Parathyroid Cancer

- Introduction
  - Rare, accounts for 0.5–5% of cases of primary hyperparathyroidism.
  - Morbidity and mortality is from symptomatic hypercalcemia and hypercalcemic crisis, not tumor burden.
  - Surgery with R0 resection is the only potentially curative treatment option.
  - Parathyroid carcinoma is radio-resistant and no cytotoxic chemotherapy has been proven effective.
- Diagnosis [45, 46]
  - High index of suspicion based on clinical presentation and imaging:
    - Calcium >12mg/dL (and especially if calcium >14mg/dL), markedly elevated PTH, rapidly progressive course (rather than the indolent course typically seen with primary hyperparathyroidism).
    - Symptoms may be severe including weakness, weight loss, confusion, polydipsia, polyuria, and dehydration; life-threatening hypercalcemic crisis may occur.
    - Parathyroid tumors >3cm should be considered suspicious.
    - Imaging may demonstrate evidence of invasion and loss of plane between parathyroid and adjacent thyroid tissue.
- Surgical management
  - En bloc resection of parathyroid with ipsilateral thyroid lobe and any involved structures.
  - Involved lymph nodes should be resected, but prophylactic central neck dissection is controversial as nodal disease is rare [45] and does not independently predict prognosis [47]:
    - Tumor size >3cm is associated 7.5 times (21% vs 2.8%) increased risk of nodal metastasis [47]
      - Possible benefit of prophylactic central neck dissection for tumors >3cm
  - R0 resection is the only potentially curative treatment option [45]:
    - Role of intraoperative PTH (IoPTH) in parathyroid carcinoma:
      - >50% drop in IoPTH is less predictive of postoperative eucalcemia for carcinoma than for benign sporadic primary hyperparathyroidism [48]:
        - IoPTH drop >50% and into the normal range predictive of an R0 resection in 92.9% of cases compared to R0 resection in 50% of cases with >50% drop but not into the normal range [49]
- Difficult to confirm diagnosis histologically:
  - Evidence of invasion or metastasis confirms diagnosis [50]
  - Suspicious findings include necrosis, nuclear atypia, mitotic figures, and fibrosis.
  - Loss of the tumor suppressor parafibromin (CDC73) portends more aggressive clinical course and occurs in a majority of parathyroid cancers [51].
    - Tumor size >4cm is associated with decreased cancer-specific survival [52]
  - AJCC staging [53]
    - Prognostic stages are not defined due to lack of data

- Tumor
  - Tis: atypical parathyroid neoplasm
  - T1: confined to the thyroid
  - T2: invasion to other adjacent structures
  - T3: invasion to major vascular structures or spine
- Nodes
  - N1a: Level VI or VII involvement
  - N1b: Any lateral cervical chain involvement (levels I–V) or retropharyngeal
- Metastasis:
  - M1: Presence of distant metastasis

– Postoperative surveillance [54]
  - PTH serves as a tumor marker
  - Calcium, PTH should be monitored at least every 6–12 months.
  - In cases of biochemical recurrence, imaging is preformed to assess for structural recurrence. Sensitivity data for detection of recurrence is lacking due to rarity of disease. Combination of ultrasound and CT features may facilitate early detection of local recurrence [46]
    - Ultrasound
      - >90% of recurrence demonstrated solid hypoechoic nodule, 81.8% of which had increased vascularity
    - Sestamibi/spect/ct
    - 4DCT
    - F18-choline PET
  - Resection is the preferred treatment for structural local recurrence
    - Must balance risk/benefit of reoperative neck surgery

- Adjuvant therapy
  – Calcimimetics are used to control calcium levels in inoperable parathyroid carcinoma
    - Cinacalcet reduced serum calcium in two-thirds of patients with inoperable disease [55].
    - May be titrated to high doses up to 90 mg four times daily.
    - Gastrointestinal side effects are not uncommon and may limit ability to treat.
      - Bisphosphonates and denosumab (monoclonal against RANK ligand) are alternatives when cinacalcet is not tolerated.
  – Radiotherapy is controversial.
  – Cytotoxic chemotherapy is generally not effective:
    - Case reports note partial response
    - No standardized regimens
    - Recent studies have suggested a role for genetic profiling to assess potentially actionable mutations [56, 57]; however, data regarding specific agents and response rates are limited to case reports such as the following:

- Sorafenib in a patient with a CDC73 germline mutation [58]
- One of two patients treated with sorafenib experience regression of metastatic lesions, the other died of progression [59]
- Compassionate use pembrolizumab for abdominal nodal metastasis with biochemical remission [60]

References

1. Haugen BR, Alexander EK, Bible KC, Doherty GM, Mandel SJ, Nikiforov YE, Pacini F, Randolph GW, Sawka AM, Schlumberger M, Schuff KG, Sherman SI, Sosa JA, Steward DL, Tuttle RM, Wartofsky L. 2015 American Thyroid Association Management Guidelines for adult patients with thyroid nodules and differentiated thyroid cancer: the American Thyroid Association Guidelines Task Force on Thyroid Nodules and Differentiated Thyroid Cancer. Thyroid. 2016;26(1):1–133. https://doi.org/10.1089/thy.2015.0020. PMID: 26462967; PMCID: PMC4739132
2. Bible KC, Kebebew E, Brierley J, Brito JP, Cabanillas ME, Clark TJ Jr, Di Cristofano A, Foote R, Giordano T, Kasperbauer J, Newbold K, Nikiforov YE, Randolph G, Rosenthal MS, Sawka AM, Shah M, Shaha A, Smallridge R, Wong-Clark CK. 2021 American Thyroid Association Guidelines for Management of Patients with Anaplastic Thyroid Cancer. Thyroid. 2021;31(3):337–86. https://doi.org/10.1089/thy.2020.0944. Erratum in: Thyroid. 2021 Oct;31(10):1606–1607. PMID: 33728999; PMCID: PMC8349723
3. Wells SA Jr, Asa SL, Dralle H, Elisei R, Evans DB, Gagel RF, Lee N, Machens A, Moley JF, Pacini F, Raue F, Frank-Raue K, Robinson B, Rosenthal MS, Santoro M, Schlumberger M, Shah M, Waguespack SG. American Thyroid Association Guidelines Task Force on Medullary Thyroid Carcinoma. Revised American Thyroid Association guidelines for the management of medullary thyroid carcinoma. Thyroid. 2015;25(6):567–610. https://doi.org/10.1089/thy.2014.0335. PMID: 25810047; PMCID: PMC4490627
4. Boucai L, Zafereo M, Cabanillas ME. Thyroid cancer: a review. JAMA. 2024;331(5):425–35. https://doi.org/10.1001/jama.2023.26348. PMID: 38319329
5. de Mul N, Damstra J, Nieveen van Dijkum EJM, Fischli S, Kalkman CJ, Schellekens WM, Immink RV. Risk of perioperative thyroid storm in hyperthyroid patients: a systematic review. Br J Anaesth. 2021;127(6):879–89. https://doi.org/10.1016/j.bja.2021.06.043. Epub 2021 Aug 11. PMID: 34389171
6. Mistry R, Hillyar C, Nibber A, Sooriyamoorthy T, Kumar N. Ultrasound classification of thyroid nodules: a systematic review. Cureus. 2020;12(3):e7239. https://doi.org/10.7759/cureus.7239. PMID: 32190531; PMCID: PMC7067371
7. Tessler FN, Middleton WD, Grant EG, Hoang JK, Berland LL, Teefey SA, Cronan JJ, Beland MD, Desser TS, Frates MC, Hammers LW, Hamper UM, Langer JE, Reading CC, Scoutt LM, Stavros AT. ACR thyroid imaging, reporting and data system (TI-RADS): white paper of the ACR TI-RADS Committee. J Am Coll Radiol. 2017;14(5):587–95. https://doi.org/10.1016/j.jacr.2017.01.046. Epub 2017 Apr 2. PMID: 28372962
8. Cibas ES, Ali SZ. The 2017 Bethesda system for reporting thyroid cytopathology. Thyroid. 2017;27(11):1341–6. https://doi.org/10.1089/thy.2017.0500. PMID: 29091573
9. Nikiforov YE, Seethala RR, Tallini G, Baloch ZW, Basolo F, Thompson LD, Barletta JA, Wenig BM, Al Ghuzlan A, Kakudo K, Giordano TJ, Alves VA, Khanafshar E, Asa SL, El-Naggar AK, Gooding WE, Hodak SP, Lloyd RV, Maytal G, Mete O, Nikiforova MN, Nosé V, Papotti M, Poller DN, Sadow PM, Tischler AS, Tuttle RM, Wall KB, LiVolsi VA, Randolph GW, Ghossein RA. Nomenclature revision for encapsulated follicular variant of papillary thyroid carcinoma: a paradigm shift to reduce overtreatment of indolent tumors. JAMA Oncol. 2016;2(8):1023–9. https://doi.org/10.1001/jamaoncol.2016.0386. PMID: 27078145; PMCID: PMC5539411

10. Baloch ZW, Asa SL, Barletta JA, Ghossein RA, Juhlin CC, Jung CK, LiVolsi VA, Papotti MG, Sobrinho-Simões M, Tallini G, Mete O. Overview of the 2022 WHO classification of thyroid neoplasms. Endocr Pathol. 2022;33(1):27–63. https://doi.org/10.1007/s12022-022-09707-3. Epub 2022 Mar 14. PMID: 35288841
11. Mazeh H, Sippel RS. Familial nonmedullary thyroid carcinoma. Thyroid. 2013;23(9):1049–56. https://doi.org/10.1089/thy.2013.0079. Epub 2013 Aug 3. PMID: 23734600
12. Capezzone M, Fralassi N, Secchi C, Cantara S, Brilli L, Pilli T, Maino F, Forleo R, Pacini F, Cevenini G, Cartocci A, Castagna MG. Long-term clinical outcome in familial and sporadic papillary thyroid carcinoma. Eur Thyroid J. 2020;9(4):213–20. https://doi.org/10.1159/000506955. Epub 2020 Apr 28. PMID: 32903994; PMCID: PMC7445652
13. Porterfield JR, Factor DA, Grant CS. Operative technique for modified radical neck dissection in papillary thyroid carcinoma. Arch Surg. 2009;144(6):567–74. https://doi.org/10.1001/archsurg.2009.89. discussion 574. PMID: 19528391
14. Araque KA, Gubbi S, Klubo-Gwiezdzinska J. Updates on the management of thyroid cancer. Horm Metab Res. 2020;52(8):562–77. https://doi.org/10.1055/a-1089-7870. Epub 2020 Feb 10. PMID: 32040962; PMCID: PMC7415555
15. Kazaure HS, Roman SA, Sosa JA. Aggressive variants of papillary thyroid cancer: incidence, characteristics and predictors of survival among 43,738 patients. Ann Surg Oncol. 2012;19(6):1874–80. https://doi.org/10.1245/s10434-011-2129-x. Epub 2011 Nov 8. PMID: 22065195
16. Ruel E, Thomas S, Dinan M, Perkins JM, Roman SA, Sosa JA. Adjuvant radioactive iodine therapy is associated with improved survival for patients with intermediate-risk papillary thyroid cancer. J Clin Endocrinol Metab. 2015;100(4):1529–36. https://doi.org/10.1210/jc.2014-4332. Epub 2015 Feb 2. PMID: 25642591; PMCID: PMC4399282
17. Chow SM, Yau S, Kwan CK, Poon PC, Law SC. Local and regional control in patients with papillary thyroid carcinoma: specific indications of external radiotherapy and radioactive iodine according to T and N categories in AJCC 6th edition. Endocr Relat Cancer. 2006;13(4):1159–72. https://doi.org/10.1677/erc.1.01320. PMID: 17158761
18. Podnos YD, Smith DD, Wagman LD, Ellenhorn JD. Survival in patients with papillary thyroid cancer is not affected by the use of radioactive isotope. J Surg Oncol. 2007;96(1):3–7. https://doi.org/10.1002/jso.20656. PMID: 17567872
19. Brose MS, Nutting CM, Jarzab B, Elisei R, Siena S, Bastholt L, de la Fouchardiere C, Pacini F, Paschke R, Shong YK, Sherman SI, Smit JW, Chung J, Kappeler C, Peña C, Molnár I, Schlumberger MJ, DECISION investigators. Sorafenib in radioactive iodine-refractory, locally advanced or metastatic differentiated thyroid cancer: a randomised, double-blind, phase 3 trial. Lancet. 2014;384(9940):319–28. https://doi.org/10.1016/S0140-6736(14)60421-9. Epub 2014 Apr 24. PMID: 24768112; PMCID: PMC4366116
20. Cabanillas ME, Ryder M, Jimenez C. Targeted therapy for advanced thyroid cancer: kinase inhibitors and beyond. Endocr Rev. 2019;40(6):1573–604. https://doi.org/10.1210/er.2019-00007. PMID: 31322645; PMCID: PMC7341904
21. Schlumberger M, Tahara M, Wirth LJ, Robinson B, Brose MS, Elisei R, Habra MA, Newbold K, Shah MH, Hoff AO, Gianoukakis AG, Kiyota N, Taylor MH, Kim SB, Krzyzanowska MK, Dutcus CE, de las Heras B, Zhu J, Sherman SI. Lenvatinib versus placebo in radioiodine-refractory thyroid cancer. N Engl J Med. 2015;372(7):621–30. https://doi.org/10.1056/NEJMoa1406470. PMID: 25671254
22. Brose MS, Worden FP, Newbold KL, Guo M, Hurria A. Effect of age on the efficacy and safety of Lenvatinib in radioiodine-refractory differentiated thyroid cancer in the phase III SELECT trial. J Clin Oncol. 2017;35(23):2692–9. https://doi.org/10.1200/JCO.2016.71.6472. Epub 2017 Jun 14. PMID: 28613956
23. Brose MS, Robinson B, Sherman SI, Krajewska J, Lin CC, Vaisman F, Hoff AO, Hitre E, Bowles DW, Hernando J, Faoro L, Banerjee K, Oliver JW, Keam B, Capdevila J. Cabozantinib for radioiodine-refractory differentiated thyroid cancer (COSMIC-311): a randomised, double-blind, placebo-controlled, phase 3 trial. Lancet Oncol. 2021;22(8):1126–38. https://doi.org/10.1016/S1470-2045(21)00332-6. Epub 2021 Jul 5. PMID: 34237250

24. Busaidy NL, Konda B, Wei L, Wirth LJ, Devine C, Daniels GA, DeSouza JA, Poi M, Seligson ND, Cabanillas ME, Sipos JA, Ringel MD, Eisfeld AK, Timmers C, Shah MH. Dabrafenib Versus Dabrafenib + Trametinib in BRAF-mutated radioactive iodine refractory differentiated thyroid cancer: results of a randomized, Phase 2, open-label multicenter trial. Thyroid. 2022;32(10):1184–92. https://doi.org/10.1089/thy.2022.0115. Epub 2022 Jul 5. PMID: 35658604; PMCID: PMC9595631
25. Waguespack SG, Drilon A, Lin JJ, Brose MS, McDermott R, Almubarak M, Bauman J, Casanova M, Krishnamurthy A, Kummar S, Leyvraz S, Oh DY, Park K, Sohal D, Sherman E, Norenberg R, Silvertown JD, Brega N, Hong DS, Cabanillas ME. Efficacy and safety of larotrectinib in patients with TRK fusion-positive thyroid carcinoma. Eur J Endocrinol. 2022;186(6):631–43. https://doi.org/10.1530/EJE-21-1259. PMID: 35333737; PMCID: PMC9066591
26. Chou R, Dana T, Haymart M, Leung AM, Tufano RP, Sosa JA, Ringel MD. Active surveillance versus thyroid surgery for differentiated thyroid cancer: a systematic review. Thyroid. 2022;32(4):351–67. https://doi.org/10.1089/thy.2021.0539. Epub 2022 Mar 17. PMID: 35081743
27. Asimakopoulos P, Nixon IJ, Shaha AR. Differentiated and medullary thyroid cancer: surgical management of cervical lymph nodes. Clin Oncol (R Coll Radiol). 2017;29(5):283–9. https://doi.org/10.1016/j.clon.2017.01.001. Epub 2017 Jan 13. PMID: 28094086; PMCID: PMC5541897
28. Konstantinidis A, Stang M, Roman SA, Sosa JA. Surgical management of medullary thyroid carcinoma. Updat Surg. 2017;69(2):151–60. https://doi.org/10.1007/s13304-017-0443-y. Epub 2017 Apr 13. PMID: 28409442
29. Tuttle RM, Ganly I. Risk stratification in medullary thyroid cancer: moving beyond static anatomic staging. Oral Oncol. 2013;49(7):695–701. https://doi.org/10.1016/j.oraloncology.2013.03.443. Epub 2013 Apr 16. PMID: 23601563
30. Meijer JA, le Cessie S, van den Hout WB, Kievit J, Schoones JW, Romijn JA, Smit JW. Calcitonin and carcinoembryonic antigen doubling times as prognostic factors in medullary thyroid carcinoma: a structured meta-analysis. Clin Endocrinol. 2010;72(4):534–42. https://doi.org/10.1111/j.1365-2265.2009.03666.x. Epub 2009 Jun 26. PMID: 19563448
31. Gawlik T, d'Amico A, Szpak-Ulczok S, Skoczylas A, Gubała E, Chorąży A, Gorczewski K, Włoch J, Jarząb B. The prognostic value of tumor markers doubling times in medullary thyroid carcinoma—preliminary report. Thyroid Res. 2010;3(1):10. https://doi.org/10.1186/1756-6614-3-10. PMID: 21047422; PMCID: PMC2987862
32. Wells SA Jr, Robinson BG, Gagel RF, Dralle H, Fagin JA, Santoro M, Baudin E, Elisei R, Jarzab B, Vasselli JR, Read J, Langmuir P, Ryan AJ, Schlumberger MJ. Vandetanib in patients with locally advanced or metastatic medullary thyroid cancer: a randomized, double-blind phase III trial. J Clin Oncol. 2012;30(2):134–41. https://doi.org/10.1200/JCO.2011.35.5040. Epub 2011 Oct 24. Erratum in: J Clin Oncol. 2013 31(24):3049. PMID: 22025146; PMCID: PMC3675689
33. Schlumberger M, Elisei R, Müller S, Schöffski P, Brose M, Shah M, Licitra L, Krajewska J, Kreissl MC, Niederle B, Cohen EEW, Wirth L, Ali H, Clary DO, Yaron Y, Mangeshkar M, Ball D, Nelkin B, Sherman S. Overall survival analysis of EXAM, a phase III trial of cabozantinib in patients with radiographically progressive medullary thyroid carcinoma. Ann Oncol. 2017;28(11):2813–9. https://doi.org/10.1093/annonc/mdx479. PMID: 29045520; PMCID: PMC5834040
34. Wirth LJ, Sherman E, Robinson B, Solomon B, Kang H, Lorch J, Worden F, Brose M, Patel J, Leboulleux S, Godbert Y, Barlesi F, Morris JC, Owonikoko TK, Tan DSW, Gautschi O, Weiss J, de la Fouchardière C, Burkard ME, Laskin J, Taylor MH, Kroiss M, Medioni J, Goldman JW, Bauer TM, Levy B, Zhu VW, Lakhani N, Moreno V, Ebata K, Nguyen M, Heirich D, Zhu EY, Huang X, Yang L, Kherani J, Rothenberg SM, Drilon A, Subbiah V, Shah MH, Cabanillas ME. Efficacy of Selpercatinib in RET-altered thyroid cancers. N Engl J Med. 2020;383(9):825–35. https://doi.org/10.1056/NEJMoa2005651. PMID: 32846061; PMCID: PMC10777663

35. Are C, Shaha AR. Anaplastic thyroid carcinoma: biology, pathogenesis, prognostic factors, and treatment approaches. Ann Surg Oncol. 2006;13:453–64. https://doi.org/10.1245/ASO.2006.05.042.
36. Subbiah V, Kreitman RJ, Wainberg ZA, Cho JY, Schellens JHM, Soria JC, Wen PY, Zielinski C, Cabanillas ME, Urbanowitz G, Mookerjee B, Wang D, Rangwala F, Keam B. Dabrafenib and Trametinib Treatment in Patients With Locally Advanced or Metastatic BRAF V600-Mutant Anaplastic Thyroid Cancer. J Clin Oncol. 2018;36(1):7–13. https://doi.org/10.1200/JCO.2017.73.6785. Epub 2017 Oct 26. PMID: 29072975; PMCID: PMC5791845
37. Pembrolizumab, Dabrafenib, and Trametinib Before Surgery for the Treatment of BRAF-Mutated Anaplastic Thyroid Cancer. https://clinicaltrials.gov/study/NCT04675710
38. Xiang J, Wang Z, Sun W, Zhang H. A relook at the 8th edition of the AJCC TNM staging system of anaplastic thyroid carcinoma: a SEER-based study. Clin Endocrinol. 2021;94(4):700–10. https://doi.org/10.1111/cen.14371. Epub 2020 Dec 26. PMID: 33368530
39. Glaser SM, Mandish SF, Gill BS, Balasubramani GK, Clump DA, Beriwal S. Anaplastic thyroid cancer: prognostic factors, patterns of care, and overall survival. Head Neck. 2016;38(Suppl 1):E2083–90. https://doi.org/10.1002/hed.24384. Epub 2016 Feb 19. PMID: 26894506
40. Pezzi TA, Mohamed ASR, Sheu T, Blanchard P, Sandulache VC, Lai SY, Cabanillas ME, Williams MD, Pezzi CM, Lu C, Garden AS, Morrison WH, Rosenthal DI, Fuller CD, Gunn GB. Radiation therapy dose is associated with improved survival for unresected anaplastic thyroid carcinoma: outcomes from the National Cancer Data Base. Cancer. 2017;123(9):1653–61. https://doi.org/10.1002/cncr.30493. Epub 2016 Dec 27. PMID: 28026871; PMCID: PMC5906051
41. Ain KB, Egorin MJ, DeSimone PA. Treatment of anaplastic thyroid carcinoma with paclitaxel: phase 2 trial using ninety-six-hour infusion. Collaborative Anaplastic Thyroid Cancer Health Intervention Trials (CATCHIT) Group. Thyroid. 2000;10(7):587–94. https://doi.org/10.1089/thy.2000.10.587. PMID: 10958311
42. Prasongsook N, Kumar A, Chintakuntlawar AV, Foote RL, Kasperbauer J, Molina J, Garces Y, Ma D, Wittich MAN, Rubin J, Richardson R, Morris J, Hay I, Fatourechi V, McIver B, Ryder M, Thompson G, Grant C, Richards M, Sebo TJ, Rivera M, Suman V, Jenkins SM, Smallridge RC, Bible KC. Survival in response to multimodal therapy in anaplastic thyroid cancer. J Clin Endocrinol Metab. 2017;102(12):4506–14. https://doi.org/10.1210/jc.2017-01180. PMID: 29029287
43. Maniakas A, Zafereo M, Cabanillas ME. Anaplastic thyroid cancer: new horizons and challenges. Endocrinol Metab Clin N Am. 2022;51(2):391–401. https://doi.org/10.1016/j.ecl.2021.11.020. Epub 2022 May 4. PMID: 35662448
44. Maniakas A, Dadu R, Busaidy NL, et al. Evaluation of overall survival in patients with anaplastic thyroid carcinoma, 2000–2019. JAMA Oncol. 2020;6(9):1397–404. https://doi.org/10.1001/jamaoncol.2020.3362.
45. Rodrigo JP, Hernandez-Prera JC, Randolph GW, Zafereo ME, Hartl DM, Silver CE, Suárez C, Owen RP, Bradford CR, Mäkitie AA, Shaha AR, Bishop JA, Rinaldo A, Ferlito A. Parathyroid cancer: an update. Cancer Treat Rev. 2020;86:102012. https://doi.org/10.1016/j.ctrv.2020.102012. Epub 2020 Mar 19. PMID: 32247225
46. Eldaya RW, Calle S, Wong FC, Learned KO, Wintermark M. Parathyroid carcinoma: imaging features of initial presentation and recurrence. A single center experience. Neuroradiol J. 2024;37(1):92–106. https://doi.org/10.1177/19714009231212361. Epub 2023 Nov 7. PMID: 37934201; PMCID: PMC10863576
47. Hsu KT, Sippel RS, Chen H, Schneider DF. Is central lymph node dissection necessary for parathyroid carcinoma? Surgery. 2014;156(6):1336–41. https://doi.org/10.1016/j.surg.2014.08.005. discussion 1341. Epub 2014 Nov 11. PMID: 25456903; PMCID: PMC4254726
48. Solórzano CC, Carneiro-Pla DM, Lew JI, Rodgers SE, Montano R, Irvin GL 3rd. Intraoperative parathyroid hormone monitoring in patients with parathyroid cancer. Ann Surg Oncol. 2007;14(11):3216–22. https://doi.org/10.1245/s10434-007-9590-6. Epub 2007 Sep 6. PMID: 17805932

49. Armstrong VL, Vaghaiwalla TM, Saghira C, Chen CB, Wang Y, Anantharaj J, Ackin M, Lew JI. A >50% intraoperative parathyroid hormone decrease into normal reference range predicts complete excision of malignancy in patients with parathyroid carcinoma. J Surg Res. 2023;S0022-4804(23):00646–7. https://doi.org/10.1016/j.jss.2023.11.074. Epub ahead of print. PMID: 38155027
50. Erickson LA, Mete O, Juhlin CC, Perren A, Gill AJ. Overview of the 2022 WHO classification of parathyroid tumors. Endocr Pathol. 2022;33(1):64–89. https://doi.org/10.1007/s12022-022-09709-1. Epub 2022 Feb 17. PMID: 35175514
51. Gao Y, Wang P, Lu J, Pan B, Guo D, Zhang Z, Wang A, Zhang M, Sun J, Wang W, Liang Z. Diagnostic significance of parafibromin expression in parathyroid carcinoma. Hum Pathol. 2022;127:28–38. https://doi.org/10.1016/j.humpath.2022.05.014. Epub 2022 May 30. PMID: 35654240
52. Sun XM, Pang F, Zhuang SM, Xie LE, Zhong QY, Liu TR. Tumor size rather than the thyroid invasion affects the prognosis of parathyroid carcinoma without lymph node or distant metastasis. Eur Arch Otorrinolaringol. 2022;279(9):4587–94. https://doi.org/10.1007/s00405-022-07403-w. Epub 2022 May 21. PMID: 35596806
53. Landry CS, Wang TS, Asare EA, Grogan RH, Junt JL, Ridge JA, Rohren E, Shah JP, Subramaniam RM, Brierley JD, Seethala RR, Perrier ND, "Chapter 75. Parathyroid" American College of Surgeons, and American Joint Committee on Cancer. Collaborative Staging Task Force. Ajcc cancer staging system (version Version 9). In: Mahul B, editor. Amin and Stephen B Edge Version. 9th ed. Chicago, IL: American College of Surgeons; 2022.
54. Thwin M, Mihai R. Parathyroid cancer: updates and postoperative surveillance imaging. Surg Oncol Clin N Am. 2023;32(2):271–8. https://doi.org/10.1016/j.soc.2022.10.004. PMID: 36925184
55. Silverberg SJ, Rubin MR, Faiman C, Peacock M, Shoback DM, Smallridge RC, Schwanauer LE, Olson KA, Klassen P, Bilezikian JP. Cinacalcet hydrochloride reduces the serum calcium concentration in inoperable parathyroid carcinoma. J Clin Endocrinol Metab. 2007;92(10):3803–8. https://doi.org/10.1210/jc.2007-0585. Epub 2007 Jul 31. PMID: 17666472
56. Teleanu MV, Fuss CT, Paramasivam N, Pirmann S, Mock A, Terkamp C, Kircher S, Landwehr LS, Lenschow C, Schlegel N, Stenzinger A, Jahn A, Fassnacht M, Glimm H, Hübschmann D, Fröhling S, Kroiss M. Targeted therapy of advanced parathyroid carcinoma guided by genomic and transcriptomic profiling. Mol Oncol. 2023;17(7):1343–55. https://doi.org/10.1002/1878-0261.13398. Epub 2023 Apr 11. PMID: 36808802; PMCID: PMC10323885
57. Kutahyalioglu M, Nguyen HT, Kwatampora L, Clarke C, Silva A, Ibrahim E, Waguespack SG, Cabanillas ME, Jimenez C, Hu MI, Sherman SI, Kopetz S, Broaddus R, Dadu R, Wanland K, Williams M, Zafereo M, Perrier N, Busaidy NL. Genetic profiling as a clinical tool in advanced parathyroid carcinoma. J Cancer Res Clin Oncol. 2019;145(8):1977–86. https://doi.org/10.1007/s00432-019-02945-9. Epub 2019 Jul 15. PMID: 31309300
58. Rozhinskaya L, Pigarova E, Sabanova E, Mamedova E, Voronkova I, Krupinova J, Dzeranova L, Tiulpakov A, Gorbunova V, Orel N, Zalian A, Melnichenko G, Dedov I. Diagnosis and treatment challenges of parathyroid carcinoma in a 27-year-old woman with multiple lung metastases. Endocrinol Diabetes Metab Case Rep. 2017;2017:16–0113. https://doi.org/10.1530/EDM-16-0113. PMID: 28458892; PMCID: PMC5404464
59. Akirov A, Asa SL, Larouche V, Mete O, Sawka AM, Jang R, Ezzat S. The clinicopathological spectrum of parathyroid carcinoma. Front Endocrinol (Lausanne). 2019;10:731. https://doi.org/10.3389/fendo.2019.00731. PMID: 31708875; PMCID: PMC6819433
60. Lenschow C, Fuss CT, Kircher S, Buck A, Kickuth R, Reibetanz J, Wiegering A, Stenzinger A, Hübschmann D, Germer CT, Fassnacht M, Fröhling S, Schlegel N, Kroiss M. Case report: abdominal lymph node metastases of parathyroid carcinoma: diagnostic workup, molecular diagnosis, and clinical management. Front Endocrinol (Lausanne). 2021;12:643328. https://doi.org/10.3389/fendo.2021.643328. PMID: 33833736; PMCID: PMC8021949

Surgical Oncology: Review Questions and Suggested Answers

Review Questions

1. A 55-year-old healthy woman presents with jaundice (total bilirubin of 12 mg/dL). She undergoes ERCP and EUS showing a mass in the head of pancreas with abutment along the portal vein around 60 degrees. Cytology confirms adenocarcinoma. The Ca 19-9 is 1900 U/mL and bilirubin is now 1.0 mg/dL after biliary stent placement. Describe any further workup and initial treatment plan with rationale.
2. A 55-year-old healthy woman is diagnosed with a new pancreatic head adenocarcinoma that appears resectable by initial imaging. During operation for planned pancreatoduodenectomy procedure (Whipple), the surgeon discovers involvement of the first jejunal vein branch during dissection. The patient did not receive chemotherapy or radiation prior to operation. Describe intraoperative decision-making given this unexpected finding.
3. A 75-year-old man with history of coronary artery disease is diagnosed with a new pancreatic head adenocarcinoma that appears resectable by initial imaging and undergoes operation for planned pancreatoduodenectomy procedure (Whipple). During the porta hepatis dissection, a test clamp is placed across the gastroduodenal artery (GDA) resulting in loss of pulse in the proper hepatic artery. Describe the next steps of operation given this unexpected finding.
4. A 55-year-old healthy woman is diagnosed with a new pancreatic head adenocarcinoma. Two weeks after pancreatoduodenectomy procedure (Whipple), she presents to the Emergency Department with three episodes of bloody emesis. A surgical drain remains in place with gray, cloudy fluid consistent with pancreatic leak. Hemoglobin and vitals are stable. Describe workup and management of this patient.
5. A 65-year-old healthy man has distal gastric cancer with obstructive symptoms and node-positive disease by clinical staging (uT3N1 by EUS). Describe next steps in management with rationale.

6. A 65-year-old healthy man has distal gastric cancer with node-positive disease by clinical staging (uT3N1 by EUS). During the first two cycles of FLOT chemotherapy, he requires increasingly frequent transfusions due to anemia and associated melena. Repeat upper endoscopy confirms slow bleeding from the tumor. What are next steps in management with rationale?
7. A 56-year-old man with no significant medical history undergoes right hepatectomy and porta hepatis lymphadenectomy for intrahepatic cholangiocarcinoma. Margins are negative and there is one of four porta hepatis lymph nodes positive for adenocarcinoma. Describe next steps in management for the patient with rationale.
8. A 70-year-old woman presents with painless jaundice. On CT scan she is found to have intra- and extrahepatic biliary dilation without pancreatic ductal dilation. There are indeterminate hypodense lesions in segments II and VI. Describe the next steps in management of the patient.
9. A 65-year-old woman undergoes laparoscopic cholecystectomy for acute cholecystitis. Pathologic examination shows adenocarcinoma invading the perimuscular connective tissue on a cauterized surface (the specimen was not oriented). Review of preoperative imaging shows enlarged lymph nodes near the portal vein and no liver lesions. Describe next steps in management.
10. A 73-year-old man without cirrhosis presents with abdominal pain and weight loss. RUQ ultrasound shows a liver mass, and MRI liver protocol confirms a LIRADS-5 mass in the right liver measuring 6 cm in diameter involving segments 6 and 7. AFP level is 568. Describe next steps in management with rationale.
11. A 73-year-old man without cirrhosis presents with abdominal pain and weight loss. RUQ ultrasound shows a liver mass, and MRI liver protocol confirms a large infiltrating mass in the right liver with tumor invasion into the right portal vein and four small satellite tumors around the primary mass. AFP level is 2350. Describe next steps in management with rationale.
12. A 58-year-old man with cirrhosis undergoes surveillance ultrasound showing a liver mass. RUQ ultrasound shows a liver mass, and MRI liver protocol confirms a LIRADS-5 mass in the right liver measuring 6 cm in diameter involving segments 6 and 7. AFP level is normal, total bilirubin is 0.8, INR and Cr are 1.0, albumin is 3.6, and platelet count is 57,000. Describe next steps in management with rationale.
13. A 39-year-old average-risk woman presents to discuss breast cancer screening. She has no family history of breast cancer. When should she begin image screening for breast cancer and what information would you tell her about screening imaging?
14. A 37-year-old woman presents to discuss breast cancer screening. Her mother was diagnosed with breast cancer at age 46. When should she begin image screening and what information would you tell her about screening imaging?
15. An 18-year-old woman wishes to discuss breast cancer screening. She received thoracic radiotherapy for Hodgkin's lymphoma at age ten and has no family history of breast cancer. When should she begin image screening for breast cancer and what information would you tell her about screening imaging?

16. A 30-year-old average-risk transgender woman presents to discuss breast cancer screening. She has received seven years of hormone therapy. At what age should image screening begin and what else would you tell her about image screening?
17. A 31-year-old woman undergoes mammogram for a palpable unilateral mobile breast mass demonstrating BIRADS-3 characteristics. She has no other symptoms. What is the next best step?
18. A 55-year-old woman presents with unilateral nipple inversion and retraction without palpable mass on physical exam. Diagnostic mammogram demonstrates a BIRADS-4 lesion. What is the next best step?
19. A 65-year-old woman undergoes unilateral skin-sparing mastectomy with SLN biopsy for a 2 cm invasive ductal carcinoma. The nodes are not palpable however pathology returns one-fourth lymph nodes positive. Margins are negative. What is the next best step in management?
20. A 59-year-old woman undergoes unilateral skin-sparing mastectomy with SLN biopsy for DCIS. Pathology returns a 1.0 cm invasive ductal carcinoma, ER/PR+ and HER2+, and nodes negative. What is the next best step in management?
21. A 35-year-old woman undergoes unilateral SSM with SLN biopsy for DCIS. Pathology returns a 1.5 cm IDC ER/PR- and HER2+. pN0. OncotypeDX is 26. What is the next best step in management?
22. A 75-year-old woman undergoes right mastectomy and SLN biopsy for IDC. She is stage IIA with high-risk features and is advised to undergo adjuvant chemotherapy. She refuses. One year later, she develops a large painful, immobile mass in the ipsilateral axilla. Core biopsy demonstrates benign lymphoid tissue. What is the next best step in management?
23. A 55-year-old healthy patient is referred from the plastic surgeon after a skin graft for a 3 cm squamous cell carcinoma (SCC), poorly differentiated, with lymphovascular invasion. Margins are negative. They are concerned that the patient needs further care. On physical exam, there is no lymphadenopathy. What other considerations should you have for the patient?
24. A 72-year-old woman with a 4 cm Merkel cell carcinoma (MCC) of the leg has palpable lymphadenopathy. Staging imaging is without distant disease and biopsy proves MCC in the palpable nodes. The patient receives neoadjuvant immunotherapy with an excellent response on PET. She undergoes a wide local excision and inguinal node dissection. Final pathology reveals a complete pathologic response (pCR). Should this patient get any further therapy?
25. A 90-year-old man with an extensive history of sun damage presents with multiple lesions on his scalp. Two of the lesions are biopsy-proven well-differentiated squamous cell carcinoma (SCC). The Mohs surgeon removes both of those, and there is now a 10 × 8 cm (large) defect on the apex of the patient's scalp with persistent positive margins. How do you advise this patient?
26. A 55-year-old woman with a history of right breast cancer 7 years ago (partial mastectomy, sentinel lymph node biopsy, and radiation) presents with a bruise on the right outer breast. A dermatologist does a biopsy showing high-grade angiosarcoma. How would you manage this patient?

27. A 75-year-old-woman is four weeks after completion of chemoradiation for moderately differentiated anal squamous cell carcinoma. While the lesion appears to be smaller, it is still there. How long would you wait to consider surgical resection?
28. The patient from question 27 has residual local disease at 6 months. They also have biopsy-proven inguinal nodal disease on the right which was also radiated. There is still palpable nodal disease and repeat biopsy shows residual disease. Staging imaging has no distant disease. How would you treat this patient?
29. A 60-year-old man is sent to medical oncology a month after a sigmoid resection for a T3N2M0 grade 2 neuroendocrine tumor. Postoperative somatostatin PET shows a pelvic lymph node near the anastomosis that is 1.5 cm in size with a high SUV, suggestive of residual nodal disease. Medical oncology would like you to take out this lymph node so the patient is disease free.
30. A 72-year-old woman has a growing pigmented lesion of the back. Biopsy shows a melanoma with a depth of 2.2 mm transected at the base, with ulceration, mitotic rate 3/mm^2, and presence of regression. A wide excision and sentinel lymph node biopsy are done. In the left axilla, two of three sentinel nodes are positive, the largest measuring 0.4 mm. In the right axilla, all nodes were negative. What is the next treatment plan?
31. A 54-year-old woman has a history of melanoma excised from the pretibial area three years ago with wide excision and sentinel lymph node biopsy. Final path was pT2aN0Mx. She now presents with raised, pigmented lesions in the lower thigh. What is the initial workup? What is the treatment if biopsy shows intransit lesion? How does the treatment plan change if the amount of disease is not resectable?
32. A patient is referred after laparoscopic appendectomy for acute appendicitis. Pathology shows a low-grade appendiceal mucinous neoplasm. What further information or workup is needed, and how would you evaluate for treatment options?
33. Ten years following distal gastrectomy for a gastric antral GIST, a 75-year-old man presents with multiple (six total) peritoneal masses. Biopsy confirms recurrent, metastatic GIST with an exon 9 mutation. What treatment modifications are necessary in this patient?

Suggested Answers

1. The patient has a persistent elevation of CA 19-9 after resolution of jaundice. At a minimum, CT CAP with contrast is needed for complete staging as well as further characterization of tumor as resectable, borderline, or locally advanced. If the CT scan confirms less than 180-degree abutment of the vein, the mass is resectable. CT/PET scan is a reasonable adjunct to evaluate for occult metastatic disease given the high CA 19-9, especially if any indeterminate areas show on CT CAP. If no metastatic disease is found, up-front surgical resection followed by adjuvant therapy with mFOLFIRINOX should be the goal. Given

the high CA 19-9 and vein abutment, neoadjuvant chemotherapy or a perioperative chemotherapy approach with either mFOLFIRINOX or gemcitabine and nab-paclitaxel is also an acceptable treatment plan.
2. Involvement of the first jejunal branch by tumor is considered locally advanced unresectable. In this case, the surgeon must determine if ligation of the branch is feasible without need to resect SMV within the deep mesentery. Resection of the distal SMV is often not feasible as there remains no adequate distal target for venous reconstruction. If the vein can be ligated with preservation of the SMV, this is reasonable to do. It is also reasonable to abort the operation with this finding and plan for chemotherapy or chemoradiation.
3. This situation usually arises in the setting of celiac artery stenosis. Ligation of the GDA may result in diminished or loss of flow within the proper hepatic artery. This can result in liver ischemia or poor healing of the biliary anastomosis postoperatively. Options are to abort this operation which must be considered in more frail patients or those less likely to survive serious postoperative complications. Another option is to ligate the GDA and plan for arterial bypass if proper hepatic arterial blood flow is compromised. In that case, one should consider total pancreatectomy especially if the pancreas gland is soft or pancreas duct small, increasing the risk of postoperative pancreatic leak. A pancreatic leak with arterial bypass can result in graft injury leading to major postoperative hemorrhage.
4. One of the most serious complications after Whipple operation is hemorrhage from the gastroduodenal artery stump. This is most common in the setting of pancreatic leak. The bleeding may manifest as either intraperitoneal blood or upper gastrointestinal bleeding. In this patient, the authors recommend admission to an intensive care unit, large bore IV access, and urgent consultation with both gastroenterology and interventional radiology. CT angiogram in a hemodynamically stable patient is a reasonable first study. In hemodynamically unstable patients, we prefer emergent abdominal angiography. Upper endoscopy has a role, and given bleeding ulcer and gastritis are also in the differential diagnosis.
5. One should consider up-front surgical resection in a patient with gastric cancer and obstructive symptoms without metastatic disease. Since perioperative chemotherapy is associated with superior outcomes, another consideration may be feeding jejunostomy and neoadjuvant chemotherapy. For the latter, the surgeon must be thoughtful about placement of the j-tube in terms of distance from the ligament of Treitz since eventual reconstruction may require Roux-en-Y gastrojejunostomy or esophagojejunostomy.
6. It is reasonable to proceed with operation at this point if anemia is complicating perioperative chemotherapy. In the metastatic disease setting, radiation oncology should evaluate to see if palliative radiation can slow or stop bleeding from the primary tumor.
7. Assuming the patient made adequate recovery from operation, referral to medical oncology is appropriate to evaluate for adjuvant therapy options. At the time of this publication, adjuvant therapy for six months with oral capecitabine is

appropriate. Regimens like gemcitabine, cisplatin, and durvalumab are appropriate for locally advanced or metastatic disease.
8. Endoscopic retrograde cholangiopancreatography with brushings and stent placement is appropriate in this patient with jaundice and concern for malignant etiology. A liver protocol MRI with MRCP reconstruction may help define the level of stricture and further characterize the liver lesions.
9. The patient has an indication for second operation, specifically segment IVb/V hepatectomy with porta hepatis lymphadenectomy.
10. If the patient is a candidate for major hepatectomy, surgical resection is the preferred therapy for this patient without cirrhosis. The surgeon should determine the volume of the future liver remnant to be sure it is adequate if right hepatectomy will be needed. In this patient with a mass in segments 6/7, a right posterior sectorectomy may be feasible.
11. This patient has a diffusely infiltrating tumor with multiple nodules and portal vein invasion. This is an advanced stage C hepatocellular carcinoma by BCLC criteria. Recommended initial treatment is with systemic therapy (atezo/bev or durvalumab/tremelimumab). In this case, regional therapy options may be feasible since the tumor is limited to the right liver.
12. This patient has cirrhosis with portal hypertension and compensated liver function. The HCC is early stage (A) by BCLC criteria. The patient should be evaluated for liver transplant. Since the mass is 6 cm in size, initial therapy with chemoembolization may be best as a bridging therapy even if transplant is the ultimate goal.
13. The patient should begin annual screening mammography at age 40. Historically, age 40–50 was a common recommendation. Currently, many guidelines recommend age 40 for an average risk patient.
14. The patient should begin annual screening mammography whenever her age is ten years younger than her mother (age 36), unless another first-degree relative was diagnosed at a younger age. If her mother was premenopausal at age 46, genetic counseling should be done.
15. The patient should begin annual screening mammography at age 25. Annual screening mammogram with tomosynthesis is indicated eight years after radiation to the chest but not prior to age 25.
16. The patient should begin annual screening mammography at age 40 because more than five years of hormone use increases the risk of developing breast cancer.
17. The patient should have a physical exam in six months with diagnostic mammogram or ultrasound. It is not necessary to proceed with core needle biopsy for a BIRADS-3 lesion.
18. The patient should undergo a core needle biopsy of the concerning area.
19. The patient should undergo regional node radiation and adjuvant chemotherapy.
20. The patient should undergo adjuvant therapy with trastuzumab and endocrine therapy with anastrozole.

21. This premenopausal patient should be treated with adjuvant chemotherapy and trastuzumab with ovarian suppression/ablation.
22. The physician should discuss the biopsy result with breast radiology. If the biopsy is discordant, an excisional biopsy should be done next.
23. Sentinel lymph node biopsy (SLNB) is preferred but not always possible at the time of index operation. High-risk SCC should offer SLNB, especially in younger, healthy patients.
24. As of this publication, there is no role for further therapy. Radiation is a consideration for some patients with MCC; however, it is not indicated in this patient with a complete pathologic response after immunotherapy.
25. It is ill-advised to continue to resect more scalp tissue. One should consider shave biopsies a few centimeters away from the lesions to prove there is a larger field defect. One option is skin graft followed by definitive radiotherapy.
26. All sarcoma patients should be discussed at a multidisciplinary tumor board. For angiosarcoma, disease often extends microscopically past the visualized area of discoloration. An MRI should be obtained for planning purposes. While radiation is not generally used for secondary angiosarcoma, it can be for primary angiosarcoma. Recent data suggests the use of neoadjuvant chemotherapy (such as paclitaxel) can reduce local recurrence rates after resection.
27. Waiting six months for complete response is advised. If the disease begins to grow, consider restaging and APR or second-line therapy if metastatic disease. There is no role for sentinel lymph node biopsy.
28. Both APR and inguinal lymph node dissection are recommended. This can be at the same time as the APR or staged depending on patient's functional status. Even if the primary responds and the nodal basin does not, resection is recommended, with close monitoring of the primary and for metastatic disease.
29. While waiting for the patient to recover from the initial operation, it is reasonable to consider systemic therapy. It is important to consider this may not be a lymph node but rather peritoneal disease.
30. This patient has a stage IIIC (pT3bN2aM0) melanoma. They need full-body staging (we prefer CT-PET and brain MRI) and a referral to medical oncology to evaluate for adjuvant immunotherapy. Surveillance should also include ultrasound of the nodal basin (left axilla) every four months for two years and then every six months.
31. First, she needs a complete physical exam and biopsy. If biopsy is positive for melanoma, the patient needs complete staging imaging, perhaps CT-PET and brain MRI. If no other diseases, resection with adjuvant therapy is the ideal treatment. If the recurrence is a single, resectable lesion, then consider repeat sentinel lymph node biopsy. In the setting of a large area of disease, neoadjuvant immune checkpoint blockade and BRAF/MEK inhibition are options with later attempt at resection depending on response. For unresectable disease, options include LAG3 inhibition, T-vec, limb infusion, and limb perfusion. Referral to a tertiary center with experience treating intransit disease is a high priority.

32. Review of the operative and pathology reports is the first step to know margin status, whether the appendix was perforated and if the surgeon saw any other mucinous lesions. If this LAMN did not penetrate to the serosa or mesoappendix, margins are negative and have no perforation; the original operation was likely curative. Consider colonoscopy after recovery. If any of the above risk factors are present, follow national guidelines for surveillance. For a positive margin, consider ileocecectomy. Right hemicolectomy is not required as this disease does not spread to lymph nodes. If in the presence of residual or recurrent peritoneal disease, evaluate for cytoreduction and heated intraperitoneal chemotherapy (HIPEC). There is no good data to support prophylactic HIPEC in the absence of known disease.
33. The presence of an exon 9 mutation means the patient should get a higher dose of imatinib (800 mg/day) and that response rate is lower. There is a role for cytoreduction if the metastases are resectable. In general, we recommend imatinib in the neoadjuvant setting initially; however, operation may be indicated for other reasons besides cancer control, such as palliation of symptoms or tumor complication like bowel obstruction.

Index

A
Abdominal recurrence-free interval (AFRI), 302
Abdominal recurrence-free survival (ARFS), 302
Abdominoperineal resection (APR), 151, 365
Ablation, 139
Abnormal lymph nodes, characteristics of, 165
ACTICCA-1 trial, 37
Active surveillance, 171
Adenocarcinoma (AC), 71, 331–333, 359
   choice of therapy, 332
   diagnosis, 331
   evaluation and clinic stage, 332
   surveillance, 333
   polyp, 156
   risk factors for, 71
Adenoma, 32
Adenomyomatosis, 32
Adjuvant immunothcrapy, 365
Adjuvant systemic therapy, 170, 178
Adjuvant therapy, 37, 66, 73, 86, 87, 141, 153, 191, 235–237, 349
Adrenal adenoma, 123
Adrenal tumors
   ACC, 5
      American Joint Commission on Cancer 8th edition Staging, 7
      evaluation, 6, 7
      histology/pathology, 7
      incidence, 5
      presentation, 5
      prognosis, 8
      risk factors, 5
      surveillance, 8
      TNM categories, 7
      treatment, 8
   incidentalomas, 1
      borders, 3
      density, 2
      functional evaluation, 3
      growth rate, 3
      imaging, 1, 2
      laterality, 2
      size, 2
   pheochromocytoma, 9
      American Joint Commission on Cancer 8th edition Staging for, 12
      evaluation, 10, 11
      histology, 11
      presentation, 9
      prognosis, 14
      risk factors, 9
      surveillance, 14
      TNM Categories, 11
      treatment, 12, 13
Adrenal venous sampling, 4
Adrenocortical carcinoma (ACC), 5
   American Joint Commission on Cancer 8th edition Staging, 7
   evaluation, 6, 7
   histology/pathology, 7
   incidence, 5
   presentation, 5
   prognosis, 8
   risk factors, 5
   surveillance, 8
   TNM categories, 7
   treatment, 8
Adrenocorticotropic hormone, 6
Advanced Liver Cancer Prognostic System (ALCPS), 140
Aldosterone, 4, 6
Alpha-adrenergic blockade, 12, 13
Alpha blockade, 12
Alpha-fetoprotein, 136

Anal adenocarcinoma, 25
Anal canal, 20, 21
Anal cancer
  anal adenocarcinoma, 25
  anatomy, 21, 22
  choice of therapy, 150
  evaluation and staging, 149
  incidence rates, 22
  locoregional disease, 23, 25
  melanoma, 25
  metastatic disease, 25
  perianal basal cell carcinoma, 26
  radiotherapy, 155
  surgical therapy, 151
  verrucous carcinoma, 26
  workup and staging, 22
Anal squamous cell carcinoma (ASCC), 21, 147, 148, 150
Anal verge, 21
Anaplastic thyroid cancer, 347, 350
Anastrozole, 364
Angiosarcoma, 280, 286, 365
Aspiration, 45
Atezolizumab plus bevacizumab, 140
Atypical lipomatous tumors (ALT), 285
Avapritinib, 108

B

Barcelona Clinic Liver Cancer (BCLC) staging, 137
BARD1 mutation, 120
Basal cell skin cancer, 195, 201–202
  adjuvant therapy, 200
  choice of therapy, 198–203
  diagnosis, 195
  evaluation, 197
  management of recurrence, 203
  neoadjuvant therapy, 202
  nonoperative therapy, 198
  surgical therapy, 199, 200
Benign incidentalomas, 2
Beta-adrenergic blockade, 12
Bevacizumab, 141, 154
Bilateral adrenalectomy, 4
Bilateral salpingo-oophorectomy (BSO), 120, 121
Biliary tract cancers (BTCs), 29
  diagnosis
    anatomic classification, 32
    clinical presentation, 31
    genetics, 31
    histology, 32
  epidemiology, 30, 31
  evaluation and staging, 33–35

  initial therapy, 36, 37
  locoregional therapies
    hepatic artery infusion pump, 38
    radiation, 38
    transarterial therapies, 38
  surveillance, 39
  systemic therapy
    adjuvant therapy, 37
    neoadjuvant therapy, 38
    options, 37
Binimetinib, 178
Biomarkers, 110
Bismuth-Corlette classification, perihilar cholangiocarcinoma, 33
BRCA1 mutation, 121
BRCA 2 mutation, 121
Breast cancers, 47–51, 54–64, 120, 360, 364
  adjuvant therapy, 66
  choice of therapy, 56
  diagnosis, 41, 43, 45, 52
    biopsy, 45
    clinical examination, 43
    environmental risk factors, 45
    familial risk factors, 46
    imaging, 43–45
    pathologic principles, 46, 52, 53
    screening, 42
  evaluation and clinical stage, 53, 54
  locally advanced and recurrent/metastatic disease, 66
  NAT, 65, 66
  radiation therapy, 67
  surgical therapy, 65
  surveillance, 67
Breast guidelines, 117–118
Breast Imaging Reporting and Data System (BIRADS), 44
Breast screening, 121
Bronchial/thymic carcinoid, 123
Buschke-Lowenstein tumor, 26

C

Cabozantinib, 141, 346, 349
Calcium channel blockade, 12
Cancer of Liver Italian Program (CLIP), 137
Cardiotoxicity, 67
Catecholamines, 4, 5
CDH1 mutation, 122
CDKN2A mutation, 122
Celiac artery stenosis, 363
Cervical dysplasia, 26
Cetuximab, 153, 154
Checkpoint inhibition, 171, 173
CHEK2 mutation, 122

Chemical shift analysis, 2
Chemoembolization, 364
Chemoradiation, 73, 362, 363
Chemotherapy, 13, 300, 303
ChemoXRT, 26
Cholangiocarcinoma, 32
Cholesterol polyp, 32
Cirrhosis, 133
Cisplatin, 13, 364
c-KIT mutation, 109
Clamp gastroduodenal artery (GDA), 230
Clear cell renal cell carcinoma, 130
Clinically positive node, 173
Clinically suspicious lymph nodes, biopsy of, 164
Cobimetinib, 178
Colon adenocarcinoma, 119, 128
Colon cancer, 150
   choice of therapy, 150
   evaluation and staging, 148
   surgical therapy, 151
Colon guidelines for testing, 118
Colonoscopy, 148, 156
Colorectal cancer (CRC), 147
   evaluation and staging, 149
   screening for, 148
Completion lymph node dissection (CLND), 171
Computed tomography (CT), 1, 6, 10, 101
Contralateral gland, 3
Contrast-enhanced mammography (CEM), 44
Core needle biopsy, 45, 364
Cushing's syndrome, 3
Cutaneous lichens amyloidosis, 123
Cutaneous melanoma
   advanced disease, 173
   clinical presentation and prognostication, 161–163
   epidemiology, 161
   evaluation and clinical staging
      diagnostic tests, 163–165
      imaging, 165
      lab tests, 165
   local disease
      adjuvant systemic therapy, 170
      surgery, 168, 169
   locally advanced disease, 170, 171
   local satellite/transit recurrence, 177
   metastatic disease, treatment, 178
   nodal recurrence, 177, 178
   RCT for surgical margins in, 169
   regional therapy, 176, 177
   survival, 168
   targeted therapy, 171, 172
   unresectable disease, treatment, 175
   WLE scar recurrence, 177
Cytoreduction, 366
Cytoreduction and heated intraperitoneal chemotherapy (CRS/HIPEC), 85
Cytoreductive surgery, 267, 272, 274
Cytotoxic chemotherapy, 351

D

Dabrafenib, 172, 178, 346
Dacarbazine, 13
Dasatinib, 108
Dermatofibrosarcoma protuberans (DFSP), 211, 288
   adjuvant therapy, 213
   choice of therapy, 212
   diagnosis, 211
   evaluation and clinical stage, 212
   neoadjuvant therapy, 214
   surgical therapy, 213
Dermatologic Cooperative Oncology Group—Selective Lymphadenectomy Trial (DeCOG-SLT), 171
Desmoids, 120, 280, 288, 320–322
Disease surveillance after chem-radiation, 24
Distal cholangiocarcinoma, 29
Distal extrahepatic cholangiocarcinoma (ECC), 35
   definition of, 32
   surgical principle, 36
Distal gastrectomy, 362
Distal gastric cancer, 359, 360
Distant metastasis, 56
Dostarlimab-gxly, 141
Dotatate PET, 2
Doxazosin, 12
Duodenal adenocarcinoma, 119
Duodenal screening, 124
Durvalumab, 140, 364
Dutch D1D2 lymphadenectomy trial, 85
Dysphagia, 76

E

Encorafenib, 178
Endocrine guidelines for genetic testing, 119–130
Endometrial carcinoma, 129
Endoscopic mucosal resection (EMR), 82
Endoscopic retrograde cholangiopancreatography (ERCP), 34, 364
Endoscopic submucosal dissection (ESD), 82
Endoscopic treatment for GIST, 106
Endoscopic ultrasound (EUS), 34, 72, 81, 97

Endoscopy, 96
Entrectinib, 108, 347
Epithelioid GISTs, 98
Epithelioid sarcoma, 281
Esophageal cancer
  complications after esophagectomy, 76
  management, 73
  palliative options for dysphagia, 76
  pretreatment evaluation, 72–73
  surgical management, 74–75
  surveillance, 76
  TNM Staging, 72
Esophagojejunostomy, 363
Ewing's sarcoma, 281
Excisional biopsy, 45
Extent of lymphadenectomy, 84, 152
External beam radiotherapy (EBRT), 13, 140
Extrahepatic cholangiocarcinoma (ECC), 29
  diagnosis, 31
  distal, 35
    definition of, 32
    surgical principle, 36
  epidemiology, 30
  perihilar
    definition of, 32
    liver transplantation, 37
    surgical principle, 36

F

Familial adenomatous polyposis (FAP), 119, 148
Familial papillary thyroid carcinoma, 343
Familial paraganglioma syndromes, 9
Fibrosarcoma, 281, 287
Fine-needle aspiration (FNA), 164, 341
5-fluorouracil (5-FU), 23, 152
Floxuridine (FUDR), 38
FOLFIRI (5-FU, Leucovorin, Irinotecan), 153
FOLFIRINOX, 154
FOLFOX, 37, 150, 153
Follicular cell-derived carcinoma, 343

G

Gallbladder adenocarcinoma (GC), 30
  diagnosis
    anatomic classification, 32
    clinical presentation, 31
    histology, 32
  epidemiology, 30, 31
  surgical principle, 36
  T stage, 35
Gastric adenocarcinoma, 120
Gastric cancers, 122, 363
  adjuvant therapy, 86, 87
  choice of therapy, 82
  diagnosis, 79
    environmental risk factors, 79, 80
    familial risk factors, 80
    pathologic principles, 80
  endoscopic therapy, 82
  evaluation and clinical stage, 81
  immunotherapy and biologic therapy, 88
  locally advanced and metastatic disease, 87
  radiation therapy, 88
  staging modalities, 81
  surgical therapy, 83, 85
  survival by clinical stage, 82
  TNM staging, 81
Gastric carcinoid, 123
Gastric conduit, 75
Gastric guidelines for genetic testing, 118–119
Gastric ulcers, 80
Gastrointestinal stromal tumors (GISTs), 283
  diagnosis, 97
    endoscopy, 96, 98
    histology, 98, 99
    imaging, 101
    immunohistochemistry, 100
    molecular analysis, 100
    symptoms, 95
  epidemiology, 94–95
  evaluation and clinical stage, 101
    follow-up, 105
    pathologic stage classification, 102, 103
    risk stratification, 103
  location of, 93
  pathophysiology, 95
  prognosis, 103, 104
  size, 94
  treatment
    endoscopic, 106
    medical, 106–110
    surgical, 105, 106
Gemcitabine, 364
Gene expression profile (GEP), 163
Genotyping, 100
GRETCH score, 139

H

Heated intraperitoneal chemotherapy (HIPEC), 155, 366
Hepatectomy, 36, 360, 364
Hepatic artery infusion chemotherapy, 141
Hepatic artery infusion pump, 38
Hepatocellular carcinoma (HCC), 134, 137, 138
  adjuvant therapy, 141

clinical trials for, 141–143
diagnosis
  biopsy, 136
  imaging, 135
  serum markers, 136
  staging, 136, 139
  symptoms, 135
epidemiology, 134, 135
hospice, 141
locoregional therapies, 139
staging, 137
surgical resection, 139
systemic therapy, 140
transplantation, 139
Hereditary diffuse gastric cancer (HDGC), 80
Hereditary nonpolyposis colorectal cancer (HNPCC), 80, 148
High-intensity focused ultrasound ablation (HIFU), 140
Hirschsprung disease, 123
Histotripsy, 140
Hospice, 260–261
Human papilloma virus (HPV), 19, 20
Hypercortisolism, 3, 4
Hyperproliferative cutaneous adverse events, 172
Hypertension, 9
Hyperthermic intraperitoneal chemotherapy (HIPEC), 267

I
ICC, 35
IL-2, 176
Ileal pouch – anal anastomosis, 119
Ileocecectomy, 366
Ileorectal anastomosis, 119
Imatinib, 366
Imatinib therapy, 107–109
Immunohistochemistry, 100
Immunosuppression, 162
Immunotherapy, 88
Immunotherapy trials, 170
Incidentalomas, 1
  borders, 3
  density, 2
  functional evaluation, 3
  growth rate, 3
  imaging, 1, 2
  laterality, 2
  size, 2
Inguinal lymph node dissection, 365
Intensity-modulated RT (IMRT), 23
Intraarterial chemotherapy (IACT), 140
Intraarterial radiotherapy, 140

Intrahepatic cholangiocarcinoma (ICC), 30, 35
diagnosis
  anatomic classification, 32
  clinical presentation, 31
epidemiology, 30
liver transplantation, 37
surgical principle, 36
Intralesional injection, 175
Intransit disease, 175
In-transit metastases, 174
Intraoperative decisions, 306
Intraoperative PTH (IoPTH), 352
Intraoperative radiation (IORT), 233
Iodine-123 (^{123}I)–labeled metaiodobenzyl guanidine (MIBG), 10
Iodine-131 meta-iodobenzylguanidine (^{131}I-MIBG), 13
Ipilimumab, 176, 178
Isolated limb infusion (ILI), 177
Isolated limb perfusion (ILP), 176, 177
Ivor Lewis esophagogastrectomy, 74

J
Jaundice, 359
Juvenile polyposis, 128

K
Kinase inhibitors, 346

L
Laparoscopic appendectomy, 362
Laparoscopic cholecystectomy, 360
Laparoscopic distal gastrectomy, 85
Laparoscopic techniques, 105
Large intestinal neuroendocrine tumors, 156
Large intestine cancers
  choice of therapy, 150, 151
  colorectal cancer, 148
  diagnosis
    risk factors, 148
    symptomatic cases, 147
  evaluation and staging, 148, 149
  metastatic cancer, management of, 153, 154
  peritoneal metastases, surgical resection of, 154, 155
  radiotherapy, 155
  surgical resection of liver and lung metastases, 154
  surgical therapy, 151, 152
  systemic therapy for nonmetastatic cancer, 152

Lauren classification system, 80
Leather-bottle-like stomach, 80
Leiomyosarcoma (LMS), 280, 285
Lenvatinib, 140, 141, 346
Leucovorin, 152
LiFraumeni, 129
Limited resectable disease, 175
Liposarcoma, 284–285
Liver-directed therapy, 38
Liver Imaging Reporting And Data System (LI-RADS) criteria, 135
Locally advanced disease, 66
Locoregional disease, 73
 chemotherapy, 23
 management of, 23, 25
Locoregional lymphadenectomy, 8
Locoregional therapies, 38, 139
Low-dose dexamethasone suppression test, 3
Lymphadenectomy, 308
Lymphatic mets, 174
Lymphoma, 336–338
Lynch syndrome, 80, 119, 125

M

Magnetic resonance imaging (MRI), 2, 6, 10, 44, 101
Malignant cutaneous adnexal tumors, 214, 215
Malignant fibrous histiocytoma (MFH), 284
Malignant melanoma, 161
Malignant peripheral nerve sheath tumors (MPNSTs), 288
Malignant pheochromocytoma, 10–12
Mammogram, 43
Mammography, 364
Mayo protocol, 37
McKeown esophagogastrectomy, 74
Medullary thyroid carcinoma (MTC), 339, 347
Melanoma, 25, 122, 161, 162, 166–168
 margins for wide local excision of, 169
 treatment, 362, 365
 see also Cutaneous melanoma
MelMarT-II, 168
MEN1 mutation, 122
MEN2A mutation, 123
MEN2B mutation, 124
Merkel cell carcinoma (MCC), 206, 210, 361
 adjuvant therapy, 208, 209
 choice of therapy, 205
 diagnosis, 203
 evaluation and clinical stage, 204, 205
 neoadjuvant therapy, 211
 nonoperative therapy, 207

 surgical therapy, 207, 208
Merkel cell polyomavirus (MCPyV), 204
Metastasectomy, 310–312
Metastatic cutaneous squamous cell carcinoma, 193–194
Metastatic directed therapy, 178
Metastatic disease, 25, 178
Metastatic GIST, 105, 109
mFOLFIRINOX, 363
MicroGISTs, 94
MicroRNAs, 110
Microsatellite-instability high (MSI-H), 151
Microsatellites, 174
Microscopic satellites, 175
Miettinen and Lasota risk classification, 107
Milan criteria, 139
Minimally invasive gastrectomy, 85
Minimally invasive surgical technique, 164
Mitomycin, 23
Mitotane, 8
MLH1 mutation, 125
Molecular Breast Imaging (MBI), 44
MRI, *see* Magnetic resonance imaging
MSH2 mutation, 126
MSH6 mutation, 127
Multicenter Selective Lymphadenectomy Trial-I (MSLT-I), 170
Multiple Endocrine Neoplasia Type II, 9
Multivisceral disease, 178
MUTYH mutation, 124
Myxofibrosarcoma, 287

N

Necrotic conduit, 76
Neoadjuvant chemotherapy, 363, 365
Neoadjuvant rectal cancer trials, 155
Neoadjuvant therapy (NAT), 38, 65, 174
Neoadjuvant treatment, 229
Neuroendocrine
 choice of therapy, 335
 diagnosis, 333, 334
 evaluation and clinic stage, 334, 335
 surveillance, 336
 tumor, 335
Neurofibromatosis 1 (NF1), 9, 124
Nigro protocol, 23
Nilotinib, 108
Nivolumab, 25, 140, 141, 172, 178
Nivolumab plus ipilimumab, 141
Nonmelanoma skin cancer, 185
Nonresectable disease, 14

O

Okuda system, 137
Oligometastatic disease, 178
Ongoing Optimal Perioperative Therapy for Incidental Gallbladder Cancer (OPT-IN) trial, 38
Open approach, 8
OPTiM study, 176
Oxaliplatin, 153, 155

P

P14ARF mutation, 122
PALB2 mutation, 124
Palliative care, 247, 248
    barriers, 248
    chronically ill, 249–251
    delivering serious news, 256–258
    opportunities and roles, 248
    REMAP, 257
    resources, 262
Palliative radiation, 363
Pancreas guidelines for genetic testing, 118
Pancreatic adenocarcinoma (PDAC), 225–227
Pancreatic cancer, 122, 234, 240
    adjuvant therapy, 235–237
    complications, 234–235
    diagnostic workup, 225–228
    metastatic, 237–240
    neoadjuvant treatment, 229
    primary tumor, 228–229
    surgical technical approach, 230–234
Pancreatic/duodenal neuroendocrine tumor, 123
Pancreatic head adenocarcinoma, 359
Pancreatic neuroendocrine tumors, 130
Pancreaticoduodenectomy, 230–235, 359
Panitumumab, 153, 154
Papillary thyroid carcinoma (PTC), 343
Paraganglioma, 130
Parathyroid adenoma, 123
Parathyroid cancer, 352, 353
Pembrolizumab, 25, 140, 141, 172, 178
Perianal basal cell carcinoma, 26
Perianal HSIL, 20
Perianal skin, 21
Perihilar cholangiocarcinoma, 29, 33
Perihilar extrahepatic cholangiocarcinoma (ECC), 35
    definition of, 32
    treatment
        liver transplantation, 37
        surgical principle, 36
Peritoneal cancer index (PCI), 154, 269
Peritoneal carcinomatosis index (PCI), 272
Peritoneal metastases, surgical resection of, 154, 155
Peritoneal surface disease severity score (PSDSS), 269
Peritoneal surface malignancies (PSM), 267
    diagnosis and workup, 268–270
    follow-up, 274
    primary peritoneal tumors, 271
    surgical treatment, 271–274
    treatment, 270–271
Persistent disease, 165
Phenoxybenzamine, 12
Pheochromocytoma, 4, 5, 9, 123, 130
    American Joint Commission on Cancer 8th edition Staging for, 12
    evaluation, 10, 11
    histology, 11
    presentation, 9
    prognosis, 14
    risk factors, 9
    surveillance, 14
    TNM Categories, 11
    treatment
        surgical resection, 12, 13
        systemic therapy, 13
Pheochromocytoma of the Adrenal gland Scaled Score (PASS) score, 11
Pituitary adenomas, 123
Plasma metanephrines, 4
Platelet-derived growth factor receptor alpha (PDGFRA), 95
PMS2 mutation, 127
Polypectomy, 156
Porta hepatis lymphadenectomy, 36, 360
Positron emission tomography (PET), 101
Post colectomy, 119
Postresection Evaluation of Recurrence-free Survival for Gastrointestinal Stromal Tumors With 5 Years of Adjuvant Imatinib (PERSIST-5) clinical trial, 107
Prague classification, 72
Premalignant neoplasms, 19, 20
Primary aldosteronism, 4
Prophylactic total gastrectomy, 122
Pseudomyxoma peritonei, 267, 268
PTEN (Cowdens), 125

R

RAD51C/D mutation, 128
Radiation therapy, 8, 23, 38, 67, 88, 170, 173, 177, 351, 365

Radiopharmaceutical therapy, 13
Ramucirumab, 141
Reconstruction, 232
Rectal adenocarcinomas, 149
Rectal cancer
  choice of therapy, 150
  evaluation and staging, 149
  radiotherapy, 155
  surgical therapy, 151
Regional therapy, 176, 177
Regorafenib, 141
Regorafenib larotrectinib, 108
Resectability, 228
Resectable disease, 14
Resectable nodal disease, 173
Retroperitoneum, 279, 284, 285, 291
Rhabdomyosarcoma (RMS), 281, 289
Risk of malignancy (ROM), 342
Risk reduction, 120, 130
Roux-en-Y esophagojejunostomy, 83
Roux-en-Y gastrojejunostomy, 363

S

Sarcoma guidelines for genetic testing, 119
Satellite metastases, 174
Self-expanding metal stent (SEMS), 230
Selpercatinib, 141, 349
Sentinel lymph node biopsy (SLNB), 164, 168, 169, 307, 365
Serum markers, 136
177-Lutetium-DOTATATE (^{177}Lu-DOTATATE), 13
Sex cord stromal tumors, 129
Siewert classification, 72
Single nucleotide polymorphisms (SNPs), 130
Sintilimab, 141
Skin cancer, 162
Skin punch biopsy, 45
SLNB, *see* Sentinel lymph node biopsy
SMAD4 mutation, 128
Soft tissue sarcomas (STS), 279, 283, 301–302
  characteristics, 280–282
  classification, 283–289
  clinical evaluation, 289–291
  diagnosis, 291–292
  extremity and trunk, 290, 306–307
  multidisciplinary management, 297–305
  radiation therapy, 312–313
  retroperitoneum, 291
  stage and grade, 293–297
  subtype special considerations, 292–293
  surgical technique, 305–312
Somatostatin receptor scintigraphy, 2
Sorafenib, 108, 140, 141, 346
Spindle-cell GISTs, 98
Squamous cell carcinoma (SCC), 19, 71, 361
Squamous cell skin cancer
  adjuvant therapy, 191
  choice of therapy, 190
  diagnosis, 185, 186
  evaluation, 187
  management of recurrence, 195
  neoadjuvant therapy, 195
  nonoperative therapy, 190
  surgical therapy, 190
Squamous intraepithelial lesions (SIL), 19
Stereotactic body radiation therapy (SBRT), 233
STK11, 128
Stomach adenocarcinoma, 128, 129
STORM trial, 143
Subtotal and distal gastrectomy, 83
Succinate dehydrogenase (SDH)-deficient GISTs, 100
Succinate dehydrogenase B subunit (SDHB), 14
Sunitinib, 13, 108, 109
Superficially invasive, 23
Suspicious metastases, 164
Suspicious skin lesions, 163
Sympathetic paraganglioma, 11, 12
Symptomatic metastatic disease, 178
Symptom management, 256
Synovial sarcoma, 281, 285
Systemic therapy, 8, 13, 25, 31, 140, 153–154, 173, 175, 178, 313–319, 364, 365

T

Talimogene laherparepvec (T-VEC), 175
Targeted therapy, 171, 172
Terazosin, 12
Therapeutic lymph node dissection (TLND), 173
Thyroid cancer, 339–342
Thyroid carcinoma, 120
Todani classification of choledochal cysts, 30
Tokyo score, 139
Topical imiquimod, 176
Total gastrectomy, 83
TP53, 129
Tracheoesophageal fistula, 76
Trametinib, 172, 178

Transarterial chemoembolization (TACE), 38, 139, 141
Transarterial radioembolization (TARE), 38
Transarterial therapies, 38
Transcutaneous electrical nerve stimulation (TENS), 251
Transhiatal esophagogastrectomy, 75
Trastuzumab, 364, 365
Tremelimumab plus durvalumab, 140
Trichloroacetic acid (TCA), 20
Triple-negative breast cancer (TNBC), 65
T-VEC, 175, 176, 365

U
Ultrasound (US), 1, 43, 165
Unilateral skin-sparing mastectomy, 361
Unresectable disease, 175
Urine metanephrines, 5

V
Vandetanib, 349
Variants of undetermined significance (VUS), 131
Vascular anatomy, 151
Vasopressors, 13
Vein resection, 232
Vemurafenib, 172, 178
Venodilation, 176
Verrucous carcinoma, 26
Vinblastine, 13
Von Hippel-Lindau disease, 9, 130

W
Weiss criteria, 7
Whipple operation, 363
Wide local excision (WLE), 164
Wild-type GISTs, 100

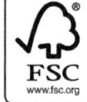

MIX
Papier aus verantwortungsvollen Quellen
Paper from responsible sources
FSC® C105338

If you have any concerns about our products,
you can contact us on
ProductSafety@springernature.com

In case Publisher is established outside the EU,
the EU authorized representative is:
Springer Nature Customer Service Center GmbH
Europaplatz 3, 69115 Heidelberg, Germany

Printed by Libri Plureos GmbH
in Hamburg, Germany